Wave Length and Action Potentials: History of the International Federation of Clinical Neurophysiology

Wave Length and Action Potentials: History of the International Federation of Clinical Neurophysiology

BY

MARC R. NUWER
Department of Neurology, David Geffin UCLA School of Medicine, and Department of Clinical Neurophysiology, Ronald Reagan UCLA Medical Center, Room 1194, 710 Westwood Plaza, Los Angeles, CA 90095, USA

AND

CARL H. LÜCKING
Professor and Chairman Emeritus,
Department of Neurology and Clinical Neurophysiology, Albert-Ludwigs-Universität, D-79106 Freiburg, Germany

SUPPLEMENTS TO CLINICAL NEUROPHYSIOLOGY
VOLUME 61
2010

ELSEVIER

ELSEVIER B.V.
Radarweg 29
1043 NX Amsterdam
The Netherlands

ELSEVIER Inc.
525 B Street, Suite 1900
San Diego, CA 92101-4495
USA

ELSEVIER Ltd.
The Boulevard, Langford Lane
Kidlington, Oxford OX5 1GB
UK

ELSEVIER Ltd
84 Theobalds Road
London WCIX 8RR
UK

First edition 2010

Library of Congress Cataloging in Publication Data
A catalog record is available from the Library of Congress.

British Library Cataloguing in Publication Data
A catalogue record is available from the British Library.

ISBN-10: 0-444-53475-X (this volume)
ISBN-13: 978-0-444-53475-0 (HB)
ISBN-13: 978-0-444-53476-7 (PB)
ISSN (Series): 1567-424X

∞ The paper used in this publication meets the requirements of ANSI/NISO Z39.48-1992 (Permanence of Paper).
Printed in The Netherlands.

Preface

Archives are the pillar of the history of each society. Since 1968 the Federation Executive Committee has discussed the necessity of creating a professionally maintained archive. No final solution was found about where to deposit Federation documents. In the early eighties William Cobb, then having just finished his term as Past-President, was given the task of writing a Federation history book. This was published with the title *Wave Length: a History of the IFSECN*. The book was given to all registrants at the Federation's 1985 London Congress.

Documents of the first 30 years of the Federation have been preserved only sparsely. This is also true for records about the journal since Elsevier had not kept records from the early decades. By the mid-nineties these archive issues again arose when the Executive Committee sought to know when and under what conditions certain rules were drawn up, or when named lectures or special meetings were held. Attempts again then to establish a Federation archives were side-tracked by a belief that General Assembly minutes were published and that the *EEG Journal* represented the IFCN archives. That resource, however, was fragmented and incomplete. Many minutes published in the journal were incomplete, mentioning reports as attachments to the original meeting materials, but attachments that were not incorporated into the formally printed minutes in the journal. Many past printed congress programs are lost, along with information about their key speakers, scientific and educational emphasis, venue and registration details, and social events. Deliberations of committees were lost over time. The journal sources were insufficient, scattered and fragmented as was noted very clearly in preparing this book.

Later the Executive Committee suggested that archiving might be a responsibility assumed by the successive Past-Presidents. The Long Range Planning Committee sought to preserve the documents accordingly at a formal professional archive institution that was prepared to maintain materials and make them available as needed. No institution yet was identified. A Permanent Executive Secretariat was considered as an alternate place for an archive, but those firms were more expert in organizing activities than in archiving per se.

For the present, the Executive Committee decided to compile an updated history book. In 2007, we two authors were asked to write this book because of our long experiences within the Federation. Both of us have served the Federation for more than 20 years as President, Past-President and Committee members. Our personal files contain many documents from Fiscal Periods since 1985. Additional source materials were obtained from other Presidents, Executive Committee members, Chapter officers and Congress conveners.

This history book aims to add the most recent 30 years to the history of the first three decades as written previously in *Wave Length*. The text of Cobb's book, with minor editing, is included here to complete this as a comprehensive historical overview. This certainly is in accord with the idea of the late William Cobb who himself wrote asking one of us (CHL) in 1996: "I wonder if you would like to consider a second edition of '*Wave Length*,' bringing it up to date."

This book is written by three authors, if one includes Cobb who was the original author of the first set of chapters. Each has brought different writing styles and individual approaches to the material. All have tried to be as objective as possible, but could not totally eliminate some subjectivity and story telling in selecting the presented facts and telling about events. In one sense, the book aims not just to tell the what, where and when, but also the how and why of Federation history.

The authors wish to give a historical background for the decision-making of the Federation officers and for all those who are interested in the history of the Federation. The book will be presented as a gift to the participants of the International Congress in Kobe, 2010. That followed the suggestion of W. Cobb as he expressed it in the same 1996 letter encouraging that an updated history book be "a gift at a congress" so that all who are interested can share in the story and facts behind the Federation and how it came to be as it is now. We hope this book meets those goals.

Marc R. Nuwer
Los Angeles, CA, USA

Carl H. Lücking
Freiburg, Germany

Acknowledgements

The authors wish to thank all those who made this work possible and those who helped us in our Federation service.

In preparation of this work, we thank the many individuals who contributed information. The list is too many to enumerate, but it includes many chapter officers, congress organizers, journal editors, Past-Presidents, and Executive Committee members from the past 30 years. Robert Ellingson, Federation President in 1981–1985, sent his boxes of Federation files dating from his service as President and Past-President and some from his three terms as Federation Secretary. Many other individuals also contributed details, documents, and recollections, and answered our emailed pleas for information and photographs. Andrew Eisen was very helpful in increasing our own collection by the number of photographs he contributed, and many others also generously sent electronic photographs from other activities.

We also thank those who brought us into Federation activity by giving us the opportunity to serve. This included Mary A.B. "Molly" Brazier, a Federation President and Editor-in-Chief, and an early mentor to one of us (MRN). Federation President John Desmedt appointed one of us (MRN) to serve as committee chairman for a series of practice guidelines. He also appointed one of us (CHL) as a member of the Rules Committee in his term. During the next fiscal period Federation President Jun Kimura appointed both of us to serve the Federation on the Rules Committee, increasing our activities and introducing us to many more individuals in the Federation.

William Cobb wrote the first Federation history, *Wave Length: A History of the IFSECN*. That work is reprinted here as the first set of chapters with minor new editing. His work in synthesizing and memorializing Federation history is not only highly appreciated but also a key to our ability to present here a history that included those first 35 years. The title of this book is based on his title.

We thank the Federation Delegates who placed their trust in us by the honor of electing us to serve as a Federation President. We thank the members of the Federation Executive Committees who served during our own terms in office, who made our service so much easier and effective.

The current Executive Committee, under the leadership of President Hiroshi Shibasaki, also deserves our thanks for their commission for us to write this work, as well as their sponsorship of making this book a gift to the attendees at the 2010 Kobe Congress.

We wish to thank the UCLA staff member, Sylvia Fong, who helped with much of the research and preparation work to actually compile and publish this volume.

Without the contributions and help of all these individuals, this book could not have been written.

Marc R. Nuwer
Los Angeles, CA, USA

Carl H. Lücking
Freiburg, Germany

Foreword to the 1983 *Wave Length* book

The 11th International Congress of Electroencephalography and Clinical Neurophysiology held in London on 25–30 August 1985 marks a return after 38 years to the site of the meeting now called the 1st International Congress, and the return of its sponsor, the International Federation of Societies for Electroencephalography and Clinical Neurophysiology, to the place of its conception. Fortunately, many of "The Founders", those who attended the 1st International Congress, are still active and will attend the 11th.

Since almost two generations have passed, the Executive Committee of the International Federation decided that it was none too soon to record the history of the Federation and of its better known organ, the journal *Electroencephalography and Clinical Neurophysiology,* in some formal and permanent fashion. This book is the result.

No better choice of author could have been made than William A. Cobb, who was present at the conception and has been continuously active in Federation affairs ever since, serving as a member of the early organizing and planning groups; as Treasurer of the Federation from 1957 to 1962; Chairman of the Committee on amendment of the Statutes of that Fiscal Period and principal author of the 1961 Constitution; variously as European Editor, Managing Editor, Publications Manager, and Publications Editor of The EEG Journal from 1961 until 1985, save for the 4 years of his Presidency of the Federation, 1973–1977. No one has more firsthand knowledge of the business of the Federation and of the Journal over the years, and he is in possession of the bulk of the Federation's archives. Indeed, no one can be said to have contributed more to the Federation and to the Journal, as will be evident by reading this book, despite Bill Cobb's rather matter-of-fact references to his own role(s). This history will be of value as a contribution to the broader history of the biomedical sciences and to future officers and members of the Federation, who will gain a deeper understanding of its traditions and how it all came about. The value of his narrative is strengthened by the author's frankness, his unwillingness to gloss over the difficulties, disappointments, and human controversies that are inevitable in the development of complex organizations. I believe you will find it a balanced account, brief but thorough, and felicitously embellished here and there by personal touches.

We are grateful to Dr. Cobb for yet another of his many contributions to the Federation.

R.J.Ellingson
President, IFSECN
25 April 1985

Preface to the 1983 *Wave Length* book

In the course of a long association with the Federation and its Journal I have accumulated a considerable bulk of publications and correspondence. Since retirement I have had leisure — surprisingly little — to put them in some sort of order and remove the purely trivial. On a number of occasions, from 1968 onwards, the Executive Committee has discussed the possibility of forming an archive of the Federation, of which my material could form at least the skeleton; while the idea has always found favour the problems of where to keep it, at what cost and by whom maintained have so far prevented its realization.

However, at the request of the Executive Committee, I have made use of the material in two ways: first, a collection of those reports and Statutes, at present current, that have been published in the Journal, together with the unpublished report of the Magnus Committee; this appeared in 1983 as "*Recommendations for the Practice of Clinical Neurophysiology*" in the *Supplement* series. Secondly, the present book; the first International Meeting in 1947 was in London and it seemed particularly appropriate that the book should be ready for the return to London in 1985. This period of 38 years is perhaps the "Wave Length" of the title, the first cycle of the Federation; certainly it is the period of my own association with it.

My sources for the initial meeting are partly memory but largely an almost complete typescript put together by Geoffrey Parr, the secretary of the EEG Society at that time, and never published. Material for the next few years is scanty as it had not yet become customary to publish regular reports in the Journal and I only began to get all the correspondence on becoming Treasurer in 1957. After that the major sources are the published reports and editorials from the Journal (these are listed in Appendix 4), amplified by the correspondence of the Executive Committee and Editorial Board.

Some gaps in the early record have been filled from the files of Herbert Jasper and, particularly, of Mary Brazier, and nearly all the pictures come from the San Diego Congress of 1969, provided by Bob Ellingson. For all these I am most grateful.

Most of this material could have been available to several others and this history might have been put together by an American or a Frenchman; no doubt it would then have been to some extent a different story. This one is necessarily somewhat personal and Anglocentric and if some events and personalities have not received their due, I can only apologize and disclaim any intentional slight. This is not to say that there have been no omissions; brevity has demanded them and prudence has sometimes counselled that the more colourful correspondence was best forgotten.

W.A.Cobb
Beaulieu, UK
1985

Contents

Section I

Chapters

Wave Length and Action Potentials: History of the IFCN
(Supplements to Clinical Neurophysiology, Vol. 61)
By: M.R. Nuwer and C.H. Lücking

Chapter 1

1947–1949

The founding years

International contacts among the few EEG workers had hardly begun before the Second World War put a virtual stop to them. They began to be made again when the war ended and by 1947 it seemed possible to arrange an international gathering. The driving force was W. Grey Walter, assisted by Denis Hill, George Dawson, Geoffrey Parr and others, acting through The (British) EEG Society, which was already some 5 years old.

1. The founding meeting in 1947

The meeting took place in the National Hospital for Nervous Diseases in Queen Square, London, UK on July 14–16, under the chairmanship of Prof. Edgar D. Adrian, the President of The EEG Society.

He delivered the following opening address to the assembled clinical neurophysiologists:

"In opening the first International Congress of Electroencephalography I wish to express on behalf of the EEG Society our great appreciation of the position we have been allowed to assume. Wherever the Congress had been held it would have been a pleasure to meet our colleagues from other countries to compare notes, to renew old friendships and make new ones; but in allowing us to act as hosts our colleagues have given us an extra pleasure which we appreciate very highly. So that in greeting those who have come from abroad I must extend not only the warmest welcome from the British Society but also their sincere thanks for the honour of your visit.

We are proud of our position as hosts and we appreciate also the responsibilities it brings – responsibilities which cause us some uneasiness. We should have liked to welcome you to a nice clean city with all the comforts of modern civilization. Unfortunately, modern civilization has not quite the comfort of civilization seven years ago. We are conscious of our shabby streets, our buildings which need a coat of paint, our antique railway stations and our meals which recall the poem on Nebuchadnezzar when he lived on grass and said as he munched the unaccustomed food: "it may be wholesome but it is not good".

But I must not emphasize the difficulties we feel in entertaining you properly, for these material shortcomings are almost worldwide and we have no right to make ourselves out as worse off than any other country, when we have suffered so little in comparison with much of Europe. Because our scars are visible on the surface we must not pretend that they are deeper than yours.

However, the difficulties with which we have all been faced may make us all the more gratified that this new branch of medical science has progressed so well. It was an adolescent before the war, not quite certain of itself or of its reception by its elders and certainly not ready for a full fledged international Congress. It has grown up in the period of intense strain and inadequate material of the past seven years. It has been helped, I think – certainly helped in this country – by the transference of interest from the sick civilian to the relatively healthy member of the armed forces. There have been greater opportunities for control, for the comparison of different temperaments, for investigating head injuries and so on. And the result has been that the science has grown up to a much better realisation of its position.

Some of the dreams of the adolescent have been abandoned: the EEG is not the sure guide to the state of the brain that we may have hoped it would become, but we now know far better what it can show and what it cannot and the physician and surgeon have far better reason to trust the advice you can give them. I say you and not we, for I have to confess to an almost complete lack of first-hand acquaintance with the clinical uses of the EEG. To the physiologist like myself it is still a fascinating manifestation of something going on in the brain, but naturally the war years have not brought a corresponding advance on the academic side and it cannot be said that we have a very clear idea of what we are recording, where it comes from or what part these electrical oscillations play in the brain mechanism generally.

It is a satisfactory state for the physiologist to have such a problem, such obvious phenomena waiting to be fitted into the picture, just as it is satisfactory to the clinical scientist to have a record which he can correlate with cerebral abnormalities; but naturally the position is only satisfactory as a transient stage. I suppose I am one of the few people here old enough to have seen the introduction of the electrocardiogram into medicine. The recording of the human heart currents seemed at first little more than a technical tour de force, *and we thought of Einthoven as the designer of a remarkable galvanometer and not much more. It was not until he and Thomas Lewis had established the physiological analysis that the pathological changes in the electrocardiogram became of such importance to the heart specialist, and then they became of such importance that he was in danger of neglecting everything else. I do not think the electroencephalogram is ever in danger of becoming too exclusive a guide to the neurologist or the psychiatrist – he has so many more symptoms to deal with than shortness of breath and anginal pain – but we cannot go wrong in trying to develop the full possibilities of the EEG and we cannot do this without a clear understanding of what we are measuring, without the analytical approach which Thomas Lewis brought to bear on the electrocardiogram.*

Perhaps I speak too much as a physiologist, but our programme for this meeting shows that we are all fully aware of the need for this kind of approach. It is a programme full of important communications on the physiological, just as much as on the clinical, side and the sooner we get down to it the better. But as I have the floor for an unspecified time, I cannot refrain from abusing my position by showing you two slides from a recent experiment which seem to me to make a rather pretty commentary on the records we make from our heads. This one looks familiar enough: there is a series of large potential waves at 12 c/s (Hz), stopped by a short period of sensory stimulation and building up again when the stimulus is over. It might be a record of the alpha rhythm when the eyes are opened and shut, but in fact it comes from the olfactory bulb of the rabbit and the pause coincides with the drawing of air through the nose and the consequent olfactory stimulation. The rabbit was under Nembutal and so the tendency to synchronised activity is probably exaggerated, but it is interesting to find the electrical behaviour of the human cerebrum echoed by the simpler mechanism of the olfactory bulb – as, in fact, it is echoed by such remotely related nerve cell systems as that in the optic ganglion of the water beetle.

But the slide comes from the end of a record after the olfactory stimulus had been withdrawn. Some residue of the smell is still about, but the sensory discharge at inspiration cannot be seen, though it is enough to break up the resting beat of the nerve cells. Here is the full record. To begin with the olfactory bulb is quiet. At the signal the nose is exposed to the smell of amylacetate, a fairly strong olfactory stimulus, and at the first inspiration there is an immediate response consisting of a fairly regular discharge at a high frequency (40 c/s or so). This activity arouses the olfactory bulb and the slow, large waves begin to appear in the intervals between inspiration, but they are broken up by each period of sensory activity. At first these periods are shown by the high frequency synchronised waves; later, as the stimulus grows less intense, there is an irregular activity with occasional large waves and later still the only sign of the olfactory stimulation is the breakdown of the slow resting rhythm. In the end that rhythm fades away and the bulb quiets down again – to remain quiescent till it is woken up by a fresh olfactory stimulus.

Although the conditions are abnormal, with an anaesthetic which favours synchronised activity, I think this gives a good picture of the effects of an afferent excitation on a mass of nerve cells which can work independently or in unison. There is the synchronisation at a high rate under an intense stimulus, at a low rate under none at all, and the failure of synchronisation when the stimulus is of the strength to cause differential activity. It illustrates some of the ways in which the alpha rhythm may be influenced, though it does not exhaust the possibilities.

Well, I must not take up your time with records which illustrate my own particular interest, for Prof. Bremer has already shown much the same thing in his records from the auditory cortex. I have only introduced these to emphasise the fact that the analysis of the electroencephalogram must lead us in one direction to the fundamental properties of collections of neurons, though it leads in the other direction to the highly specific patterns of activity in the human brain.

There is one more thing to add and I take the opportunity of adding it both as chairman of today's meeting and because I am on the verge of retiring from the presidency of the British Society. It is to express the deepest regret of all of us, and I am sure I speak for every country, the deepest regret that we have not been able to hold our first congress under the presidency of Hans Berger, the discoverer of the human electroencephalogram. In the early days I tried, rather unwisely, to perpetuate his name by calling his alpha rhythm the Berger Rhythm, but he would have none of it – and it was not a very good idea because in fact he had discovered the beta rhythm too. But his remarkable pioneering work needs no such advertisement nowadays. Our meeting is the direct consequence of it. Several of the new results which will be announced in our communications would probably be found anticipated in his papers if we read them carefully enough, for with far less adequate instruments and no encouragement at all he mapped out the whole territory which we have to cover."

Naturally, the majority of those present were British but 16 other countries were represented at least once among the hundred-odd participants. Subsequent recognition that it was the first of an ever-growing series has led to its being called the First International Congress though at the time modesty or prudence allowed its organizers to claim no grander title than Meeting.

However, the third item on the first morning's program was a discussion on the "Formation of a World EEG Organization and the Foundation of an International Journal", opened by W.T. Liberson of Hartford, CT, USA. Speaking of the proposed Journal he said it "should not be concerned exclusively with electroencephalography, but be devoted to all the problems of experimental and clinical neurophysiology ... many of us do not commit ourselves to the problems of the electrical activity of the brain alone, but carry on research in the fields of electromyography, electrodermography and electrodiagnosis of peripheral nervous diseases". Unfortunately, this liberal advice was to be ignored in the early days of the Federation.

The recent war was still very much in mind and Liberson said "There is no problem more significant in its implications for peace, for international solidarity, for cultural co-operation, than the study of the brain". Herbert Jasper, while in general agreement, thought that "The hope that studies of the electrical activity of the brain alone will yield much towards this end seems naive and visionary". Rather surprisingly, he also stated that "The formation of a World EEG Organization ... does not seem to me to be a practical or desirable undertaking at the present time".

Denis Hill also was opposed to the idea of an international body, partly on the grounds of impracticality but also because it "would tend to separate our studies from the main stream of physiology on the one hand and to make the results of those studies less available to medicine and surgery on the other".

H. Fischgold and Helge Hertz, while supporting some international cooperation, thought Liberson's proposals too ambitious; Moruzzi, however, was in favour of them. All three reported the imminent or completed foundation of EEG societies in their respective countries: France, Denmark and Italy.

Regarding the Journal, Jasper stated that it was something "which we can do in the very near future", while Hill was consistent in not wishing to see the best papers hidden from the general view in a specialist journal. If other speakers expressed opinions, as they no doubt did, they were not reported.

Finally, both matters were referred to an ad hoc committee — it seems never to have acquired a more formal title — set up by Grey Walter and to meet that evening.

The terms of reference of this committee no longer exist but Grey Walter's minute does and it is clear that they were wide-ranging. Under the chairmanship of Bremer (Belgium) the members were: Walter and Hill (UK), Baudouin and Fischgold (France), Schwab and Liberson (USA), Jasper (Canada), Monnier (Switzerland), Hertz (Denmark), Moruzzi (Italy) and Ten Cate (The Netherlands); most of these can be found in Fig. 1.1.

The items discussed were:

Electrode materials: It was agreed that silver–silver chloride was the best combination. A sub-committee was to be set up to review the electrochemistry of the whole subject but nothing seems to have come of this.

Electrode placement: Monopolar is a solecism, there being no truly unipolar record; intentional bipolar derivations are better than unintentional ones; the "setting up of sound and acceptable World Standards was considered a matter of urgent practical importance". Accordingly, a sub-committee was nominated, as follows: Jasper (Convenor), Abbott (USA), Cobb (UK), Dow (USA), Hertz (Denmark) and Kershman (Canada). It never met but Jasper was active in contacts and correspondence and this was in fact the genesis of the 10–20 system.

Recording equipment: Dawson and Walter had already published "Recommendations for the design and performance of EEG apparatus" (*J. Neurol. Neurosurg. Psychiat.*, 1945, 8: 61–64) and Jasper had, that morning, presented the recommendations of the American EEG society, based on those of Dawson and Walter. Again a

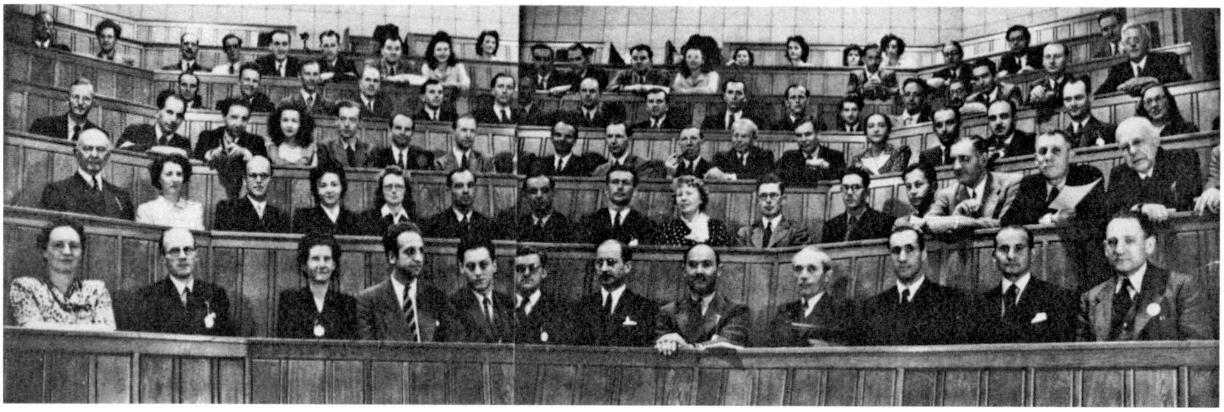

Fig. 1.1. The Founding Meeting in 1947, the first International Meeting which was held in the lecture theatre at the National Hospital for Nervous Diseases, Queen Square, London. Two photographic shots were needed because no one had thought of providing a wide angle lens. As a result of the two shots, some faces are duplicated in this composite figure. The duplicates are noted below in parentheses as "repeats". Persons who are not identified are denoted by a question mark.

- Back row: ?, D. Dow, ?, ?, J. Reynell.
- 5th row: ?, St. J. Loe, ?, ?, R.G. Kelly, M.Parsonage, P. Dell, M. Dell, (4 repeats), R. Hess, ?, ?, W. Dunham.
- 4th row: W. Langley, H.B. Morton, W.A. Cobb, W. Henderson, P. Passouant, ?, (4 repeats),?, ?, G. Moruzzi, M. Fuortes, C. Ajmone Marsan, A. Kleyntjes, J.G. Greenfield.
- 3rd row: J. Drooglever-Fortuyn, M. Roth, G. Verdeaux, J. Verdeaux, J. Dobbing, R.G. Bickford, E.E. Ponchin, (2 repeats), J. Theobald, ?, ?, Mme. Subirana, ?, H. Gastaut, J. Titeca, M.A.B. Brazier.
- 2nd row: A. Baudouin, J. Warfolk, K.-A. Melin, J. Turner, ?, C.C. Evans, (1 repeat), J. Roubicek, Mrs. Ten Cate, M.G. Saunders, N.W. Ellis, S.L. Last, J. Lefèvre, H. Fischgold, J. Ten Cate.
- Front row: M. Heppenstall, D. Hill, A. Lérique, A. Rémond, A. Übersfeldt, J. Lérique, H. Jasper, R. Schwab, F. Bremer, S. Obrador, ?, W.T. Liberson.
- Missing from this picture are, among others: E.D. Adrian, G.C. (Lairy) Bounes, G.D. Dawson, H. Hertz, G. Parr, W. Storm van Leeuwen and W.G. Walter.

Reprinted from "Handbook of EEG and Clinical Neurophysiology", Vol. 1A, p. 30, where other early photographs can be found.

sub-committee was proposed, to collect and test new proposals, with the hope that ultimately "world agreement could be attained".

Terminology: The variety and ambiguity were unanimously deplored. Hertz was commissioned to collate the various systems, with such help as he needed. This was a much more difficult task than the committee perhaps envisaged and it was to be another 11 years before a Terminology was published.

An international journal: No details are given of the resumed discussion and one wonders that agreement seems to have been reached fairly quickly. Most probably this was because Jasper had gone beyond the stage of dreaming and had given some thought to the practical details. No doubt the committee was ready enough to agree with someone who was himself willing to take the initiative. At any rate, Jasper was appointed Editor and an Editorial Board was chosen to represent as many countries as possible — perhaps a good way to emphasize the international character of the new journal but hardly the most efficient way to conduct its affairs. The committee then discussed the title of the journal and decided on that by which it has been known ever since, fortunately abbreviated when possible to *The EEG Journal*.

An international EEG organization: I cannot do better than quote in full the convener's minute, a typical piece of Grey Walter's writing:

> *"This subject evoked an energetic, candid and tiring discussion. Every shade of opinion was represented; some held that electroencephalography could have no possible relation to the putative social or political scope of an international organization, others considered that since electroencephalography is one of the most successful methods of studying the human brain, nothing human should be thought alien to it.*
>
> *It was pointed out that although these various opinions could be stigmatised as reactionary, cynical, pessimistic, sentimental, romantic, or fantastic, the fact remained that an international committee was actually in session and had already performed certain useful functions. It was agreed that in so far as continuation of these functions requires the survival of some effective body, the present* ad hoc *committee should continue in a state of suspended animation, so that it could be revived whenever further action is required of it. It was proposed and agreed that when other national or regional EEG Societies were formed, their Foreign Secretaries should become* ex officio *members of the International Committee, so that arrangements for the presentation of the reports from special sub-committees and plans for the proposed II International Congress in 1949 could be made with continuity and efficiency. It was suggested that the present Convenor should continue to act as Secretary until such time as a more formal election of Officers and a more detailed constitution could be undertaken."*

Although agreement was not reached on this last point the achievements of this committee in two evening sessions were remarkable and of lasting importance, not least the decision to hold a Second Congress in 2 years time. This First Congress had been small and intimate, rudimentary in its organization and simple in its social affairs — it had to be when food rationing was still very much in force and a restaurant meal could not legally cost more than 5 shillings per head. Nevertheless it brought together many of the subsequent leaders in the field — the first seven Presidents of the still unborn International Federation were present — some for the first time, and the bonds made at this meeting were perhaps as important for the future as were the decisions made by its *ad hoc* committee.

2. The Second International Congress, Paris

As agreed in London the second congress was planned to take place only 2 years later in Paris; the reason for this rather short interval was probably to get into step with the International Neurological Congresses, the fourth of which was to be held in Paris in 1949.

An organizing committee was set up under the presidency of Prof. A. Baudouin and with a wide international membership. Doubtless the real organization and hard work were done by the three French secretaries: H. Fischgold, H. Gastaut and A. Rémond and the treasurer, G. Verdeaux.

The Congress took place in the old "Faculté de Médicine de Paris" on September 1st–5th; each morning and afternoon session began with a report on a particular subject by a well-known scientist, followed by open discussion — there was nothing quite like the round tables and symposia which have since been the rule. Otherwise there were only free communications, all on EEG topics; in fact, the title of the congress was "Congrès International d'EEG" and there was no suggestion as yet that "Clinical Neurophysiology" might be of interest. However, the final day was a joint one with, and organized by, the Neurological Congress and one of the topics there was electromyography, presented by Fritz Buchthal.

This second Congress was much larger and altogether more organized than the first, very amateur, meeting. A fee of $10 was charged, the accommodation was excellent and the hospitality was memorable; the last included a banquet on the terrace of the Eifel Tower and a reception in the Hôtel de Ville.

The proceedings of the Congress were published in diverse ways: Brazier wrote her "Impressions", summarizing the scientific content of the Congress (The EEG Journal, 1949, 1: 509–512) and the abstracts of the Communications were published as Society Proceedings (The EEG Journal, 1950, 2: 103–114); the Reports of the principal speakers were edited by H. Fischgold and published (1951) by Masson et Cie. as the 2nd Supplement of the Journal.

3. The International Federation

Walter's *ad hoc* committee of 1947 had been active and the doubts expressed at that time seem to have evaporated; in the documents that exist there is no question of whether a federation should be formed, only of how this should be done. Gastaut acted as secretary and his unpublished report he listed a number of people who met as delegates of the various national societies: some may indeed have been delegated though others were not and the two English men, at least, insisted that any decisions reached must be ratified by their society. The subsequent report of the meeting in the Journal (1949, 1: 508) spoke of the "executive council", though it was surely not constituted by any accepted democratic process; it was as much *ad hoc* as the previous committee had been.

This group comprised:

S. Last (UK)	K. Melin (Sweden)
W. A. Cobb (UK)	T. S. von Frey (Sweden)
R. S. Schwab (USA)	H. Hertz (Denmark)
A. E. Walker (USA)	A. Subirana (Spain)
A. Baudouin (France)	M. Monnier (Switzerland)
H. Gastaut (France)	M. Gozzano (Italy)

together with H. Jasper representing the Journal, G. Zhukova of UNESCO and three of the Congress organizers: H. Fischgold, A. Rémond and G. Verdeaux. They met on September 1st in the Salon des Goncourt of the Restaurant Drouant, over a meal the like of which some of us had not enjoyed for years (see the comment above on London restaurant food in 1947) and it was not until 10.30 p.m. that the real business of the evening began.

Gastaut had prepared two drafts of a constitution of the Federation, with the help of Baudouin, Walter and Schwab, representing the first three national societies, and an international lawyer. The second of these drafts was presented to the "Council", which made further modifications and the French text was finally agreed 20 min after midnight, after the constitution had been read in its entirety and discussed paragraph by paragraph.

It is interesting to follow the changes of title of the Federation. In the first two drafts it is called "Féderation Internationale d'Electroencéphalographie et de Neurophysiologie Appliquée", the last word being changed to "Clinique" in the third draft. In the report in the Journal (1949, 1: 508) it is called, obviously incorrectly, "The International Federation of EEG Societies". In February 1951 Jasper objected that "it is not possible to federate a science. A federation is of people or societies of people". Accordingly a poll was taken by letter and several of the extant votes favour the short title quoted above, no doubt because of its brevity. Among them, surprisingly, was that of Grey Walter, who had always insisted that EEG was a technique and that our true business was neurophysiology, whether basic or clinical. However, "Clinical Neurophysiology" was retained and, in the version of the Statutes finally printed, the present cumbersome form was reached.

The General Assembly, as defined by this Constitution, met at 9 a.m. the following morning and elected the first group of Officers, consisting of:

Edgar D. Adrian	Honorary President	UK
Herbert H. Jasper	President	Canada
Robert S. Schwab	Vice Presidents	USA
W. Grey Walter		UK
Fritz Buchthal		Denmark
Henri Gastaut	Secretary	France
Antoine Rémond	Treasurer	France

The Executive Committee comprised the above together with the president and secretary of each Member Society.

It was also decided that the next congress should be in America in 1952, leaving the place and the organization to the American EEG Society.

A further meeting of the General Assembly at 9 a.m. on September 3rd discussed and formalized the affairs of the Journal. It was decided that:

(1) The Editor and Editorial Board should be appointed by the General Assembly;
(2) Questions concerning the interior organization of the Journal should be submitted to the International Federation;
(3) The Federation would not have any responsibility for the debts of the Journal but would receive any profit which might arise.

Understandably the last was accepted unanimously and it has proved to be of far reaching importance. The first two, however, also accepted unanimously, were totally impractical since the General Assembly was to meet only briefly in 3 years time. Experience has shown that appointing an editor is not a matter of election but of finding someone of known ability and dedication who is willing to accept the task.

Why the publication of the Constitution was delayed is a mystery, perhaps an oversight, but its terms remained unknown to all but a few for over 2 years. The text published (Journal, 1951, 3: 519–522) was that agreed in Paris, with some minor modifications, side by side with an English translation under the title of "Bye-Laws" (French "Statutes").

This Constitution proved to be a good basis for development but already contained the seeds of future problems. An Executive Committee (Article V) consisting of six officers elected by the General Assembly (at unspecified intervals) and one member (the original document had two) of each society elected annually by his society was hardly a working proposition even in these early days when member societies were few (12 are listed at the date of publication). In addition, Article VII states that the Executive Committee "may also meet at any time at the request of *one* of its members" (my italics). Since a meeting of the Executive Committee has usually involved about half of its members crossing the Atlantic this was an expensive privilege to put in the keeping of any single member. Fortunately it was never exercised.

3.1. Electroencephalography and Clinical Neurophysiology

Having been given the go-ahead Jasper assembled his team of helpers, most significantly his Managing Editor. The Journal's debt to the extrovert enthusiasm of Bob Schwab is incalculable; from an attic office in the Massachusetts General Hospital, with the dedicated assistance of Mary Brazier, he set up the necessary organization and negotiated a contract with Williams and Wilkins. However, the cost of printing in French and Spanish as well as in English proved prohibitive and the contract was amicably dissolved. In Canada printing in French and English presented no problem or additional expense (in practice, Spanish was never used) and Jasper was able to make a new contract with Thérien Frères of St. Laurent, Quebec, to print the Journal. Jasper was fortunate in finding an assistant, Mrs. M. Prados, who prepared all the manuscripts, supervised the printing and corrected the proofs, aided by his wife Margaret.

Grey Walter was co-editor for Europe, John Knott looked after the Society Proceedings, E.J. Baldes in America and Geoffrey Parr in England edited Technical Notes and Charles Henry painstakingly collected and arranged an Index of Current Literature. Despite this varied assistance the load on Jasper must have been a heavy addition to a busy professional career.

Although the intention was, and has remained, that the Journal should contain only original articles it was necessary at first to solicit them from colleagues — a problem which must be common to most new ventures of this sort. Jasper was fortunate in being able to start his first issue, in February 1949, with a symposium on the "Physiological Basis of Epileptic Discharge" in which the speakers were Gerard, Penfield, Jasper, McCulloch, Darrow, Elliott, Toman and Lennox. Later pages included the names of Walter, Hallowell Davis, Bremer, Brazier, Gastaut, Gibbs and Knott. The last issue of the year contained papers by Moruzzi and Magoun and by Lindsley, Bowden and Magoun, on the brain-stem reticular formation, which were to influence thought on cerebral activation for years to come.

Thus, the Journal made a good start and established for itself a secure position, providing about equal proportions of clinical and experimental results and, in its Society Proceedings, a forum for brief reports of current work. Authors' Instructions in the first issue (Journal, 1949, 1: 135–136) state that these Proceedings should not exceed 100 words (250 for annual meetings and congresses, with an additional 100 words for discussion). In fact, many of them were much longer than this and as early as February 9, 1949, which must have been within a few days of the appearance of the first issue, the Managing Editor, Schwab, was writing to society secretaries "we have had to reduce the size of the abstract of each communication from 200 to 150 words and no discussion will be included". By the following year discussions had disappeared but many of the abstracts were longer than ever, in which the Editors seem to have acquiesced, since the next Authors' Instructions (Journal, 1962, 14: 159–160) accepted 250 words.

When the International Federation was founded in September 1949, Jasper handed to it the ownership of the Journal with "full authority over its management, policy and selection of members of its editorial board", while retaining responsibility for its debts. This generous offer was made the sweeter by the promise to hand over any future profits to the Federation, though in fact it was many years before this had any significant effect. At this time expenditure greatly exceeded income, partly because of difficulties, due to currency restrictions, in collecting subscriptions from outside North America.

Wave Length and Action Potentials: History of the IFCN
(Supplements to Clinical Neurophysiology, Vol. 61)
By: M.R. Nuwer and C.H. Lücking

Chapter 2

1949–1953

President: H.H. Jasper

At this time financial problems played a major role. The Journal was struggling to reach profitability, hindered by the difficulty of collecting and transmitting subscriptions from Europe to Boston, and transatlantic travel was beyond the reach of the majority. Although a fair number of Americans had been able to get to Paris the reverse journey from Europe to America for the next congress seemed likely to present greater difficulties. For this reason an early decision was taken to postpone the congress by one year, to 1953, and associate it in time with the International Physiological Congress, to be held in Montreal in September, in the hope that this would improve the attendance. Thus the four yearly cycle of congresses and later the Fiscal Period of the Federation were established.

All the affairs of the Federation had to be conducted by letter and there was much correspondence between the President Herbert Jasper (Fig. 2.1) and the Secretary Henri Gastaut, culminating in three important events. The applications for membership of the so-called affiliated societies were accepted; they were the Spanish, Italian, Danish, Dutch, Swedish, Belgian, Swiss, Japanese, German (FRG) and South (later called Latin) American societies. Memories of the World War were still strong five years after its end and the admission of the German and Japanese societies was not unopposed but the majority view was that the Federation was concerned only with Science and Medicine, not with politics.

The Constitution as published in 1951 (Journal, 3: 519–522) incorrectly states "Incorporated, Paris 1949". In fact the Federation was a Registered Charity, and registration took place with the deposition in 1951 of the Statutes in the Préfecture de Bouches du Rhône. For a long time the legal address of the Federation was that of the Secretary, Gastaut's house on the Promenade de la Corniche in Marseilles. It remained so after he had ceased to be secretary and after he had left it; this anomaly was corrected only fairly recently, when tax avoidance compelled a more realistic arrangement. In 1950 the Federation became a founder member of the Council for the Coordination of International Congresses of Medical Sciences (CCICMS, later CIOMS) and the change in date of the next congress was in part a first fruit of this. Modest financial support was also provided by CIOMS for some of the Federation's activities.

Gastaut's report to the General Assembly of 1953 states that "Article VI (of the Statutes) was changed at the meeting of CIOMS", but it is difficult to see how this could have been done constitutionally nor is there any indication of the nature of the change. Subsequent correspondence, however, indicates that the phrase "The General Assembly is composed of all the officers of the member societies" was dropped as it had become impractical with the growth of the Federation (though the phrase remains unchanged in the version of the Statutes published in the Journal, 1958, 10: 381–384). Instead each society was invited to name one delegate and these, with the officers, formed the General Assembly.

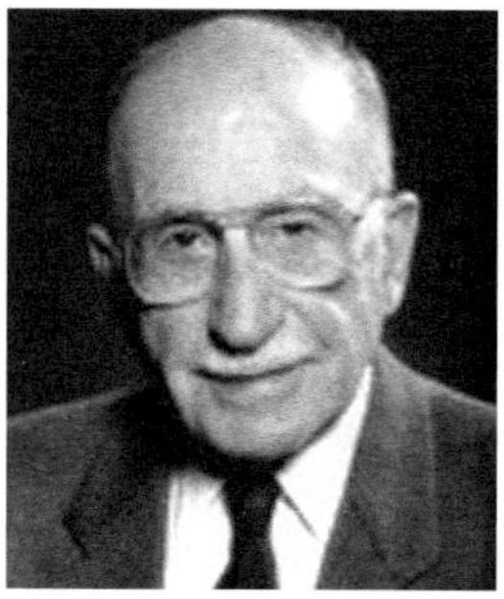

Fig. 2.1. Herbert H. Jasper of the Montreal Neurological Institute, first Federation President, proponent of the International 10–20 system, founder and first editor of *Electroencephalography and Clinical Neurophysiology*.

In June 1952 Jasper convened a meeting of these national delegates in Brussels and 13 of the societies were represented, only Japan being absent. This was, I think, the only occasion on which such a meeting, apart from those associated with congresses, was held; how it was financed is not apparent. The major topic was the provisional program of the coming congress made by the American organizers; Journal affairs were also discussed.

In May 1950 Jasper had proposed setting up three committees, on Apparatus, Clinical Techniques and Terminology. Gastaut objected that the Statutes allowed only two, though Statute X says "Special committees, in unlimited numbers, may be appointed." The reason for the misunderstanding is not evident but it seems to have been resolved and the committees were appointed.

Although Statute IX says that "Each member association shall pay to the Federation an annual assessment . . .", no serious attempt seems to have been made to collect any dues until September 1952, when the Treasurer, Rémond, sent out a circular letter proposing annual contributions from the various societies, ranging from $100 (USA) to $10; the societies were invited to object if they thought these arbitrary assessments were wrong. There is no evidence that they did so and by the end of the period the majority of dues had been paid and the Treasurer had a small sum to pass on to his successor.

1. The EEG Journal

In March 1951 negotiations were opened with the American Physiological Society to take over the publication of the Journal. This body already published a number of well known journals, including the *American Journal of Physiology* and *Physiological Reviews*, and so had the necessary organization to be able to take one more journal in its stride. The Society was helpful but made conditions which, though acceptable to Jasper and Schwab, those most closely concerned, must have been rejected by the majority since no agreement was reached.

Instead, the business affairs of the Journal were moved later in 1951 from Boston to Montreal, where a Managing Secretary was appointed. This does not seem to have been entirely successful because Jasper reports later that "the business management of our affairs was badly handled in 1953" but things were finally sorted out by a new Managing Secretary, Mrs. L. Denton, with the help of Margaret Jasper.

Meanwhile the Journal continued to grow, both in number of pages (632 in 1953) and in subscriptions, nearly 2000. Costs, however, were continually rising and the Journal had not quite reached profitability nor had most of the starting loans, intended to be for not more than 3 years, been paid off.

The continuing debt was in part due to an over estimate of the sales of *Supplement 1*. This was a "Bibliography of Electroencephalography" by Mary Brazier, published in 1950, which covered the period to 1948 and was to prove invaluable to EEG workers for many years to come. However, it was a financial burden on the struggling Journal and Jasper tried to shift the load of $1566 to the Federation; not having anything like that amount of money the Federation declined.

In his first annual report of January 1950, after the publication of the first four quarterly numbers, totalling 524 pages, Jasper was able to report 1350 subscriptions, about double the more pessimistic estimates. Despite all the voluntary help the expenses of starting up the Journal had been heavier than expected and the necessary finances had been generously provided by interest-free loans from some American and Canadian colleagues to the extent of $5500; they were to be repaid within 3 years. The subscription was $8; $5 to society members!

Supplement 2, the *Proceedings of the Second Congress*, after much discussion, was published by Masson in Paris. The main reason for this seems to have been that a substantial French government grant to the Congress would have been withdrawn if the publication had not been in France. Several later supplements were published under the same imprint though their association with the Federation seems to have been of the slightest and did not include either editorial control or financial interest.

2. The Third International Congress, Boston

Under the presidency of Alexander Forbes the third Congress was held in Radcliffe College, Cambridge, MA from 17 to 22 August, 1953. A complete list of the officers can be found in *Supplement 3* of the Journal from which it may be supposed that the indefatigable Bob Schwab, assisted by Mary Brazier, Earl Walker, Charles Henry and Jerome Merlis, were the chief organizers. This publication also has a list of societies which made financial contributions and one wonders who it was persuaded the College of Chest Physicians that it had an interest.

There were six symposia, each with three main speakers; these were later published, with the discussions, as *Supplement 4* of the Journal. The free communications were given in the form of panel presentations and 300 word abstracts of these, with one figure, were prepared for distribution at the congress, forming *Supplement 3* of the Journal. The cost of this was defrayed by including advertisements.

A meeting of the so-called General Assembly took place on the Sunday before the Congress opened, with Jasper in the chair. Twenty people were present, seven of them from the host country and the remainder from 11 member societies. It is doubtful if all of them were truly delegates though a great effort had been made that every society should be represented. Minutes of the meeting were kept by Schwab, the secretary of the Congress, rather than by Gastaut, the secretary of the Federation, probably because the meeting was conducted largely in English, though Gastaut read his report in French. A typescript of these minutes exists but it was never published.

Gastaut described the development of the Federation during the preceding 4 years, the development of its Constitution and its relations with CIOMS. He also mentioned that he had organized transport to the Congress for 64 Europeans, a number which had been whittled away by cancellations and an air transport strike to zero. Other Europeans had of course made their own arrangements and many had succeeded in reaching Boston.

One of the victims of these disasters was the Treasurer, Rémond, and his report was read and discussed in his absence. The problems of transmitting funds from one country to another at this time were still considerable and it was proposed to set up the treasury permanently in the USA, though it is hard to see how this would have helped; it was pointed out that the country of the Treasurer would change every 4 years and the site of the treasury must necessarily change with him. A committee of five national treasurers was set up to discuss the problems of the international transfer of funds and the avoidance of liability to taxation.

Two small changes in Statute V were then made, making it possible for the representative of each member society in the Executive Committee to be "designated" by his society rather than "elected annually" and removing the restriction on the number of Vice-Presidents.

A "slate" of officers was next presented and, after discussion in "a general and friendly way," was accepted, though in later years such a method of block election was to be heavily and rightly criticized. The number of Vice-Presidents

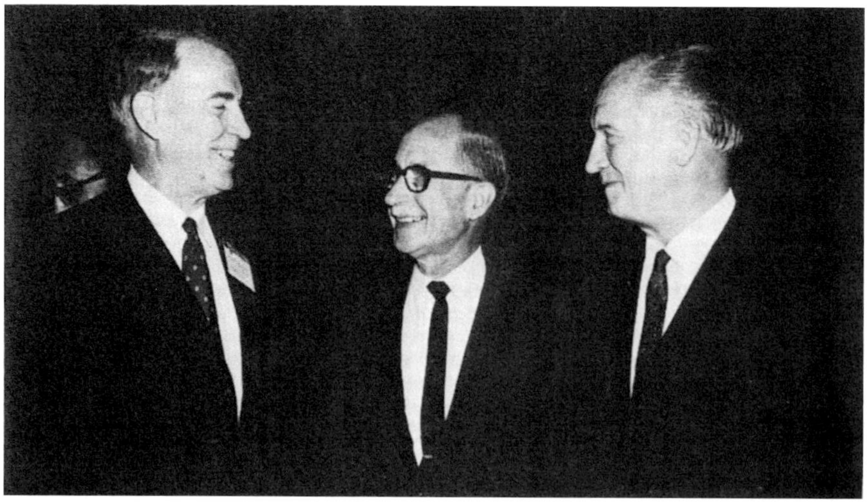

Fig. 2.2. From left to right:
- Frederick E. Gibbs, of Chicago, pioneer of clinical EEG, discoverer of the spike and wave complex, author of a famous Atlas of EEG.
- Herbert H. Jasper, first of Providence, RI, and later of the Montreal Neurological Institute (where he was responsible for the curious association of EEG with skiing). Founder and first editor of the EEG Journal. First president of the International Foundation (1949–1953).
- D.B. Lindsley, pioneer of EEG in America, whose early studies were a cornerstone of pediatric and neonatal EEG. A leading contributor to the study of cerebral electrical correlates of behaviour.

was increased to 10, evidently with the intention of widening the international representation, though this hardly seems to have been necessary when each society had its own designated member. Grey Walter was elected President, Mary Brazier, Treasurer and Henri Gastaut remained as Secretary "to ensure continuity." Thus the Executive Committee consisted of the 14 society representatives, ten Vice-Presidents and three executive officers with Herbert Jasper in the anomalous position of Honorary President, 28 members in all, surely too large a number to have any realistic executive function (Fig. 2.2).

The official party for the Congress members was a New England clam-bake at Crane's Beach. Unfortunately, the evening sky was overcast and the air none too warm; even so, one European lady was censured for the immodesty of her two-piece bathing suit — the bikini had not yet arrived in Massachusetts.

Wave Length and Action Potentials: History of the IFCN
(Supplements to Clinical Neurophysiology, Vol. 61)
By: M.R. Nuwer and C.H. Lücking

Chapter 3

1953–1957

President: W. Grey Walter

Day-to-day information on this period is slight but for the first time the Proceedings of the General Assembly at the end of the period were published (Journal, 1958, 10: 367–369) so that a good summary of the 4 years' work exists, together with the reports of the various committees. The Federation organized its activities in this term under the capable leadership of W. Grey Walter (Figs. 3.1 and 3.2).

Each of these reports opens with a statement to the effect that it is an updating of the report made to the previous General Assembly; since there is no evidence that any of the reports in 1953 were circulated they cannot have had any widespread effect. The committees, of course, worked by correspondence, with occasional contacts between individual members. However, a meeting of all the officers and committee members was arranged to occupy several days before the congress to finalize the reports; this was organized by Otto Magnus to take place in Oosterbeek, which had been the centre of the battle for Arnhem, of which it is a suburb; the weather was fine and the meetings were held on the lawns surrounding the conference house in a very relaxed atmosphere, which contributed greatly to the progress of the committees. Their reports, with lists of all the members, were published (Journal, 1958, 10: 370–389) and for the first time the Federation expressed in detail its recommendations on the conduct of clinical EEG examinations, on training and on specifications for EEG apparatus. Not all of these recommendations have had general acceptance but one which has stood the test of time is the "International 10–20 system" of electrode placement, drawn up by Jasper as the result of initiatives taken at the first congress and published now for the first time. A committee on nomenclature had evidently found its task too daunting and failed to produce a report.

During the period five new societies were admitted to membership, those of Australasia, Austria, Norway, the USSR, and Romania, and at the congress a further two, Hungary and India, bringing the total to 20 societies.

1. The EEG Journal

Herbert Jasper's report of 1954 gave great satisfaction; the circulation had passed the 2000 mark, the number of published pages was over 720, the administrative difficulties had been overcome and the Journal showed a modest profit. This last was surprising in view of an 80% increase in expenditure during the year, partly because of the increased size and circulation but mainly the beginning of the rise in costs of paper and salaries. Nevertheless, all the starting loans had been repaid and the Journal was free from debt. Even the deficit on *Supplement 1* had been almost wiped out by the successful sales of *Supplements 3* and *4*, the proceedings of the Boston Congress.

Since the beginning of 1954 Jasper had had Peter Gloor, also of the Montreal Neurological Institute, as editorial assistant, an arrangement which was evidently most successful. Less

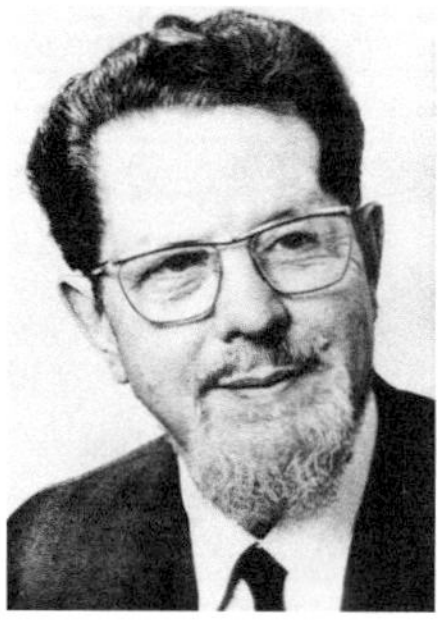

Fig. 3.1. W. Grey Walter, second Federation President and organizer of the 1947 London First Congress.

satisfactory, it seems, was an attempt to make the European editorship more active by appointing new assistant editors. However, by the following year Jasper comments that the work of H. Fischgold, F. Buchthal and H. Shipton was "becoming of increasing importance".

By 1955 subscriptions had risen to over 2200 and many of the new subscribers were buying all the back issues. This necessitated the reprinting of many of them at a cost of $6000, which put the Journal temporarily in the red again. The following year's report, however, showed a profit of a similar sum, $6000, and a further profit of $2000 on the Supplements.

By the end of 1957, after 10 years of operation, the circulation was about 2500 and still increasing. Despite great pressure on space the number of pages was held to about 750, because of the heavy and rising cost of printing. Jasper speaks of "tightening of our editorial policy" to try to reduce the publication delay and keep the costs in balance

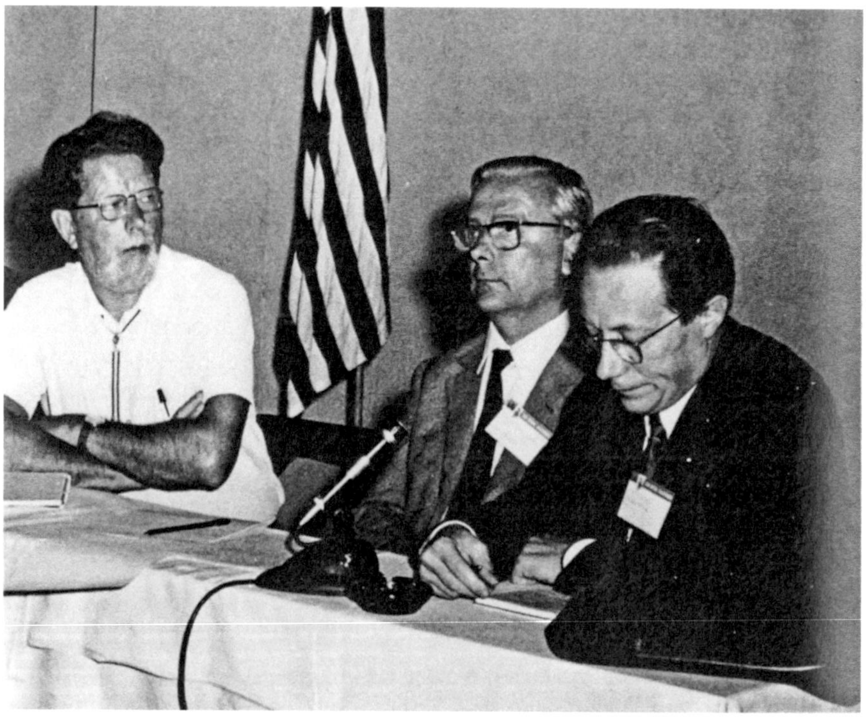

Fig. 3.2. From left to right:
- W.G. Walter of Bristol. Pupil of E.D. Adrian and the first English clinical EEGer. Named delta and theta waves. Discovered the Contingent Negative Variation. Organizer of the first International Meeting in London. Co-founder of the Federation and its second President, 1953–1957.
- Willem Storm van Leeuwen, The Netherlands, EEG Journal editor from 1957, and Treasurer 1962–1969.
- Pierre Buser of Paris. European editor 1973–1979. Treasurer 1983–1985.

with the subscriptions. The price of the Journal was still only $10 a year.

At the Congress in 1957 Grey Walter resigned as European Editor and his place was taken jointly by Otto Magnus and W. Storm van Leeuwen in The Netherlands. John Knott retired from editing Technical Notes and was replaced by H.W. Shipton and Fritz Buchthal. Clinical and Laboratory Notes were edited in America by R.S. Schwab and in Europe by H. Fischgold.

In Brussels it was recommended that all papers should be in English if possible but that any European language could be accepted. Fortunately there was little response to this open invitation and French continued to be the only language used, apart from the majority of papers in English. A further decision was to provide summaries of all papers in German and French as well as in English. This policy seems to have been applied only to Main Articles but for them was continued for some years.

Although it had at first been a great financial worry to the editors, the "Bibliography" of Mary Brazier was now established as a most valuable tool and, at Brussels, it was decided to compile a second volume for the period 1949–1959. The obvious choice for this task was Charles Henry, who had been diligently collating and sorting references for the quarterly "Index of Current Literature" from the first issue of the Journal. He was to be assisted by Cosimo Ajmone Marsan, making his first contact with the Journal which he was later to edit with such distinction. This endeavour never reached fruition but the gap was later filled in other ways.

2. The Fourth International Congress, Brussels

This Congress was held in the week of July 22, 1957, under the presidency of Frédéric Bremer, in the Palais des Beaux-Arts in Brussels, as part of the "First International Congress of Neurological Sciences". This brought together neurology, neurosurgery, neuroradiology and neuropathology as well as EEG. In this vast gathering, opened in the presence of King Baudouin (the only time we had such patronage), well organized though it was, individuals felt lost and the intimacy of the first congress, already suffering progressive erosion in Paris and Boston, had gone forever. There were many, not only EEGers, who said never again.

Abstracts of the free communications were precirculated in the Excerpta Medica Congress series (1957) and the proceedings were published as *First International Congress of the Neurological Sciences*, Vol. 111 by Pergamon Press, edited by L. van Bogaert and J. Radermecker (1959, 707pp).

At the General Assembly (of the EEG Congress; Neurological Sciences held one as well) on July 24 the reports of the officers and of the committees were presented. The Treasurer had got her affairs in good order and provided a surplus for the 4 years of $887.

Once again a slate of officers, which had been discussed at "the preliminary Assembly", whatever that may have been, was presented. It was accepted "unanimously (with one exception)"; it is not clear whether the exception was among the electors or the elected. The new President was Henri Gastaut, the Secretary M.A.B. Brazier, and the Treasurer W.A. Cobb. Fourteen Vice-Presidents were elected, all of them different from the list of 1953 with the single exception of R.S. Schwab.

Despite the misgivings over the size of this congress it was decided to hold the next in the same place and at the same time as that of Neurology. This later turned out to be Rome in September 1961 and the neuropathologists also decided to meet then and there, so that the widespread desire for a more restricted meeting was hardly satisfied.

Wave Length and Action Potentials: History of the IFCN
(Supplements to Clinical Neurophysiology, Vol. 61)
By: M.R. Nuwer and C.H. Lücking

Chapter 4

1957–1961

President: Henri Gastaut

In retrospect, this can be seen as a period of great importance to the Federation and its Journal, of increasing maturity and expertise, perhaps springing from the comradeship and understandings of the meeting in Oosterbeek and certainly spurred on by the leadership of Henri Gastaut (Figs. 4.1 and 4.2). (A secretary once wrote his name as Gusto — mistaken or misheard but wholly appropriate.) An inhibiting factor was the very small size of the budget, $2490 from four years subscriptions, which was not enough to cover the expenses of the executive officers, small though they were: better times were in sight by the end of the period.

Five further societies were admitted to the Federation during the period: Bulgaria, Czechoslovakia, Israel, Poland and South Africa, bringing the total to 25.

In Brussels it was proposed to set up a Committee on Terminology and this was later appointed. At first efforts to bring it into action were not very successful but an independent attempt by Dutch workers was brought to the notice of Gastaut by Magnus and Storm van Leeuwen and proved to be the starting point for more productive efforts; a "Proposal for 1958" was circulated and formed the basis for discussion at a meeting on the EEG of Tumours at Wassenaar, The Netherlands, in 1959. Those present were not exactly the members of the Committee but that did not matter and many useful ideas were exchanged, leading to the "Proposal of 1959". Finally, after endless correspondence on fine points of detail a "Proposal for 1960" resulted which, after editing, was published in the Journal (1961, 13: 646–650) as a "Preliminary Proposal for an EEG Terminology".

For a number of years Gastaut, with the energetic support of Robert Naquet and others, had conducted an annual "Colloque de Marseille" in the early autumn (the 25th and last was held in 1980). These were not part of the Federation's activities but they increasingly attracted an international audience and in October 1960 the opportunity was taken by most of those closely concerned with the running of the Federation to meet for two days in Marseilles to discuss the organization of the Advanced Course and the Congress to be held in the following year. The main topic, however, was the Constitution, the deficiencies of which were becoming more and more apparent. As a consequence of this meeting a "Committee on Amendment of the Statutes" was set up consisting of H. Gastaut (Marseilles), Grey Walter (Bristol), M.A. Brazier (Boston), W. Storm van Leeuwen (Leyden), C. Henry (Hartford), O. Magnus (Wassenaar) and H. Petsche (Vienna), with W.A. Cobb (London) as chairman. It fell to the last to draft all the proposals and to collate the voluminous and often contradictory opinions expressed by his colleagues.

The administration of the Federation, as required by the Constitution of 1951 (Appendix 2), was by an Executive Committee consisting of "the President, three Vice-Presidents, the Secretary, the

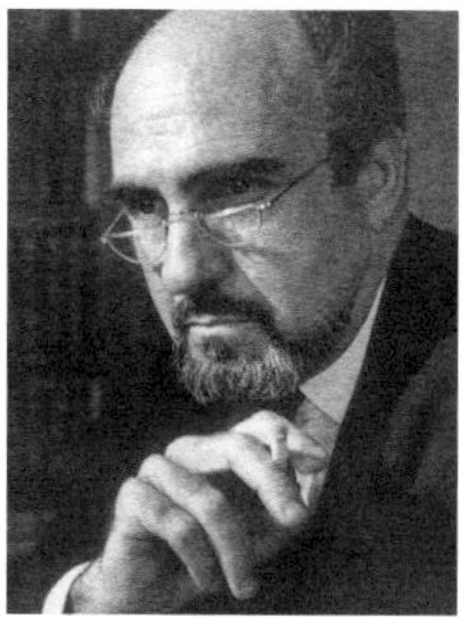

Fig. 4.1. Henri Gastaut of Marseilles, first Secretary and third IFSECN President.

Treasurer, all elected by the General Assembly, in addition to one representative from each of all the national societies who will be elected annually by his national society" (Statute V). The General Assembly, meeting only once in four years, was "composed of all the officers of the member societies" (Statute VI).

Thus at this time, if every society played its part, which was not always the case, there were 25 representatives of societies in the Executive Committee plus the six officers, elected by the General Assembly, 31 in all. Despite the fact that Statute VII permitted one of the members of the Committee to call a meeting at any time, this was clearly impossible and physical meetings could only take place at the times of Congresses, far too long an interval for effective administration. Equally, consensus by correspondence was immensely time consuming and expensive. In practice the day-to-day affairs of the Federation fell more and more into the hands of the officers.

The solution arrived at was to limit the Executive Committee to the elected officers, substituting the Past-President for the three Vice-Presidents, and adding the Editor-in-Chief of the Journal to create the closest possible liaison between it and the Federation. The old Executive Committee was renamed the Council, interposed between the Executive Committee and the General Assembly, voting by post on proposals put to it by the Executive and meeting before the General Assembly at Congresses.

Apart from requiring each society to elect a delegate the Federation rightly made no attempt

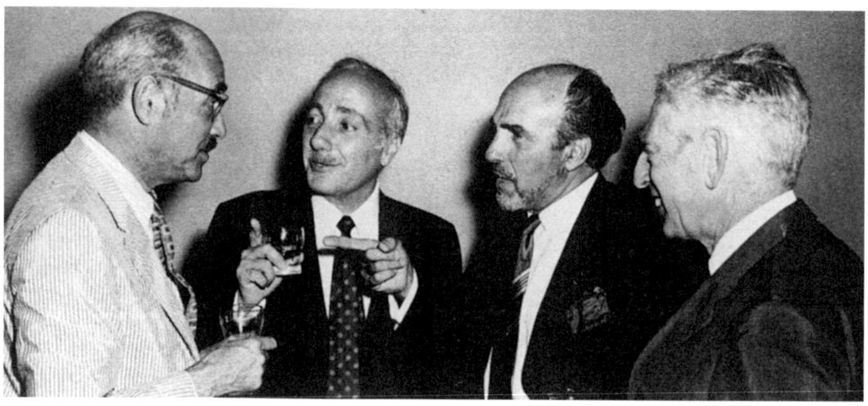

Fig. 4.2. From left to right:
- Robert (Bob) Schwab of the Massachusetts General Hospital, Boston, where he and M.A.B. Brazier organized the business side of the Journal.
- Robert (Bobby) Naquet, assistant to Gastaut in Marseilles, ubiquitous figure at the Colloquia, Secretary 1961–1969, President 1977–1981.
- Henri Gastaut of Marseilles. Dynamic leader of French EEG, Convener of the International Federation 1949, Secretary 1949–1957, President 1957–1961.
- Otto Magnus of Wassenaar, The Netherlands. European co-editor of the Journal with Storm van Leeuwen, 1957–1961. Organizer of the Advanced Courses in Marseilles, 1961 and Salzburg, 1965.

to interfere in the organization of the societies. Thus "all the officers" might be as many as a society pleased, which was felt to be inequitable. Accordingly, the General Assembly was defined as the Council and three officers, or their specified alternates, of each Member Society.

With the addition of a definition of voting rights (Statute VIII), of the Fiscal Period which fixed the term of officers and committees (Statute IX), and the setting up of a Nomination Committee (Statute XI) to conduct elections the above changes provided a workable constitution as democratic as possible within the limits set by general meetings only at four yearly intervals.

As will be described in the next section on the Journal, the Federation had suddenly become the possessor of significant capital and the potential of an appreciable annual income. It was essential to regularize the finances and protect them, so far as possible, from taxation. Statute XIV and its associated Bye-Laws set out the new financial framework.

At this time the titles of the Member Societies, with very few exceptions, mention only the EEG and this restricted interest is clearly shown by the contemporary Society Proceedings in the Journal, which rarely refer to topics other than EEG and cerebral electrophysiology. This limitation was felt by some, particularly Gastaut and Cobb, to be inimical to the healthy future of the Federation. Today most laboratories are of "Clinical Neurophysiology" and few restrict their interests to the EEG alone, but in 1960 there was considerable resistance to the idea of deliberately expanding the scope of the Federation, despite the second part of its title. The problem was of immediate consequence because electromyography and electroneurography had arranged a meeting to be held in 1961 in Pavia and there was talk of setting up their own Federation. The solution arrived at, of giving EMG its own Commission within the Federation and direct representation in the Executive, was to prove highly controversial, though finally accepted by all the members of the committee and later by the General Assembly.

Since the Statutes could only be changed at four yearly intervals it was thought desirable to add to them a set of Bye-Laws which could be changed at any time with the postal agreement of the members of the Council. The new Statutes and Bye-Laws were published later with the Proceedings of the General Assembly (Journal, 1962, 14: 935–952).

1. The EEG Journal

The circulation of the Journal continued to increase, to 2800 by the end of 1960, and so did the number of submitted papers, resulting in an alarming publication delay, despite the printing of 850 pages in 1959 and 960 in 1960. An instruction to authors to shorten their papers to not more than 4000 words and six figures was published (Journal, 1959, 11: 438), though with little noticeable effect. In spite of a deficit in 1958 of $11,000, largely due to the printing of back issues, the account was in balance again by the end of 1959. Jasper declared that it was necessary to increase the subscription to $13. It is noteworthy that after 10 years of operation the Journal had never been able to pass on any profit to the Federation, which had been the hope at the founding meeting of the latter in 1949. However, this was about to change.

In his report on 1958 Jasper announced the resignation of Pierre Gloor from the Montreal office and his own intention to resign at the end of 1961. He thought that the Journal should be handed over to a "reputable international publishing house". During the following year there was much exploration and discussion of a possible publisher and of a new editorial structure, since the "American" office would soon be vacant and in Europe Magnus and Storm van Leeuwen wished to resign.

The possibility of publishing in Europe was favoured by some on the grounds that it would be less expensive and also that it would favour the much prized international character of the Journal. A large majority of contributors and of subscribers were American and it was feared that, if the Editor-in-Chief and the publisher were also American, the claim to be international might be hard to sustain. The first mention of Elsevier occurs in a letter from Cobb to Jasper in December 1959.

However, in April 1960 Jasper reported that negotiations with The American Institute of Biological Sciences in Washington were far advanced. Why they fell through is not apparent from the correspondence, though the problem mentioned in the previous paragraph may have been one factor. At any rate, in September 1960 Jasper concluded a remarkable contract with the Elsevier Publishing Company of Amsterdam, whereby the Federation would retain control of the editing of the Journal and receive one-third of the profits, without liability in the event of loss. Furthermore, Elsevier bought the whole stock of back issues of the Journal and the Supplements for rather more than $30,000. Thus, in an instant the fortunes of the Federation were transformed. Issues in future were to be bimonthly and the first under the new imprint appeared in January 1961, with a very modest foreword from Jasper under the heading "Letter from the Editors".

Meanwhile, Jasper had been persuaded to remain for a while longer as Editor-in-Chief and Cosimo Ajmone Marsan became "Editor for the Western Hemisphere and the Far East". Not long after this Otto Magnus resigned, leaving Storm van Leeuwen alone as "Editor for Europe and the Middle East". Things did not work out too well at first and in a letter of August 1961 Jasper says: "We should not have changed the editorial board at the same time as the publisher."

Another publishing effort of this period should be mentioned, though at the time it had no direct connection with the Journal. Books on EEG were few, incomplete and partially out of date and it was felt that the Federation should produce a comprehensive text as part of its educational commitment. The two Frenchmen, Gastaut and Rémond, had been much impressed by the story behind a highly successful French mathematical text which had been apparently written by Bourbaki; apart from being that of a 19th century French general this name was unknown to mathematicians. It transpired that it was a pseudonym for a team of writers who had all corrected each other's texts until something near perfection had been achieved.

Accordingly, although discussions had begun some months before, the *éditeur fictif* came into being in July 1960 under the name of Fiseeg, and his component parts were Jasper, Walter, Gastaut, Brazier, Cobb, Fischgold, Henry, Magnus, Rémond and Storm van Leeuwen. Much as we all approved of the plan, by the time many letters had been exchanged to establish the chapter headings, their contents and their authors, the initial impetus had been lost and no one could find the time or energy to begin the serious business of writing. The project lingered on for at least two years before quietly dying, though it was to be revived again under another name some years later.

2. The Fifth International Congress, Rome

Though it was not strictly part of the Congress it is proper to mention here the Advanced Course in EEG which was held immediately beforehand. This had been conceived in Brussels and Otto Magnus had been charged with its organization, assisted by Willem Storm van Leeuwen. As soon as Marseilles had been chosen as the site it was obvious that Gastaut and Robert Naquet should join them to form an organizing committee.

Through the good offices of Gastaut the Faculté de Médecine and the Cité Universitaire were made available, making it possible to run the course very inexpensively; in fact 80 of the 420 participants, from 40 countries, were technicians. They were, as it turned out, holding their first international meeting.

The course, from August 28 to September 2, 1961, was opened by three doctors *honoris causa* of the University of Aix-Marseilles in colourful academic robes and tall hats. It consisted of lectures in the mornings and EEG interpretation sessions in the afternoons, with ample time to enjoy the pleasures of the Provence. It was voted a great success.

Planning for the congress program had begun two years before with a poll of Member Societies, which attempted to find from them the most favoured topics and structure. In October 1960 the officers and some other members of the Federation met the Italian organizers (there was no formally constituted Organizing Committee as yet) to draw up the program. They were Prof. Gozzano, Dr. Vizioli and Dr. Ricci, President, Secretary and Treasurer, respectively.

The Congress was held in the Palazzo Pio of Rome in the week of September 4 and at the same time as the Neurological Congress. The inaugural ceremony was appropriately splendid and numerous dignitaries had their say in grandiloquent phrases.

The meeting of the Executive Committee arranged to take place before the General Assembly was an object lesson on how not to do such things. It was held during lunch in a crowded restaurant, with waiters constantly moving around the tables, with the only window open to the heat and noise of the Via della Concilliazione, and with some 20 members speaking French or English, in most cases not their native languages.

At the General Assembly the Treasurer pointed out that expenditure had been rather more than income and he proposed a more rational system of contributions from the Societies, based on the numbers of their members. Initially it was agreed to pay $5 per 10 members, amounting in all to about $850 per year. The Societies had also been asked to contribute $2 per head to support the Congress and this was to continue. The new wealth provided by the sale of the Journal was, for the present at least, to be regarded as a fund for the support of the Journal and any other publications of the Federation.

The new Constitution was explained and discussed without engendering any great heat. The approval of the General Assembly is recorded as being unanimous. Three distinguished electromyographers were then proposed to form the EMG Commission. They were Fritz Buchthal (Denmark), I. Hausmanova (Poland) and Ed Lambert (USA); these names were to prove controversial, not for any personal reason, but because they were not all members of member societies; at the time they were accepted without demur.

Although strictly speaking the new Constitution would not be in force until after the Congress an attempt was made to act according to it in the election of the officers who would form the Executive Committee. A Nomination Committee had been set up under Grey Walter, the immediate Past-President. Its proposals of Mary Brazier as President, R.G. Naquet as Secretary and W.A. Cobb as Treasurer (for a second term) were accepted. The new style Executive Committee thus consisted of the above with Jasper (Editor-in-Chief), Gastaut (Past-President) and Buchthal (EMG Commission).

Wave Length and Action Potentials: History of the IFCN
(Supplements to Clinical Neurophysiology, Vol. 61)
By: M.R. Nuwer and C.H. Lücking

Chapter 5

1961–1965

President: M.A.B. Brazier

The revised Statutes introduced the term "Fiscal Period" for the interval between one congress and the next, normally four years, and firmly established it as the term of all offices and the life of all committees, so we may use it from here on.

In the present Fiscal Period four more societies joined the Federation, those of Luxembourg, Yugoslavia, Canada and Greece. There was some hesitation over accepting the first, because of its appropriately small size, but certainly there have been no regrets. The total was now 29.

It soon became apparent that some people were dissatisfied with certain aspects of the new Constitution but it was not until its publication (Journal, 1962, 14: 943–949) that things came to a head. The objections were concentrated on the EMG Commission and on the mode of election of its officers; it is evident from the letters that went to and fro at this time that the intention of welding all the various branches of Clinical Neurophysiology into a single Federation did not have universal appeal, or perhaps that too high a price was being paid for it. However, there being little chance that this line of attack would have any success, the arguments raised by the objectors were entirely of a legalistic nature.

To deal with these problems the President set up a Rules Committee in May 1963 with the widest possible terms of reference, consisting of A.E. Walker (Baltimore), A. Rémond (Paris), O. Magnus (Wassenaar) and M. Saunders (Winnipeg), under the chairmanship of W.A. Cobb (London).

The first point discussed was whether the EMG Commission had been legally constituted; to oversimplify a complex situation this depended on whether the new constitution was in force at the time, since the old one gave virtually no guidance on any procedural matters. The Rules Committee decided that the new constitution could not be considered as operative until after the end of the General Assembly and hence that the Commission was set up under the old constitution and could not be considered illegal.

A second major objection was to the mode of election of the members of the EMG Commission. Anticipating the new statutes the President had arranged for the Executive Officers to be elected by the new method and set up a Nomination Committee for the purpose; unfortunately he did not use this for the election of the members of the Commission but offered a list of names — the "slate" of former days — to the Council, which approved it. The Proceedings of the General Assembly stated that he "proposed" these names, though in fact he was reporting the decision of the Council. In American usage a president cannot himself propose a motion, though this is normal in many European countries. A further point of contention was that only one of the three commissioners was a member of a society within the Federation; in his anxiety to forestall the setting up of an EMG federation Gastaut had asked the "Pavia Committee" to propose names and naturally those suggested were not necessarily members of EEG societies.

Again the Rules Committee took the view that the election took place before the new statutes were in force and that under the old it was legitimate for the President to make the proposal. Further, there was nothing in the Statutes to prevent the election of a non-member.

The Committee finally reported to the President at some length and this report, which was a direct reply to a detailed criticism by the American delegate, was sent to the American EEG Society. In a brief formal letter of October 1963 they rejected it.

In view of this the President decided to ask all the delegates for their views on the new Constitution. The replies were almost all in favour though they raised some points for discussion and others had arisen in the extensive correspondence of the Rules and Executive Committees, so that it became clear that further modifications of the Statutes were desirable.

It was proposed to increase the size of the Executive Committee by the appointment of a Member-at-Large; the controversial membership of the Chairman of the EMG Commission was retained. The appointment of a Rules Committee at the beginning of each Fiscal Period was obligatory. Many minor points of procedure were clarified.

To remove the ambiguities of procedure which had been apparent in the previous General Assembly, it had been strongly urged that some code of practice should be adopted and, indeed, Roberts' Rules of Order had been advocated. This is a little red book which sets out American parliamentary procedure in great detail. It was not sufficiently realized that the chances of following these Rules correctly in an Assembly which met only at 4-year intervals were small indeed. Accordingly Michael Saunders, with the help of the other members of the Rules Committee, was commissioned to draw up the Federation's own Rules of Order. To provide some chance that they would be observed a Procedural Counsellor was introduced, with no other task than to guide the President in his conduct of the meeting.

By the time this work was finished (Saunders later made a simplified version for the meeting of the Council) the Rules Committee had been continuously active for 18 months. The philosophy of the chairman, at least, possibly of the other members also, was that "rules" should be as few and simple as possible, yet the Committee found itself forced by outside pressures to produce a volume and complexity of Statutes and Bye-Laws far greater than it wished.

1. The EEG Journal

As mentioned in the last chapter the Editor-in-Chief and the regional editors had all expressed the intention of resigning — Magnus had already done so — and the relationship between the two remaining regional editors was increasingly strained. A meeting of the Editorial Board had resolved nothing and the new President Mary Brazier (Figs. 5.1 and 5.2) saw it as urgent that a

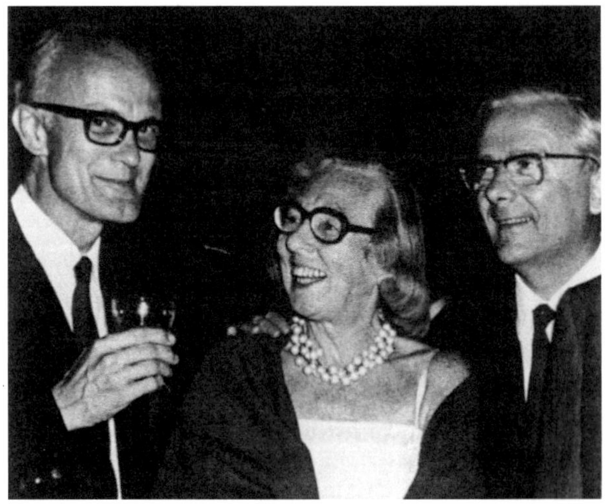

Fig. 5.1. From left to right:
- Lennart Widén of Karolinska Institute, Stockholm. Editor of Supplement 25, *Recent Advances in Clinical Neurophysiology*, 1967.
- M.A.B. Brazier, who worked with F. Golla in London, R.S. Schwab in Boston and H.W. Magoun in Los Angeles. Compiled Supplement 1, *Bibliography of EEG* (1950), Treasurer 1953–1957, Secretary 1957–1961, President 1961–1965, American Editor of Journal 1972 and Editor-in-Chief 1973–1984.
- Willem Storm van Leeuwen of Leyden and Utrecht. European co-editor of the Journal with Otto Magnus 1957–1961, Treasurer 1962–1969.

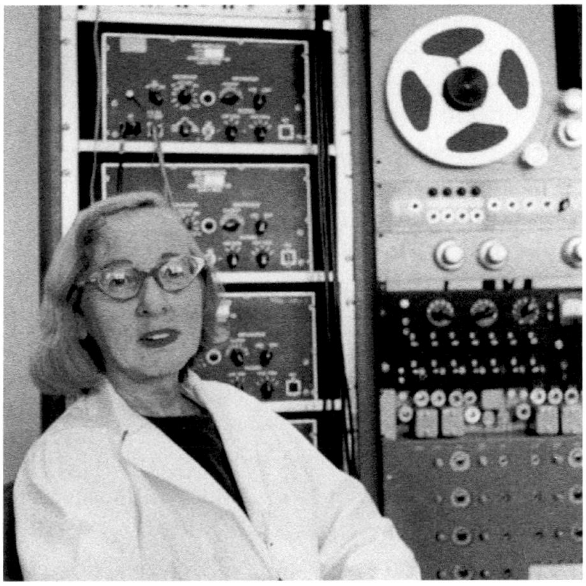

Fig. 5.2. Mary A.B. "Molly" Brazier, Federation Treasurer 1953–1957, Secretary 1957–1961, President 1961–1965, American Editor of Journal 1972 and Editor-in-Chief 1973–1984. Shown here with her laboratory equipment at the UCLA Brain Research Institute, and including the old instrument racks and tape drives used for EEG research in that era.

solution should be found. Accordingly a further meeting was convened in Amsterdam — to be near to Elsevier — in March 1962, at which it was decided that Cobb should take the place of Storm van Leeuwen as European Editor and Ajmone Marsan agreed to continue as American Editor. The post of Editor-in-Chief was replaced by Managing Editor, held by Cobb (because of his relative proximity to Elsevier). This arrangement, born out of storm and stress, was to give the Journal a long period of stability.

When the Journal was taken over by Elsevier a change was made from quarterly to bi-monthly publication. By 1964 the demand for space had become such that a new contract was made, to publish 1308 pages in monthly issues, forming two volumes. This of course necessitated an increase in the subscription rates, from $13 to $19.50, and there were fears for the effect which this might have on the circulation; in fact, it increased to its highest level so far of 3030. A further experiment at this time was to issue extra numbers as the need arose, to be paid for retrospectively; the fear that the subscribers might object or refuse to pay was not confirmed.

It had been the intention to publish the symposia of the Rome Congress as one of the Journal Supplements. For a variety of reasons great delays occurred in the collection and processing of the material and finally it became clear that a balanced symposium volume was impossible. Accordingly the authors were given the possibility of having their papers published quickly in the Journal, Elsevier offering an extra 100 pages to help absorb this extra material. Fearing a repetition of this misfortune, an editor, Lennart Widén of Stockholm (Fig. 5.1), was appointed in good time to oversee the material generated by the Vienna Congress and steps were taken to ensure that it was punctual and complete. Every subsequent Congress has been fully reported in its own Supplement.

The Vienna Supplement, when it came out in 1967, was the 25th. Of these Elsevier had produced the last six and Masson et Cie of Paris, in the rather curious arrangement mentioned earlier, six of the remainder. Only a few of the total were Federation proceedings and most were reports of limited symposia, not necessarily with Federation backing. Some, on the other hand, were monographs by one or more authors.

2. The Sixth International Congress, Vienna

Following the success of the Advanced Course in Marseilles, Otto Magnus was asked to organize a similar course to precede the Congress in Vienna. This he did in conjunction with Helmuth Petsche, one of the organizers of the Congress, and they quickly settled on Salzburg as the site, most suitable because of its excellent congress hall, its hotels and its beautiful and historic background. Like the first, this Course was meticulously planned and most successful, attended by 650 members from 49 countries, of whom 130 were technicians.

It was immediately followed by the Congress, held in all the splendour of the Hofburg of Vienna, running simultaneously with the Neurological Congress and both under the presidency of Prof. Hans Hoff. The local organization of the EEG Congress was in the hands of Kurt Pateisky and Helmuth Petsche, with the expert backing of the Medical Faculty of the University of Vienna.

The Proceedings of the General Assembly, held on September 9, are reported in great detail, together with reports of numerous committees, in the Journal (1966, 20: 293–320), which also includes the modified Statutes and Bye-Laws, and a revised version of the Terminology.

The proposed changes in the Statutes had been agreed by the postal vote of the Council but further proposals were made, and generated considerable heat, at the Council meeting held during the Congress. One, that there should be one delegate for every hundred members of a society, was rejected by the Council and not presented to the General Assembly; this was the first of several attempts to introduce a form of proportional representation. Another, accepted by the Council but failing to find the necessary support in the General Assembly, was a proposal to have three (rather than one) members-at-large.

W. Storm van Leeuwen (Fig. 5.1) had replaced Cobb as Treasurer in 1961, when Cobb became Managing Editor of the Journal. The treasurer's accounts and budget offered a very different picture from the relative poverty of former years. Apart from the capital derived from the sale of back issues the Journal had produced about $10,000 over the 4 years and there were other lesser sources of income.

The Chairman of the EMG Commission, Fritz Buchthal (Fig. 5.3), reported that it was guided by the Pavia Committee. That committee had been set up at the congress in that city in 1961, which had a wide international membership. He also mentioned that a second EMG Congress had been held in Copenhagen in 1963 under the joint auspices of the Federation and the World Federation of Neurology.

It was known that the next Neurological Congress would be in America; the General Assembly agreed to leave the place and time of the EEG Congress to the American EEG Society

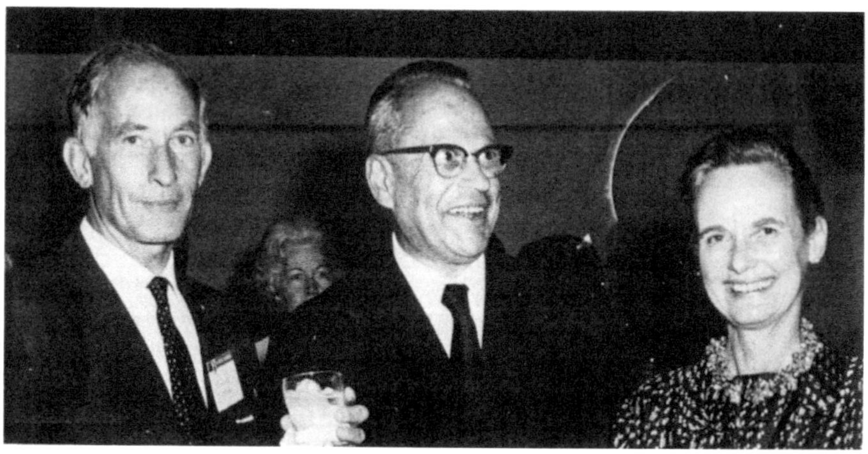

Fig. 5.3. From left to right:
- R. Hess of Zurich. Treasurer 1969–1973.
- Fritz Buchthal of Copenhagen, a founding Federation Vice-President and first Chairman of the EMG Commission 1961–1965 and again EMG Commission Chairman 1969–1973.
- Margaret Lennox-Buchthal, wife of Fritz, daughter of William Lennox. Author of Supplement 32: *Febrile Convulsions*.

"provided that the time should be close to that of the International Neurology Congress."

Thus began the relative independence of our congresses which has been maintained ever since; they have in fact been held in the week before the Neurology Congress, sometimes in the same city but sometimes as far apart as San Diego and New York.

Gastaut, as Chairman of the Nomination Committee, had scrupulously followed the procedure sketched out in the new Statutes for the election of the Executive Committee, though with some misgivings. When he came to ask those nominated if they were willing to stand for election they all refused, except one for each post. Thus it was only possible to submit to the Council for confirmation a list of single names looking remarkably like the "slate" of previous occasions, though in fact the outcome of a quite complex electoral process.

The list then submitted to the General Assembly was as follows:

President	A. Rémond
Secretary	R. Naquet
Treasurer	W. Storm van Leeuwen
Chairman of EMG Commission	E. Lambert

They would serve together with

Past President	M.A.B. Brazier
Editor of the Journal	W.A. Cobb

These Nominations were accepted by acclamation.

Wave Length and Action Potentials: History of the IFCN
(Supplements to Clinical Neurophysiology, Vol. 61)
By: M.R. Nuwer and C.H. Lücking

Chapter 6

1965–1969

President: A. Rémond

Meetings of the Executive Committee and Editorial Board had always been kept to a minimum because of the cost, since they invariably entailed at least one double Atlantic crossing, usually more. So far as possible they were arranged in association with meetings for which at least one of the members would receive travel expenses from other sources. In fact, this principle continues to be followed and has often reduced the expenses of meeting to a surprisingly small figure.

The new President, Antoine Rémond (Fig. 6.1), was in the fortunate position, as a result of working for an international airline, of being able to travel anywhere at a small fraction of the normal cost, which he did very often. Thus he was able to hold relatively frequent partial meetings of the Executive Committee, and later of the Organizing Committee of the Congress, on either side of the Atlantic; at these, useful discussions took place, though final decisions were still usually taken by postal vote.

The new post of Member-at-Large of the Executive Committee had been approved by the General Assembly and it seemed desirable that it should be filled as soon as possible. Accordingly, the Bye-Law "Executive Committee 3" was invoked, which gives the Executive Committee powers to appoint, subject to confirmation by the Council, a member to fill a gap in its members until the end of the Fiscal Period. Michael Saunders of Winnipeg (Fig. 6.2), who had worked hard as a member of the Rules Committee, was chosen and duly confirmed by the postal vote of the Council.

The early appointment of a permanent (for the Fiscal Period) Rules Committee was now statutory. Saunders, with valuable previous experience, was appointed chairman. Much time was spent and a huge correspondence was generated throughout the period to clarify numerous minor points in the Rules.

About a year after the Vienna Congress the Organizing Committee for the next congress, now defined by Statute, began to take shape; from the hosts, the American EEG Society, Herbert Jasper was elected President, Richard Walter Secretary and Robert Ellingson Treasurer. Ed Lambert represented EMG affairs and the American Association of EMG and Electrodiagnosis. These were widely scattered and all far away from San Diego; it fell to Dick Walter, by no means a "local", to make all the plans for the physical organization of the Congress, which he did with great success, assisted by Laverne Johnson, far exceeding his role of Chairman for Local Arrangements. An early decision was to hold the Congress in San Diego in the week before the Neurological Congress in New York — the same country to be sure, but almost as far apart as they could be. The actual site of the Congress was to be the El Cortez Hotel (Fig. 6.3), which rapidly came to be called in the OCIC El Cortex Hotel. In fact the hotel later agreed to this change of title for the duration of the Congress.

San Diego is the main base of the U.S. Pacific fleet and for a while there were grave doubts whether visitors from the Iron Curtain countries

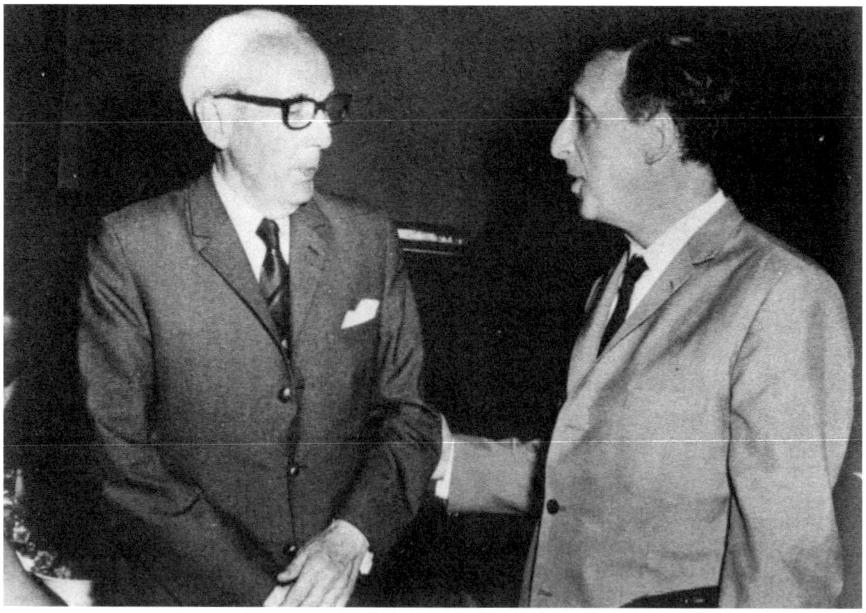

Fig. 6.1.

- Antoine Rémond (right), President 1965–1969, Editor-in-Chief of the "Handbook of EEG and Clinical Neurophysiology".
- Frédéric Bremer (left), distinguished Belgian neurologist and neurophysiologist. Founder of the Belgian EEG Society and President of the Fourth International EEG Congress, Brussels 1957.

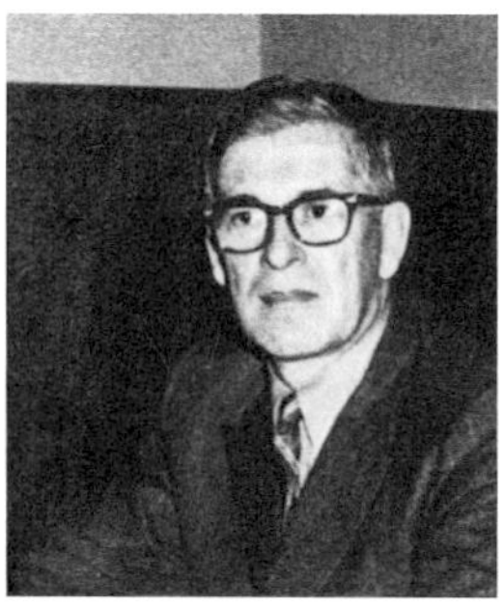

Fig. 6.2. Michael Saunders of Winnipeg. First Federation Member-at-Large (1966–1969) and Chairman of the first statutory Rules Committee. He drafted the Rules of Order for the General Assembly and Council.

would be granted visas — specifically, a reputable European scientist had been refused permission to take up a study grant to work in a San Diego laboratory. Finally, however, the difficulties were overcome and a dozen scientists from the communist countries of Europe attended. A curious sidelight on this problem will be mentioned later.

The program of the Congress was as usual in the hands of the committee led by the President, Tony Rémond. He initiated an enquiry among all interested parties as to preferred topics and methods of presentation. The same had been done before but never so elaborately; all the information was entered in a computer as it became available. Gradually the idea developed of linking the Congress program with the subsequent production of a Handbook of EEG and Clinical Neurophysiology, with some of the characteristics of the old "Fiseeg" project. For example, all the members of a Round Table at the Congress would subsequently write a section of the Handbook on the same topic, without attribution of its separate parts to individual authors. Since the Handbook would have to be all-embracing, its conjunction with the Congress added considerably to the complexity of planning the program of the latter.

All this activity, and much else, emanated from the office of Tony Rémond in La Salpêtrière,

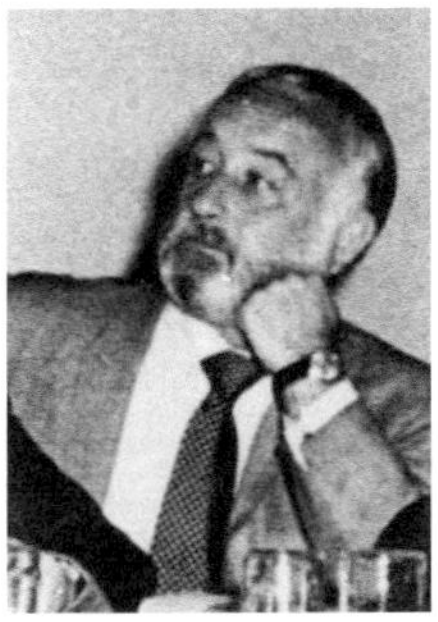

Fig. 6.3. Peter Kellaway of Houston, Texas. American Editor of the Journal 1969–1971.

Paris. Visiting him there one day in December 1968, Storm van Leeuwen and Cobb were horrified to see the state of mental exhaustion to which he had driven himself. So apprehensive were they for his health and the development of the Congress program that they called Mary Brazier in Los Angeles. She gallantly dropped everything and was in Paris within 2 days. There it was arranged that she, as the statutory deputy of the President, should take on his duties temporarily. The problems of the Congress program and, less urgently, the Handbook could be solved through a fortunate coincidence. All arrangements for the program were in the mind and files of Rémond's most competent assistant Gillian Dunkley, who had previously held a responsible post in the laboratory of Cobb in the National Hospital for Nervous Diseases in London; it was a relatively easy matter, therefore, to transfer her and the files to London, and for Cobb to guide her activities. These rescue operations were successful in that the program was completed and Rémond was able to resume his duties before long.

The Statutes allowed much freedom in the way in which elections of the officers could be conducted. The chairman of the Nomination Committee, Mary Brazier, decided to conduct the election of the President first, the rest subsequently, with the hope of avoiding some of the past difficulties. Cosimo Ajmone Marsan of Bethesda was elected President and consequently resigned as American Editor of the Journal. Later Robert J. Ellingson of Omaha, who was demonstrating his abilities most strikingly in the organizing of the Congress, was elected Secretary. The Treasurer was R. Hess of Zurich, the Chairman of the EMG Commission Fritz Buchthal of Copenhagen and the Member-at-Large, David Ingvar of Lund. The Past President, Rémond, and the Managing Editor of the Journal completed the Executive Committee for the following Fiscal Period.

During the Fiscal Period five new societies were admitted to membership, those of Turkey, Iran, Argentina, Uruguay and Mexico; shortly before the Congress a sixth was added, the American Association of Electromyography and Electrodiagnosis, bringing the total to 35. This last was made possible by a change in the Bye-Laws permitting the membership of two societies from the same country "provided that its (the second society's) main sphere of interest differs from that of the first".

This reflected the increasing acceptance that the Federation should have wider interests than in EEG alone. In June 1967 it sponsored an International EMG Congress in Glasgow and abstracts of the papers were later published in the Journal (1968, 25: 393). The Journal also contained committee reports on the "Terminology of EMG" (1969, 26: 224) and on "EMG apparatus" (1970, 28: 399).

1. The EEG Journal

The first and all subsequent issues of the Journal up to 1964 contained an Index of Literature compiled by Chuck Henry; after that they became bi-monthly. At the end of 1965 Henry indicated that he had had enough, as well he might after 16 years. Fortunately a new method of presentation was already under discussion and, after a short interval, the Index resumed as a quarterly 16-page loose leaf insert to the Journal, derived from the computer store of the Brain Information Service (BIS) of the University of California, Los Angeles, which, supported by the National Institutes of Health, provided the classified print-outs free.

Henry had also stated his wish to give up the editing of book reviews; in the hope of casting the net more widely this task was divided between a European and an American Editor, Helmuth Petsche and John Hughes, respectively, who started the work in 1967 and have conscientiously continued for 20 years. The possibility of using the Journal to speak more directly to its readers about Federation affairs had been frequently discussed and indeed it had become the practice to publish committee reports and the proceedings of the General Assembly. However, it was felt that any further extension would be an improper use of a scientific journal and, in any case, the production delay of about 5–6 months would remove any sense of immediacy. Accordingly, Rémond conceived the idea of a periodical news bulletin, which would serve to spread news and views throughout the neurophysiological world. Strictly it had nothing to do with the Journal except to complement it and was entirely the product of the President and his personal staff, but it did have the support of the Executive Committee and a grant for the first year's operation. Four numbers of "Trace" appeared in 1967 at a cost of about $4000, twice the Federation's grant. In 1968 there were six numbers but the cost was prohibitive, despite an increased grant, and the project had to be abandoned, to widespread regret.

In 1968 the Journal reached its peak of distribution, at 3400, and in 1969 increased its pages to 1400. A new contract for this number of pages included provision for a special extra issue containing the abstracts of the free communications to the Congress; everyone attending got a copy in his Congress wallet and it also had the normal Journal distribution. This scheme was most successful and it has been repeated, with minor variations, for all subsequent congresses.

Following his election as President, Cosimo Ajmone Marsan retired from the post of American Editor in July 1969, bringing to a much regretted end the 8-year collaboration with Cobb. Though differing amicably on many points, on one thing they were completely agreed, that the Journal should be as free of literal and typographical errors as possible; in this they had the staunch support of the desk editor at Elsevier, Miss Bastiaans; the text has probably never been as "perfect" as at this time.

It is no easy matter to find someone with the right qualifications to take on the time-consuming task of editing the Journal and we were fortunate to persuade, without undue pressure, Peter Kellaway of Houston, Texas (Fig. 6.3), to accept.

Although the new contract had increased the price of the Journal to $25, by the end of the Fiscal period it was becoming clear that inflation and tightening purse-strings everywhere were soon going to present the Journal, and hence the Federation, with a financial problem, which could only result in a further increase in price.

2. The Seventh International Congress, San Diego

The Congress, from September 13 to 19, 1969, took place in the excellent conference rooms of the transiently renamed El Cortex Hotel (Fig. 6.4). It had been realized that it was the 40th anniversary of the publication of Berger's first paper on the EEG and also of the Adrian and Bronk paper on the use of coaxial needles to study motor unit activity; hence the Congress theme was declared to be "Appraisal and Perspective after Forty Years of the Functional Exploration of the Nervous System". All those who registered were presented with an English translation by Pierre Gloor of Montreal of the 14 main EEG papers of Berger, beautifully produced by Elsevier as *Supplement 28* of the Journal. The Canadian EEG Society contributed substantially to the cost of its preparation.

In the same dedicatory vein the Congress opened, under the presidency of Herbert Jasper, with a session on the "Evolution of Clinical Neurophysiology since Hans Berger". Lord Adrian spoke on the ambiguously titled "Discovery of Berger", Gloor on "The work of Hans Berger", Cobb on "The past 40 years of EEG" and Grey Walter, optimistically, on "The future

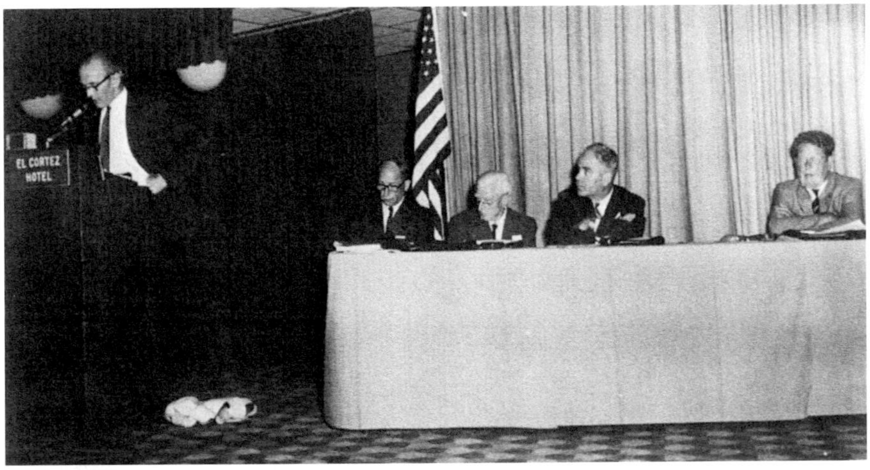

Fig. 6.4. The opening session of the San Diego Congress (1969). From left to right:
- Speaking at the lectern on "The Past 40 Years of EEG": W.A. Cobb.
- At the table: Herbert H. Jasper, E.D. Adrian (Guest of Honour), Pierre Gloor, W. Grey Walter.
- The lecture is labelled with the usual hotel name El Cortez, even though the hotel agreed to change its name to El Cortex for the week of the congress.

of EEG". In conformity with the Handbook project a large part of the Congress was taken up by a series of 13 Round Table discussions, more didactic than was usual, in which about eight speakers each dealt with one topic within a theme. A very successful innovation was the daily presentation on closed circuit television of live demonstrations of interesting observations or new techniques.

At the General Assembly it was agreed to support the Handbook project, on which a great deal of preliminary work, though no writing, had been done. Two changes in the Statutes were made, one of these defining more explicitly the composition of the Organizing Committee of Congresses. This arose largely because the organization was becoming big business (nearly 1100 members registered), involving expenses far outside the normal for the host society or the Federation. This Congress was greatly aided by a grant from the National Institutes of Health of about $42,000; nothing on this scale had been found before though every Congress had had some assistance from governmental or other official bodies; nor would it happen again, for the effects of inflation were beginning to be felt everywhere.

For entertainment San Diego has much to offer, not least the famous Zoo and Sea World, but the hosts excelled in providing a party of some kind every night. Toward the end of the evening at one of these, an open air buffet, someone said "Would you like to see the Naval Base?" This was a startling proposal in view of the secrecy in which it had appeared to be cloaked. In addition to our American driver the party finally consisted of nationals from four countries in Eastern Europe. At the gate of the Base a sentry looked briefly at the car and raised the barrier. We drove around for perhaps half an hour, seeing various ships, the crew of an aircraft carrier watching a film show, planes landing on the airstrip. When we left, the gate was again opened without any question. The explanation of this lack of the expected rigid security was that our driver had been in the naval reserve some long time before — and had never removed the pass from his car.

Wave Length and Action Potentials: History of the IFCN
(Supplements to Clinical Neurophysiology, Vol. 61)
By: M.R. Nuwer and C.H. Lücking

Chapter 7

1969–1973

President: C. Ajmone Marsan

The Federation continued its progress in representing clinical neurophysiology worldwide and sponsoring publications under the capable leadership of President Cosimo Ajmone Marsan (Fig. 7.1). The Executive Committee continued to include one Member-at-Large, in this term David Ingvar of Sweden (Fig. 7.2). Fritz Buchthal, founding Chairman of the EMG Commission in the previous decade, returned for an encore performance in that role.

Taking advantage of the change in the Statutes permitting two society members from the same country, the Belgian Society of EMG and Clinical Neurophysiology applied for membership and was accepted in 1971. The Finnish Society of Clinical Neurophysiology was accepted a little later, bringing the total of members to 37.

A change in the Bye-Laws concerned the sponsorship of meetings other than the Congress, as a result of which the Federation took a much more active part in the organization of the 4th International Congress of EMG, which was held in Brussels in September 1971. In fact, the credit for this successful meeting goes to its President, Jean Desmedt and his team, but future EMG congresses would be organized in exactly the same way as the Federation's major congress, that is, by a collaboration of designated members of the Executive Committee with the local organizers.

The Federation had had for a number of years an anomalous relationship with the Pavia Committee of EMG workers, which was already in existence when the EMG Commission was set up. Now, at the instigation of the chairman of the latter, Fritz Buchthal, a liaison group of 11 members, proposed by the Delegates, was set up. If its composition was very similar to that of the Pavia Committee that it replaced, it had gained in acceptability by being chosen from within the Federation.

The financial situation of the Federation at the end of the period seemed doubtful, though not yet alarming. The dollar, in which most of the Federation's affairs, including the collection of dues, were conducted, had been devalued; the new contract with Elsevier, mentioned later, was wrongly thought by some to be likely to reduce the income from the Journal; expenses had been greater than expected, particularly for financing the Handbook project; above all were the unpredictable effects of inflation over the coming 4 years.

A "Committee on Terminology" had been set up to update the "Proposal for an EEG Terminology" (Journal, 1966, 20: 306). Some of its proposals were controversial but none more so than that to substitute Hertz for the familiar c/s or cps. The two Editors, Brazier and Cobb, fought hard against the change, but without success. The report of this and other committees is published with the Proceedings of the General Assembly (Journal, 1974, 37: 521).

The election of the next Executive Committee was conducted as on the last occasion, that is, of the President first, the rest later. The result was: President, W.A. Cobb; Secretary, R.J. Ellingson (for the second time); Treasurer, Max Dondey (who had shown his competence as a member of

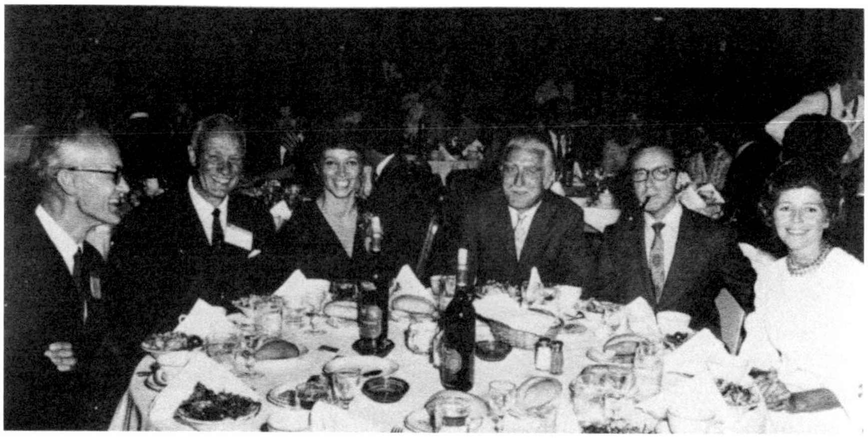

Fig. 7.1. From left to right:

- Lennart Widén, of Karolinska Institute, Stockholm. Editor of Supplement 25, *Recent Advances in Clinical Neurophysiology*, 1967.
- Arne Lundervold of Oslo. Norwegian Delegate.
- Gillian Dunkley, assistant of Cobb in London and Rémond in Paris. Much involved in the publication of *Trace*, the organization of the scientific program for San Diego and the early stages of the Handbook.
- Cosimo Ajmone Marsan of Bethesda, MD, American Editor 1960–1969, President 1969–1973.
- Dominick Purpura, a much-used Consulting Editor.
- Gabrielle Lairy of Paris, Secretary of the 1973 (Marseilles) Congress. For many years a translator of summaries for the Journal's research reports.

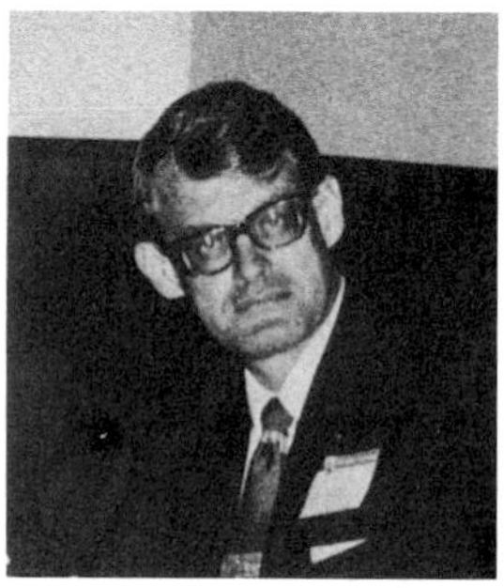

Fig. 7.2. David Ingvar of Lund, Sweden, Member-at-Large 1969–1973.

the Organizing Committee of the Congress); Chairman of the EMG Commission, A. Struppler of Munich; Member-at-Large, Helmuth Petsche of Vienna. The other members of the Executive Committee were C. Ajmone Marsan, the Past-President, and Mary Brazier, successor to Peter Kellaway, for whom the post of Editor-in-Chief was revived. The members of the EMG Commission were Jean Desmedt and Robin Willison.

1. The EEG Journal

Toward the end of the last Fiscal Period the new contract with Elsevier had given the Journal 1400 pages a year, which it seemed to need, yet very soon in the new period a falling off in the number of submissions, mainly to the American office, became apparent. By the end of 1970 the situation was so bad that one number contained only 76 pages, instead of 120, after everything available had been put into it. The reason for this remarkable swing was never clear, though less dramatic changes, both up and down, had occurred before; by the end of this period the pendulum had again swung the other way and there was so much available material that several oversize issues were necessary to reduce the surplus and the publishers suggested an increase in the total pages. Experience of the previous fluctuations, however, urged caution and nothing was done, which time showed to have been the decision.

Up to this time the agreement with Elsevier had allowed the Editorial Board to exercise some measure of control over the price of the Journal, which we had tried to keep down in the interest of the subscribers. In fact, Elsevier always had the last word, rightly, since they were the experts and bore the financial risks. It came as a complete surprise, therefore, when, at an Editorial Board meeting in Paris in November 1970, Elsevier abruptly announced that they wished to terminate the contract and draw up a new one. After a long delay a new draft contract was produced which made a number of totally unacceptable financial demands. The correspondence which followed was hampered by a prolonged postal strike in England that left the Managing Editor out of touch with his colleagues for long periods. Among other solutions that they proposed were returning to the amateur production of the Montreal days (no one offered to take on the job) and giving the Journal to another publishing house; in fact at this time, with a minimum of publishable papers, our bargaining position to do so was very weak.

Eventually, however, a new agreement was reached with Elsevier which differed little from the original though one member of the Executive Committee thought that "it means the almost inevitable loss of any future profits which the Federation might have realized from the Journal", a view shared by others though not by the Managing Editor. In fact, during the next Fiscal Period, when the effect of the new agreement was fully felt, the income from the Journal was nearly $67,000. It should be said that this was the only occasion on which we have had serious differences with Elsevier in many years association and this was due more to some clumsiness than to anything else.

These discussions evidently added to the uneasiness which Peter Kellaway felt in his work and other pressures led him to resign at the end of 1971. Fortunately Mary Brazier was persuaded to take on the task of American Editor, adding one more to her many services to the Federation; unfortunately, for her, her appointment coincided with the upsurge in submitted papers mentioned above, but she survived it with enthusiasm.

Toward the end of the period the election of Cobb as the next president led to his resignation as Editor. Once again our first choice of a replacement accepted and Pierre Buser of Paris became the European Editor from the beginning of 1973.

The computerized Index of Current Literature had developed well, growing to 48 pages per volume. From this material a new "KWIC" Index was produced, covering 1966–1969, as *Supplement 29* and then a further *Supplement 30* filled the gap from 1964 to 1966. These two, together with Brazier's original Bibliography and Bickford's KWIC Index, covered the entire field for the period of 94 years since Caton's first paper of 1875.

The demise of the "Trace" news announcement left a serious gap in communications, which the Editorial Board was loath to fill by using Journal pages. A solution came when Elsevier offered to include in each number a two-page insert, provided that the material was in the form of camera-ready copy. "News and Notes" was produced, for the first time in August 1970, by the Secretary, Bob Ellingson, and continued to provide a valuable link. Because it was printed on distinctive "Blue Pages" that was what it is usually called. It changed later to the Yellow Pages of the journal, and eventually to an on-line news section when the Federation evolved into the 21st Century.

The Handbook project was proving to be an even larger task than had been anticipated, mainly because of the difficulty of keeping the enormous team of over 200 authors up to their deadlines. At the time of the Congress only 13 parts had been published, out of a projected 48, and eight more were in press. The delay naturally increased the expenses, at first covered by advances from Elsevier and later by the Federation.

2. The Eighth International Congress, Marseilles

The Congress was held in the Faculté de Médecine in September 1973, under the Presidency of

Henri Gastaut, very much on his own ground. It was organized most imaginatively by Gabrielle Lairy, Jean Courjon and many others. Because of illness it was not intended that Robert Naquet, with the expertise of many Colloques de Marseille behind him, should have any role; in the event, as always, he became a major link in the organization.

Among the many successful ideas which were introduced the following are memorable: the highly entertaining logo which appeared on all the Congress documents; the grouping of free communications according to their related topics; simultaneous translation by scientific colleagues, under the leadership of Georges Muller of Luxembourg; the cost of this translation had become a major burden on previous congresses and the amateurs were far more effective than the professionals because they understood the topics and were familiar with the specialized vocabulary; a team of young men and girls, students and relatives of the organizers, was recruited to man the information desk, print and distribute a daily news bulletin and the didactic lectures and provide a hundred and one other useful services with, as the secretary of the Congress wrote afterwards "enfin et surtout le sourire malgré la fatigue".

A personal memory is of returning to the Faculté on the morning after the Congress and finding a number of these young girls sitting on the steps crying valedictory tears of utter exhaustion.

The Chairmen of all the committees were required to write reports of their activities; this proved most valuable to the organizers of the next congress and has been adopted as normal practice.

At the General Assembly it was agreed to consolidate the annual subscription and the contribution to the costs of the Congress, which had previously been collected separately by the Treasurer and the Treasurer of the Congress. Dues were also raised to $10/decade of members.

Some minor changes in the Statutes and Bye-Laws were made but, for the second time, the General Assembly rejected any form of proportional representation in the Council, proposed by one of the Member Societies.

A number of unusual entertainments were provided but it is the official banquet that stood out as something quite exceptional. It was held in the 14th century banqueting hall of the Palais des Papes in Avignon and commenced with the entry of a procession of medieval serving men and wenches, led by a rider on a white horse, skilfully descending the steep flight of stone stairs. Throughout the meal we were entertained by acrobats, jugglers, flame swallowers and the like, moving from table to table and all in appropriate costume. A pretentious entertainment, no doubt, but memorable nevertheless.

Wave Length and Action Potentials: History of the IFCN
(Supplements to Clinical Neurophysiology, Vol. 61)
By: M.R. Nuwer and C.H. Lücking

Chapter 8

1973–1977

President: W.A. Cobb

During the Fiscal Period, under the able leadership of President William Cobb (Fig. 8.1), three new Societies were admitted to membership, those from East Germany, Brazil and, just in time for the Congress, Chile, bringing the total to 40. This is not to say that all 40 were equally active in the membership; it was always a matter of surprise that a delegate elected for the sole purpose of keeping his society in contact with the Federation should repeatedly fail to vote or to answer requests for opinion or advice; thus, at a time when there were 38 members, only 21 made a nomination for President, and only 12 answered a ballot on an increase of the annual subscription, both matters which seem to be of some consequence. Out of 11 items submitted to the Council in a 3-year period one society never replied and several answered only two or three times. Despite many efforts to encourage or coerce the backsliders the problem still continues. Contrary to all expectation and against a background of inflation of the order of 28% for the 4 years the financial affairs of the Federation flourished. This was due to a number of factors.

1. Following the proposal of the Treasurer (Hess) in 1973 the Council agreed to increase the annual subscription by 50%. More societies paid up on time (it is not surprising that some were generally as bad at this as at voting) and the yield was $55,000, against the budgeted $32,000.
2. According to custom (and the Statutes) the two international congresses, EEG in Marseilles and EMG in Rochester, handed over their profits, which were considerably larger than anticipated ($19,000 against $11,000).
3. The Journal made a large profit ($66,000), more than double the amount foreseen.
4. The Treasurer, Max Dondey, brought to his task an expertise to which we were not accustomed, largely countering the effects of inflation and the devaluation of the American dollar and ending with a capital increase of $26,000.

From about half way through the Fiscal Period the minutes show that the President was constantly reminding his colleagues that the Federation was a non-profit making organization and that we must find ways of returning to the members the surplus, which was beginning to be substantial. A start was made with a more generous, though still very cautious, grant to the EMG Congress, and nearly $14,000 was paid in support of the Handbook office. Later, when the financial situation was more evident, the subvention to the coming Congress was increased to $55,000 and still later it was decided to remit the admission fees of invited speakers and members of Federation committees and half the fees of a number of young workers (under 35) chosen by their societies, at the rate of one grant for 20 members; the cost of these two last operations was $36,000.

A further scheme, which made a slow start but continues, was to present the Journal to impoverished libraries or departments which would not otherwise see it. This was later modified to give the Handbook, which seemed more

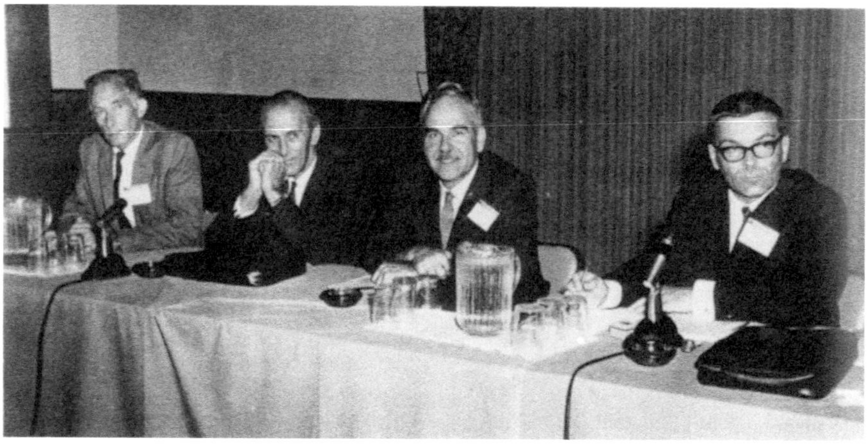

Fig. 8.1. From left to right:
- R. Hess of Zurich. Treasurer 1969–1973.
- W.A. Cobb of London. Treasurer 1957–1961, European and Managing Editor 1962–1973, President 1973–1977, Publications Manager 1977–1981, Publications Editor 1981–1985.
- Pierre Gloor of the Montreal Neurological Institute. Editorial Assistant to Jasper 1954–1958, Translator and author of "*Hans Berger on the Electroencephalogram*".
- J. Kugler of Munich. Member-at-large 1977–1981.

suited to a developing laboratory and would not involve a long-term commitment.

The Federation had always assumed itself to be tax-exempt, on the grounds of being a non-profit making body, but now that its capital had increased considerably and was invested worldwide it was found that we were paying significant taxes. Some of the money was still invested in Canada, where it had remained since the sale of the Journal stock to Elsevier; the Canadian authorities stated that it could not be tax-exempt unless it was so in France, the country in which the Federation was registered. Here it was found that our supposed registration was invalid because it had not been published initially in the "Journal Officiel". When we (that is, Boby Naquet on the Federation's behalf) tried to put that right we were told that an item in the Statutes was not acceptable, since the legal address of the Federation was not necessarily in France. Statute IV said: "The address of the Head Office of the Federation is that of the current resident." In the French version "siège social" has a rather more limited meaning than head office. Since the Statute could not be changed before the next General Assembly a new Bye-Law was passed by the Council in May 1976, followed by the definitive change in the Statute in September 1977. It stated that:

(1) "The legal address of the Federation is in France. It is specified in the Bye-Laws.

(2) The administrative address of the Federation is that of the current President."

These changes were duly registered in the "Journal Officiel" and the Federation became respectable again, at the cost of many months of effort by the Treasurer and the Rules Committee.

The EMG Commission and its various committees, under the leadership of EMG Commissioner Albrecht Struppler (Fig. 8.2), were active in gathering information on standards of training, terminology, etc., though this was not to bear fruit (i.e., reports) until the following Congress. The Fifth International EMG Congress was organized with the American Association of EMG and Electrodiagnosis at the Mayo Clinic in Rochester, MN, USA in September 1975. The President, whose right it was to be chairman of the Organizing Committee, felt that this was not very realistic at the distance involved and, as the Bye-Laws permit, deputed the task to the Secretary in

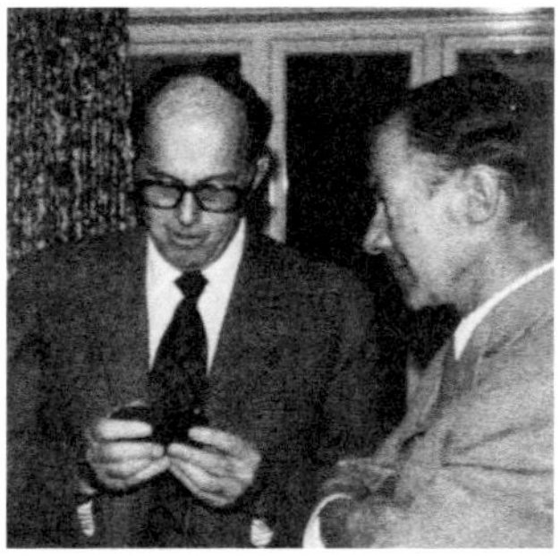

Fig. 8.2.
- Helmut Petsche (left) of Vienna. Member-at-large 1973–1977.
- Albrecht Struppler (right) of Munich. Chairman of EMG Commission 1973–1977.

Omaha, a short flight away. In fact, all arrangements were made by Ed Lambert with his usual lack of fuss and correspondence; even the secretary of the Organizing Committee said he did not know what was going on; our natural anxiety was needless and the Congress was well organized and well attended.

It was always the policy, according to the Statutes, that the Federation could recognize only one society in each country, later modified to allow a second with a different sphere of interest. The President was therefore surprised to receive, early in 1977, an invitation from the chairman of the Polish Society of EEG and Clinical Neurophysiology to its inaugural meeting; he had just checked that this was not the name of the society which had long been a member, nor were the officers the same, when he had to correct the manuscript of the proceedings of the Electrophysiological Section of the Polish Neurological Society, again bearing the name of a different secretary. Thus it seemed that there were three Polish EEG Societies, all wishing to make use of the Federation, but only one could be legitimate. A round of correspondence with those concerned, capped by personal meetings at the Congress, resolved all the problems, the members of the two sections resigning to join the autonomous new society, which in due course became the accepted member of the Federation.

For a number of years the Japanese Society had been offering to host a Congress, which we felt to be unacceptable because Japan was believed to be the most expensive country in the world and was certainly, on average, the most expensive of the member countries to reach. However, the Japanese were very persistent and perhaps the improved finances of the Federation made us more receptive; by the time of the Congress it was clear that many members of the General Assembly liked the idea but it was agreed to wait on the plans of the World Federation of Neurology.

The election of the Executive Committee was again conducted in two phases by C. Ajmone Marsan; first the President, Robert Naquet, then the Secretary and Treasurer, again the highly successful Robert Ellingson and Max Dondey respectively; the EMG chairman, J. Desmedt and the Member-at-Large, J. Kugler of Munich. The committee was completed by the Past-president W.A. Cobb and the Editor-in-Chief Mary Brazier.

1. The EEG Journal

In contrast with the previous period the story of this one is of a continuous fight against increasing publication delays, because of a backlog of papers waiting their turn. This was in part due to a change in printing method to computer type setting; though inherently quicker than more traditional methods, this at first produced rather fewer words per page and did not use a small type face for Clinical and Technical Notes and Society Proceedings, resulting in each number containing substantially fewer words than before. Combined with an increased input of papers and despite a high rejection rate this caused an ever lengthening publishing delay. A return to small print and the use of extra pages had nearly brought the situation under control again by the end of the period.

The abstracts of the Marseilles Congress had been published as an extra (13th) number, which naturally added to the cost of distribution. On this occasion the October number was used, the normal contents of which had been accommodated in extra pages in the previous three numbers, thus speeding up their publication, an arrangement which, initially, was strongly resisted by the Editor-in-Chief but ended to everyone's satisfaction.

Just before the Congress the final 39th part of the Handbook was published, leaving only the Index to be completed. No one had anticipated that it would take 8 years to finish or that the office expenses would amount to something like $40,000. Eventually all this money, which had been advanced initially by Elsevier, later by the Federation, was repaid from the profits from sales of the book, which still continue in a small way at the time of writing.

By no means all the member Societies make use of Society Proceedings though they have the right to do so. Even so, these take up a considerable amount of Journal space and at this time there was some pressure to limit them severely or even abolish the section completely. The majority opinion, however, has always been that they represent the common platform for all society members and must be retained whatever the pressure on space. Early in the Fiscal Period a compromise was reached: to reduce the words per abstract from 250 to 200 and to make a small charge to non-member societies for the inclusion of their proceedings. This last was rather with the intention of establishing that the free service was open only to Member Societies than with any hope of making a significant profit.

2. The Ninth International Congress, Amsterdam

As soon as it was known that the World Neurological Congress had chosen Amsterdam, the choice for the EEG Congress was clear; thus it was that our Congress preceded (September 4–9th) that of the International League against Epilepsy (10th) and the Neurological Congress (11–16th). Some joint sessions were held on the nineth with the epileptologists but otherwise the organizations were largely independent; that all three congresses were in the same building was particularly attractive to the commercial exhibitors. This building was the excellent RAI Congress Centre, the first time that such a purpose-built centre had been used for our Congress, which had by now outgrown the facilities that could be provided by universities and the like. However, the general organization was still provided by the local organizing committee, and it was perfect, but it did strain resources severely and in future the organization would be in the hands of professionals.

At an early date Simon Visser was chosen as Convener, Fernando Lopes da Silva as Secretary and Joost Jonkman as Treasurer. Later, as the statutes require, an honorary president had to be elected but the Dutch Society could not make a choice between Otto Magnus and Willem Storm van Leeuwen, so both were elected, to everyone's pleasure.

At the Boston congress of 1953 the use of poster presentations had been tried and largely forgotten. It was attempted again in Amsterdam to a limited extent, with very encouraging results. Of the 582 free communications actually presented 54 were on posters (and four on film). An attempt was made to group the oral presentations to form common topics to be introduced by an invited short lecture by the chairman of the session. This worked out well on the whole though the problems of making up the program were considerable, made no easier by the failure of 54 speakers to arrive.

As had been the case in Marseilles, large numbers of abstracts of free communications arrived after the deadline, but since they also represented subscriptions they had to be accepted up to the last possible moment.

Some time before the Congress it became apparent that expenses would be covered, and ways were sought of returning some of the profits to the participants, mainly in the form of free entertainment. In particular, no charge was finally made for the splendid concert by the "Concertgebouw Orkest", conducted by Bernard Haitink.

Another memorable event was a reception by the mayor and aldermen of Amsterdam in the Rijksmuseum.

In his address to the General Assembly the President drew attention to the recent deaths of Lord Adrian and Grey Walter and also, most untimely, of Michael Saunders, who had served the Federation well as its first Member-at-Large and Chairman of the Rules Committee. The invited lectures of the Congress were subsequently published as *Supplement 34, Contemporary Clinical Neurophysiology*.

Wave Length and Action Potentials: History of the IFCN
(Supplements to Clinical Neurophysiology, Vol. 61)
By: M.R. Nuwer and C.H. Lücking

Chapter 9

1977–1981

President: R.G. Naquet

During this term the Federation was under the able leadership of Robert Naquet (Fig. 9.1). In this term the other Executive Committee members were Past-President William Cobb, Secretary Robert Ellingson, Treasurer Max Dondey, Member-at-Large Johann Kugler, EMG Commission Chairman John Desmedt, and Editor-in-Chief Mary A.B. Brazier.

It has always been regarded as desirable that Member Societies should be autonomous but in some cases it has been necessary to accept as members sections of larger societies, of neurology or physiology for example. The change in status of the Polish Society, recounted in the last chapter, which was completed in July 1979, was therefore welcome. In contrast, the Indian society had long been a problem to the Executive Committee, with which it communicated on rare occasions and to which it very seldom paid dues; after personal contact with some EEG and EMG workers in India it was arranged to dissolve the old society and form a section of the Neurological Society of India, which was finally admitted to membership in February 1980. At the same time the Peruvian Society of EEG and Clinical Neurophysiology was also admitted.

The invitation of the Swedish Society to hold the Sixth International Congress of EMG in Stockholm in June 1979 was accepted. The President deputed J.E. Desmedt, the Chairman of the EMG Commission, to represent him as chairman of the organizing committee; the Convener was K.E. Hagbarth, the Secretary Anders Persson, and the Treasurer Ingemar Petersén. Over 600 people attended and the congress was reckoned to be a great success.

When it was learned that the neurologists had settled on Japan for the congress in 1981 the invitation of the Japanese Society was immediately accepted. A preliminary planning meeting was organized for September 1978 in conjunction with a scientific meeting in Vancouver, a convenient half-way point between Japan and Europe. It was also possible to arrange a nearly complete meeting of the Executive Committee at the same time. Subsequently the President and other Federation members of the Organizing Committee made a number of visits to Kyoto; the "Final Report" by the host society very truly says "the relationship among members of the two groups was marked by respect, reliability and cooperation which led to the successful conduct of the congress".

Despite continued inflation and an expenditure considerably above the budget estimate, the Federation was able to give much increased financial support to the Congress, in part resulting from the skill of the Treasurer in managing the funds and in part from the sustained profitability of the Journal. A total of US $65,000 was made available to the Japanese organizers, all of which was subsequently repaid; although the scale of this "loan" was larger than ever before it should be noted that it followed an established pattern; no congress has in fact made a loss, but the Federation's grant forms an insurance against a possible loss which an individual society could not accept.

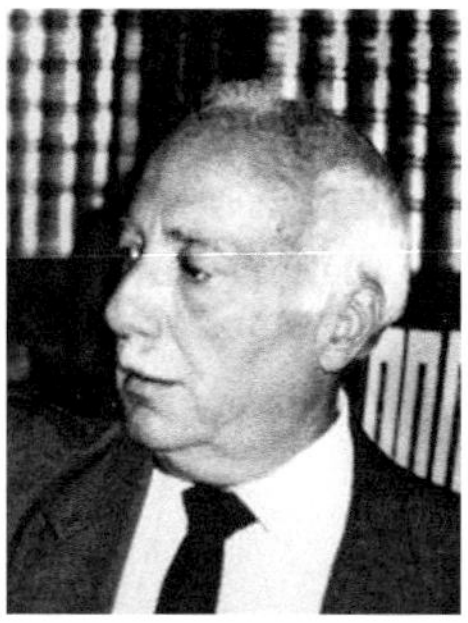

Fig. 9.1. Robert Naquet, IFSECN President 1977–1981.

The Federation also expended about US $120,000 on travel grants to invited speakers and to young scientists (selected by their own societies). This seems to be an important way of assuring the success of a congress, particularly when travel is the major item of personal expense.

Not long before the Congress a proposal was received from the Dutch Society that the title of the Federation should be changed because "it is too long for daily use and gives EEG an unrealistic priority". The suggestion had of course been made before and been rejected but this time it received a quite favourable reception from some members of the Executive Committee, though it was argued that the title of the EEG Journal could not be changed and it was not acceptable that they should be greatly different. A favoured new title was "Federation of Clinical and Experimental Neurophysiology", which certainly got nearer the truth of the matter, though no one recalled Jasper's stricture of years before, that you cannot federate a science. The proposal, in outline, was put to the Council, which rejected it; it will probably occur again.

At the last General Assembly it had been suggested that membership of the Executive Committee should be limited to one per society, to give a more equitable spread. The Committee had a good deal of sympathy for this idea but could find no practical way in which it could be implemented without possible injustice and the Rules Committee was of the same opinion, though the delegate for Uruguay wrote a dissenting report.

During the election of the President it became apparent to the Chairman of the Nomination Committee that a tie-vote was possible and he realized that such a situation was not envisaged by the Statutes; he began to enquire among his colleagues as to what to do but was spared the embarrassing situation since, at the closing date, the voting was 20–19. However, the same thing happened again in the voting for Secretary and this time it was a tie, 19–19. The chairman handed the problem to the President who decided to resolve it by a vote of the Executive Committee; it should be noted that this would not have been a practical solution of the earlier dilemma since both candidates then were members of the Committee. To resolve the problem if it should arise again the Rules Committee proposed, and the General Assembly accepted, a change in the Statutes to allow the President a casting vote in the case of any tie. Curiously, this device had been included in the first modification of the Statutes of 1961 but omitted from the next version of 1965, presumably because there were those who objected, as there were at the present time, to anyone having two votes.

The next term's Executive Committee as finally constituted was as follows: President R.J. Ellingson, Past President R. Naquet, Secretary M.D. Low of Vancouver, Treasurer M. Dondey, Chairman EMG Commission J.E. Desmedt, Editor-in-Chief M.A.B. Brazier and Member-at-Large C.A. Tassinari of Bologna.

Despite the financial success of the Fiscal Period the cautious Treasurer proposed an increase in dues (there had been none for 8 years) to $40 per decade and this was accepted by the General Assembly.

1. The Tenth International Congress, Kyoto

The Japanese appointed a very large local organizing committee of some 150 members; this did not appear to impair efficiency as might have been expected, perhaps because the basic organization was done by a highly professional company. Certainly the conduct of the Congress and all the complex arrangements associated with it left nothing to be desired. The Congress was held from September 13 to 18 in the Kyoto International Congress Hall, a most imaginative new concrete building on the outskirts of the city, in congenially landscaped surroundings. The distance from the Congress hotels was no drawback thanks to an effective shuttle service of buses. The Congress was held under the joint Presidency of N. Yoshii and K. Suhara; the Convener was Y. Shimazono, the Secretary M. Ebe and the Treasurer H. Shimazu.

Following the success of the poster presentations in Amsterdam it was decided, particularly because it was expected that language problems would be greater than usual, that all free communications should be presented as posters; incidentally, this was the first congress, except for the original London meeting, at which no simultaneous translation was provided; it had become more and more restricted over the years because of the high cost and relatively small benefit. Exactly 600 communications were offered though only 523 were actually presented, rather more than half from the host country.

Similarly, slightly more than half of the total attendance of 1550 was from Japan, a remarkable number. The total of active participants from the rest of the world was 556 which, considering the distances and expenses involved, was a very satisfactory result.

The scale which the congresses had now reached may be judged from the fact that the total cost of this one was 182 million yen; even when divided by approximately 200 to give the dollar equivalent this is still a large sum. Its provision was very different from that of recent congresses; in millions of yen the registration fees provided 59, business and other organizations contributed 101 and the members of the Japanese Society most generously donated 22 (US $110,000). The commercial exhibition, on which other congresses have relied heavily, did not contribute. The Japanese government remitted substantial taxes which would otherwise have been due.

To most of the visitors the cultural background of the Congress was entirely new and there could be no better place than Kyoto in which to experience it; our hosts went to great trouble to give and to explain to us some of its features. The entertainments provided were rightly Japanese with, no doubt, enormous concessions to Western ignorance and taste. About 1500 people attended the buffet dinner, during which two large barrels of sake were broached in the traditional, if unpracticed, manner (Fig. 9.2). The visitors had some difficulty in drinking it tidily from the square wooden boxes provided.

2. The EEG Journal

Because of tax concessions Elsevier had set up a branch at Shannon in Eire and in October 1977 the production of the Journal was moved there; naturally the move caused some confusion and delays but these appeared to be coming under control when, at Christmas time, both the general manager of the office and Mr. Cullen, in charge of the Journal, were killed in a car crash. This tragedy caused further problems which were only sorted out when the Journal was brought back to Amsterdam some months later.

This contributed to an increasing publication delay because of the build-up of papers in stock. On these occasions it is always the Society Proceedings which are blamed for taking space at the expense of original papers. They had, in fact, been increasing slightly in volume despite the reduction to 200 words per abstract of a few years before. Various solutions were mooted, including publication of separate Proceedings numbers from time to time, which would have been very expensive. Finally two proposals were accepted:

(1) to reduce the number of words to 150/abstract, which would save nearly 25%
(2) to charge the actual cost of extra pages, about US $20/abstract, to non-member societies, whose abstracts took up about 20% of the Proceedings. This proposal would affect mainly the four American regional societies

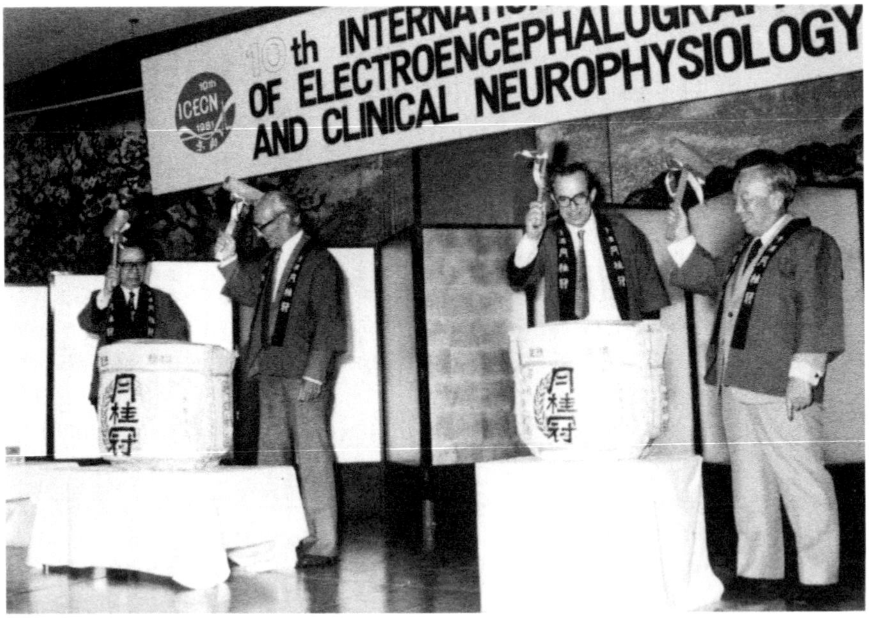

Fig. 9.2. The opening of the banquet of the Kyoto Congress, 1981. Japanese colleagues teach William Cobb and Max Dondey the art of broaching of the "*sake*" barrels.

and was strongly resisted by the American editor (i.e. the Editor-in-Chief).

For the time being, therefore, it was agreed to implement only the reduction in the number of words, from January 1979, returning to the forgotten and unworkable limit of 30 years earlier. This decision evoked a strong protest from Peter Gloor, the president of the American EEG Society, on the grounds that 150 words were insufficient to present an adequate outline of any complex investigation; as this was the view of nearly half the members of the Editorial Board (it had been a majority decision) the question was reopened. At this time more pages became available in the Journal and the proponents of the shorter abstract were induced to agree to the status quo.

For some time alarm signals had been coming from the Brain Information Service, which had freely provided the Index to Current Literature for the past 11 years. Its grant had been severely cut and it could only continue the Index with financial support from the Federation; this would have been on a scale that was thought to be greater than was justifiable and so, regrettably, the Index came to an end with the close of 1978, after nearly 30 years in one form or another. It was the pages freed by this demise which removed the pressure to shorten the Proceedings.

The first number of 1979 completed 30 years of the Journal's existence and to mark the occasion the February number came out, for the once only, in a pale green cover and contained a brief history of the Journal by Brazier and Cobb entitled *Thirty years*.

At about the same time the pressures of his university post became too much for Pierre Buser and he had to resign as European editor after six distinguished years. His replacement was quickly found in Hans van Duijn, who had collaborated with Cobb in editing the Proceedings of the Amsterdam congress as *Supplement 34, Contemporary Clinical Neurophysiology* (1978). In addition to his natural talent he had the potentially great advantage of working in Amsterdam, close to the office of Elsevier.

Sales of the Handbook had been going on steadily, both of the complete volumes and of individual parts; stocks of some of the latter were nearing exhaustion and also some of these had been written as early as 1970 and were out of date. It was decided that, while a complete rewriting was impossible and unnecessary, selected parts which were unsatisfactory should be replaced by new teams of authors. This project is going on slowly, and at the time of writing nothing has been published.

Throughout the period the excess of Journal stock, and hence the publication delay, gave constant cause for anxiety; there was never the possibility to recover from the disaster of the transfer to Shannon and the supply of new papers continued to increase despite a high rejection rate, often near to 50%. Elsevier finally offered to produce an extra volume at their own risk, as they had done for extra issues in 1964; that is, billing the subscribers retrospectively. Accordingly, the first volume of 1980 was normal while the next six numbers were twice the usual size, forming two normal volumes (49 and 50). This reduced the publication delay to under 6 months, where it has remained, and was not a financial failure as some had feared. Nor did it appear to have serious effect on the subscription list, which had already fallen somewhat from its peak of 3400. The worldwide reduction in university and library budgets caused large reductions in some Journal circulations but ours has been held at 1–2% per year, with a total hovering around 2900.

Wave Length and Action Potentials: History of the IFCN
(Supplements to Clinical Neurophysiology, Vol. 61)
By: M.R. Nuwer and C.H. Lücking

Chapter 10

1981–1985

President: Robert J. Ellingson

During this term the Executive Committee consisted of Robert J. Ellingson (President, USA) (Fig. 10.1), Robert Naquet (Past President, France), Morton D. Low (Secretary, Canada), Max Dondey (Treasurer, France) until his death in 1983, followed by Pierre Buser (France), John E. Desmedt (EMG Commission Chairman, Belgium), C.A. Tassinari (Member-at-Large, Italy), Mary A.B. Brazier (Editor-in-Chief, USA) until 1984, followed by Hans van Duijn (The Netherlands).

News of the death of IFSECN Treasurer Max Dondey saddened the Federation. He died the only victim of a tragic railway accident near Lyon in France on May 1, 1983. During his 10 outstanding years as treasurer, he successfully led the Federation through the financial troubles of the late 1970s. His friends in the Executive Committee remembered him not only as their highly competent Treasurer but for his wise council and wit, and, above all, for the warmth of his friendship. His colleagues considered that he should be remembered in a happy moment, shared here as a photograph of him broaching of the sake barrels at the 1981 Kyoto Congress and presenting at the lectern in San Diego (Figs. 9.1 and 10.2).

Past President Robert Naquet, in addition to his other duties, stepped into the gap left by Max Dondey's death and by acting as Interim Treasurer until a successor to Max Dondey was appointed and confirmed. The Executive Committee appointed Pierre Buser to serve as treasurer and the Council voted unanimously to confirm this action. This is not the first role in which Pierre Buser has served the Federation. He previously served as Editor of the *EEG Journal* for Europe, Asia, and Africa from 1973 to 1979. To honour Max Dondey, the Executive Committee designated the fellowship travel grants to the XI IFSECN in London, 1985, as Max Dondey Grants for younger scientists or students.

The Federation honoured three distinguished neurophysiologists as Honorary Fellows of the IFSECN during this term. These were William Cobb (UK), Hallowell Davis (USA) and Willem Storm van Leeuwen (The Netherlands). These were unanimously endorsed by the 1985 General Assembly.

1. Member societies

The IFSECN continued to grow with the admission of the Jordanian Society of Clinical Neurophysiology to the Federation in 1985. The EEG Society of India formally withdrew from the Federation in 1979. The Section on EEG and Clinical Neurophysiology of the Neurological Society of India applied for membership and was admitted in 1980. The EEG section of the Polish Psychiatric Association withdrew in 1977 in favour of the Polish Society of EEG and Clinical Neurophysiology. That society applied for and was admitted to membership in 1979.

The Latin American Society had been suspended in the previous Fiscal Period for persistent non-payment of dues. The Peruvian Society

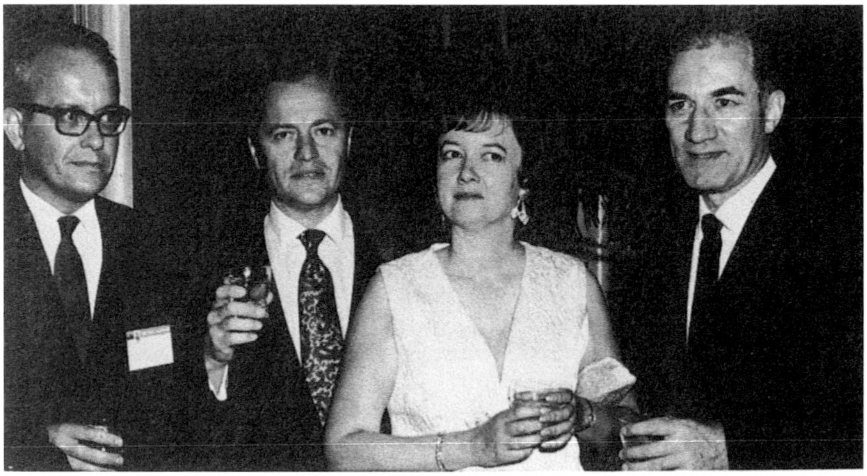

Fig. 10.1. From left to right:

- John E. Desmedt of Brussels. Member of EMG Commission 1973–1977, Chairman 1977–1985, President elect 1985.
- Robert J. (Bob) Ellingson of Omaha, NE. Treasurer 1969 (San Diego) Congress, Secretary 1969–1981, President 1981–1985.
- Marnie Ellingson, wife of Bob.
- Edward (Ed) Lambert, of the Mayo Clinic, Rochester, MN. Chairman of the EMG Commission 1965–1969.

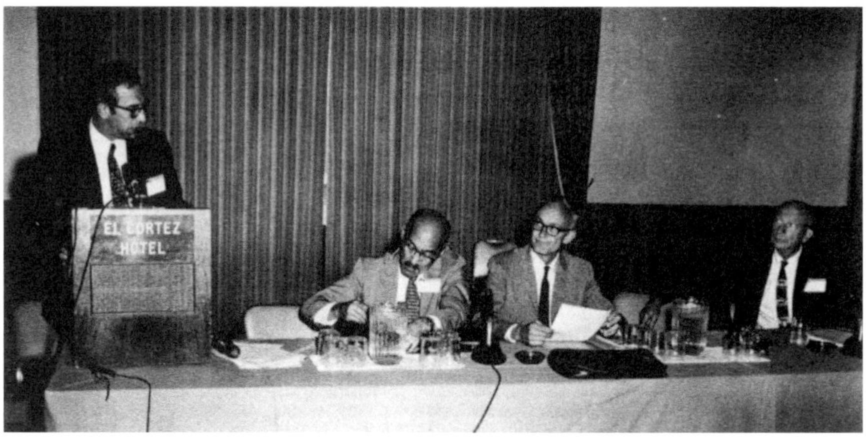

Fig. 10.2. From the previous 1969 Congress, from left to right:

- Max Dondey of Paris. Treasurer 1973–1983, who died in 1983.
- Robert S. Schwab of the Massachusetts General Hospital, Boston, MA, where he and M.A.B. Brazier organized the business side of the new Journal.
- Lennart Widén of Karolinska Institute, Stockholm. Editor of Supplement 25, *Recent Advances in Clinical Neurophysiology*, 1967.
- Charles (Chuck) Henry of Hartford, CT. Compiled the Index of Current Literature, edited Book Reviews and several supplements from 1949 to 1965.

of EEG and Clinical Neurophysiology was admitted to the Federation in June 1979. Several other Latin American nations already had national Clinical Neurophysiology societies.

The Australasian Society dissolved and was no longer a member society, replaced by a national society in Australia. It once represented Australia, New Zealand, Indonesia and the Philippines. Without much notice the Australian Association of Neurologists has been the one writing instead of the Australasian Society. The Executive Committee voted, a little reluctantly, that the EEG section of the Australian Association of Neurologists would be accepted as the member de facto representing Australian neurophysiologists. Inquiries will be made regarding the status of New Zealand and other Asian countries.

Several more societies are in arrears on their dues. Plans were made to put the societies in Turkey, Greece and Uruguay in suspension status within the Federation.

2. The EEG Journal

In 1983, the position of Editor-in-Chief is still in discussion. The proposal of two Editors appointed by the Executive Committee for a maximum of three fiscal periods is acceptable to the Rules Committee. They suggested perhaps the Editor-in-Chief be elected by the General Assembly and be re-eligible once, and be a full Executive Committee member or that the Editor-in-Chief could be appointed by the Executive Committee and be an ex-officio member of the Executive Committee.

At the beginning of this Fiscal Period, Mary A.B. Brazier served as journal Editor-in-Chief and Hans van Duijn served as journal Editor for Europe, Asia, and Africa. Because the new journal is processed in the European office there has been a considerable shift in the balance of work between the two offices. Mary Brazier therefore suggested that she should relinquish the post of Editor-in-Chief in favour of Hans van Duijn (Fig. 10.3), who was conveniently placed for

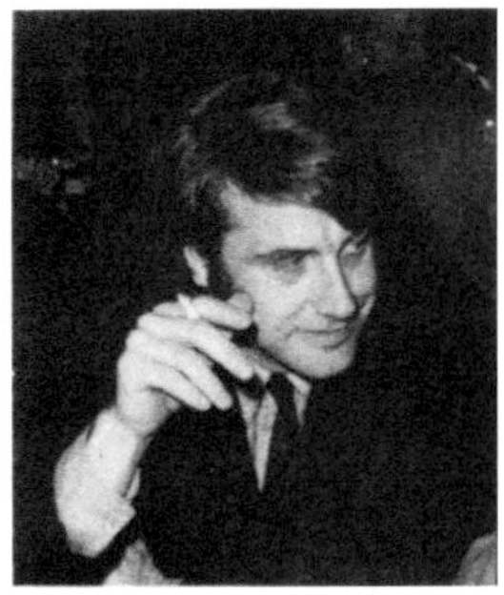

Fig. 10.3. Hans van Duijn of Amsterdam. Co-editor of Supplement 34, 1978, European Editor 1979, Editor-in-Chief 1984.

daily contact with the desk editor at Elsevier. In accepting this change, which took place on July 1st 1984, the Editorial Board felt that Mary Brazier richly deserved some respite from her heavy labours over the past 11 years. Mary Brazier continued as Editor for the Americas and the Far East.

W.A. Cobb continued to serve the Federation as Publications Editor. He was responsible for relations with the publisher, Elsevier, and for the Supplement series of book publications. He was doing the English language editing of papers submitted through the European office. He edited the book *Recommendations for the Practice of Clinical Neurophysiology* and authored the book *Wave Length, A History of the IFSECN.* He was also general editor of the Handbook series. He previously had served the Federation as the Editor-in-Chief of the EEG Journal.

After many years of slowly decreasing circulation rate, a slight but clear increase was seen during this Fiscal Period in the number of subscribers. With about 3000 subscriptions the Journal had consolidated its position in the competitive field of neuroscience publications.

The number of manuscripts received grew substantially. The American office saw the submitted manuscript number jump to 814, a 62% increase over the 504 manuscripts in the previous four years. The European office saw the submitted manuscript number jump to 612, a 37% increase over the 447 manuscripts in the previous four years. The rejection rate in both offices was over 40%. Consideration was given to expanding the number of pages published annually to accommodate the increasing number of high quality manuscripts submitted. Instead of simply increasing the pages, the editors suggested initiating a new section of the Journal dedicated to Evoked Potentials. The Executive Committee and publisher accepted this plan. Beginning in January 1985, the journal increased from 12 to 18 issues/year, with 12 issues in the traditional section and the additional six issues in the new Evoked Potential section. This will represent three volumes annually, each based on six issues.

3. Book publications

The EEG Journal Supplement book series continues to accept and publish books relevant to clinical neurophysiology. The *Handbook of Electroencephalography and Clinical Neurophysiology* has been started again as a Revised Series. This will supplement the existing Handbook by updating and including new sections. Bill Cobb invited former Federation President A. Rémond to serve as editor for initial revised series volumes on quantitative analysis, with plans for further volumes to follow on other topics that have changed significantly in the past decade. A. Rémond served as Editor-in-Chief for the original *Handbook of Electroencephalography and Clinical Neurophysiology* in the 1970s.

At the 1981 General Assembly, Otto Magnus reported on the need for a comprehensive manual on the standards of practice in clinical neurophysiology. Otto Magnus served as chair from 1979 to 1981 of the Committee on Standards of Clinical Practice of EEG and EMG. The committee prepared recommendations on the proper clinical laboratory evaluation of patients. A series of reports were published in the *EEG Journal*. To pursue that recommendation, the Executive Committee asked William A. Cobb, a past president and past editor-in-chief, to develop plans for a volume to bring together into one practical book the various Federation clinical practice recommendations. In addition, the Executive Committee commissioned further clinical guidelines to fill gaps where no guidelines had been produced to date or to update existing ones where appropriate.

The soft-covered reference book, *Recommendations for the Practice of Clinical Neurophysiology*, was published by Elsevier in 1983. William Cobb assembled the volume and guided it through publication. IFSECN was the listed author of the book. Half of the book was from Otto Magnus's Committee on Standards of Clinical Practice of EEG and EMG. It included additional reports on cessation of cerebral function and on EMG quantification as well as earlier publications on instrumentation standards, on terminology, and on the International 10–20 system. Finally the most recent version of the IFSECN Statutes and Bye-Laws from 1977 was included. The history of these clinical and technical reports should be acknowledged.

The First International Congress in 1947 recommended a standardized electrode placement system. The resulting International 10–20 system was accepted at the 1949 International Congress. That electrode placement system was included as an appendix to published IFSECN recommendations endorsed at the IV International Congress in 1957 (*Electroenceph. Clin. Neurophysiol.*, 1958, 10: 367–380). IFSECN's founding President Herbert Jasper authored this report. While these consensus recommendations were initially rather controversial, they eventually have gained essentially universal acceptance. The 1983 *Recommendations* book reprinted this International 10–20 system description.

An EEG terminology proposal was accepted to the VI International Congress in 1965 (*Electroenceph. Clin. Neurophysiol.*, 1966, 20: 306–310) and subsequently expanded to a *Glossary of Terms Commonly Used by Clinical Electroencephalographers* endorsed by the VII International Congress in 1973 and published in the Journal (*Electroenceph. Clin. Neurophysiol.*, 1973, 37: 538–548).

Contributing committee members for this report were G.E. Chatrian (Chairman), L. Bergamini, M. Dondey, D.W. Klass, M. Lennox-Buchthal, and I. Petersén. This Glossary was reprinted in the *Recommendations* book. The many terms defined in this Glossary continue to be in general use in routine clinical EEG, and familiar to the clinical EEG community of physicians and technologists. It remains an excellent teaching tool for physician and technologist trainees.

Recommendations to manufacturers about clinical EEG equipment were endorsed first at the VI International Congress (*Electroenceph. Clin. Neurophysiol.*, 1958, 10: 378–380), later expanded upon at the VIII International Congress in 1973 (*Electroenceph. Clin. Neurophysiol.*, 1974, 37: 549–553), and updated for the IX International Congress in 1977 (*Electroenceph. Clin. Neurophysiol.*, 1978, 45: 144–150). This EEG Instrumentation Standard was reprinted in the *Recommendations* book. Contributors drafting this were J.S. Barlow (Chairman), A. Kamp, H.B. Morton, A. Ripoche, H. Shipton, and D.B. Tchavdarov. Although these recommendations pertained originally to analogue EEG equipment, they mostly remain relevant as standards for the digital EEG equipment. These standards cover amplifiers, visual presentation of tracings, channel cross-talk and other issues that remain even with digital techniques.

The Committee on the Cessation of Cerebral Function reported briefly in 1969 at the VII International Congress (*Electroenceph. Clin. Neurophysiol.*, 1970, 28: 36) and in 1973 at the VII International Congress (*Electroenceph. Clin. Neurophysiol.*, 1974, 37: 530–531). The opinion report to the General Assembly of the X International Congress (*Electroenceph. Clin. Neurophysiol.*, 1982, 54: 9–10) was included in the 1983 *Recommendations* book. Contributing to this report were A.E. Walker (Chairman), D.R. Bennett, A. Bricolo, L. Cigánek, A.M. Gurvich, and N. Chiofalo. Even with standards considered by today's standards, this report has had longstanding influence as a basis cited for early brain death legal statutes and medical guidelines in various states, leading to later more modern legal and medical standards essential for transplantation medicine. In contrast to most IFSECN recommendations, this report pertains to clinical cerebral function and brain death without specifically covering clinical neurophysiology techniques.

A Committee on Methods of Clinical Examination in EEG reported to the IV International Congress in 1957 (*Electroenceph. Clin. Neurophysiol.*, 1958, 10: 370–375). Two decades later, a committee was established on Standards of Clinical Practice in EEG and EMG. That committee presented a series of clinical recommendations adopted at the X International Congress in 1981. The report included five standards for EEG, one for evoked potentials, and three for EMG. The main committee was composed of O. Magnus (Chairman) J. Daube, S. Gomes Lins, I. Hausmanowa-Petrusewicz, F. Isch, D. Klass, St. Kubicki, J. Kugler, K. Mechelse, J. Payan, G. Scollo-Lavizzari, and E. Stålberg. In addition, expert advisors were invited to contribute to drafting certain clinical recommendations: C. Dreyfus-Brisac for neonatal EEG, A.J.R. Simons for cardiac and carotid surgery, G. E. Chatrian for cerebral death EEG, A.M. Halliday for evoked potentials, and A. Rosenfalck, P.R. Styles and R. Willison for EMG instrumentation. The nine particular clinical standards from the Magnus committee are on the topics of clinical EEG, neonatal EEG, intensive care unit EEG, EEG monitoring in cardiac and carotid surgery, EEG in suspected brain death, evoked potentials, clinical EMG, EMG instrumentation, and EMG terminology. Many basic rules for clinical recording and interpretation are set forth here. The neonatal EEG section sets forth the 12.5–25% system for neonatal EEG electrode placement. The EMG terminology section builds upon and superseded the previous 1969 EMG terminology report. Only the introductory section of the Magnus committee report was published in the journal (*Electroenceph. Clin. Neurophysiol.*, 1982, 53: 9–10). Most of the Magnus committee report was published originally in the 1983

Recommendations book. These reports constitute about one-half of that book. As with other sections of the book, these portions are still excellent teaching material for physician and technologist trainees even today.

In addition to the clinical, technical and terminology in EMG reports from the Magnus committee, the 1983 *Recommendations* book includes the EMG instrumentation and quantification as well. Two of these reports were presented to the VII and VIII International Congresses in 1969 and 1973 (*Electroenceph. Clin. Neurophysiol.*, 1970, 28: 399–433; 1974, 37: 532–534). Those two older reports by C. Guld, A. Rosenfalck and R.G. Willison were considered still valid and were reprinted in the *Recommendations* book.

One further EMG report was included, a report by the Committee on Quantification in EMG drafted by R.G. Willison (Chairman), I. Petersén, P. Pinelli, J.E. Desmedt, K. Kunze, R.G. Lee, I. Hausmanowa-Petrusewicz, F. Isch, and A. Arrigo. This EMG quantification report had been presented in 1981 to the X International Congress (*Electroenceph. Clin. Neurophysiol.*, 1982, 53: 12–14).

The book was widely used for many years as a practical handbook for clinical, technical and terminology standards in clinical neurophysiology. Publication as a soft-covered book helped to keep the price of the book moderate. This 1983 *Recommendations* book continued to be the standard reference until the next federation recommendations book was published 16 years later.

4. Practice committees

Practice Committees work on a variety of topics. This extended and updated work in the previous Fiscal Period by the Magnus and other committees. The work in this Fiscal Period included EEG committees on clinical practice, instrumentation standards, training, qualifications, and paediatric EEG terminology. In EMG, the work included methodology and quantitative analysis. The reports of these committees were endorsed by the 1985 XI International Congress General Assembly. They were not published in book form, as had been done in the 1983 *Recommendations* book that compiled reports from the previous Fiscal Periods.

The Committee on Standards of Practice in EEG was charged with preparing statements on standards of practice for monitoring applications. Committee members were D.W. Klass (Chairman), B. Bergamasco, M. Biliard, A. Bricolo, R. Broughton, G.E. Chatrian, J.D. Frost, R.J. Gumnit, Y. Hishikawa, J.R. Ives, J.W. Osselton, R. Porter, P.F. Prior, R.A.F. Pronk, and W. Storm van Leeuwen. This forward looking action evaluated areas that did indeed greatly expand over the next two decades: polysomnography, operating room monitoring, long-term monitoring for epilepsy, and intensive care monitoring. The committee report was intended to supplement the work of the previous Fiscal Period's Magnus committee, which covered more routine aspects of practice in EEG and EMG.

Four Standards of Practice in EEG subcommittees each coordinated efforts with other professional organizations and consulted individual experts outside the committee, who made exceptionally important contributions. The Committee's report to the XI International Congress provided information about the state of current methods and practice standards rather than defining a set of rules. The Committee noted that many of the techniques and practices described in the report were in rapid evolution. The report sounded a word of caution about monitoring, specifically that to conduct and interpret monitoring requires considerable special training and experience for proper use of many procedures and, in some cases, teams of experts are required. Careful consideration was needed to determine appropriate indications for monitoring, and to apply the more complex, difficult, and costly of these techniques.

The Committee on Training and Qualifications in EEG was appointed in 1977 to survey internationally about EEG training programs and to propose minimal criteria for training and qualification of clinical electroencephalographers and EEG technologists. The committee was composed of C. Ajmone Marsan (Chairman), D. Battye, C. Bradshaw, M. Ebe, O. Eeg Olofsson, A.J. Gabor, J. Gaches, A.M. lvanitsky, J. Kugler, G. Pampiglione, M. Turner, and R. Zappoli. They were charged evaluating with the quality of training and the qualifications necessary to become a clinical electroencephalographer in different Federation member countries. A parallel survey evaluated the training of EEG technologists. The committee obtained the requested information from 27 countries, but did not include the United Kingdom, Spain, France, Australia, or Israel. Based on the results obtained, the different countries clearly had great variability of standards for training and the competency examinations required to perform or interpret EEGs.

The legal designation of "clinical electroencephalographer" is accepted in only some countries. In some nations, the standards are at a much higher level. In some countries, subspecialties of clinical neurophysiology are recognized, such as differentiating those who are credentialed for the central testing of EEG and evoked potentials as opposed to others who are credentialed for peripheral and neuromuscular system testing. EMG and EEG are considered completely separate subspecialties in some countries with separate training programs. Given this situation, it seemed impractical for the IFSECN to develop standard training syllabi or examinations at this time. Some minimal EEG training standards were reported to the General Assembly. A questionnaire was distributed during the previous fiscal period. The work of the committee would be facilitated by dividing the committee into two work groups, one for each of the Eastern and Western hemispheres. C. Ajmone Marsan will serve as co-chairman of the Western and Elmqvist for the Eastern hemisphere.

The Committee on New Applications, Methods, and Quantitative Analysis of EMG originally was formed in 1977 and chaired by R.G. Willison. A preliminary report was submitted to the X International Congress in 1981. The new expanded committee consisted of R.G. Lee (Chair), A. Arrigo, C.J. De Luca, J.E. Desmedt, P. Guiheneuc, I. Hausmanowa-Petrusewicz, M. Hayward, F. Isch, K. Kunze, L. Lindstrom, M. Meyer, I. Petersén, and H. Shimazu. Additional experts were consulted in electronics and engineering. The committee noted that many medical and non-medical specialists now use a wide variety of EMG techniques. The committee focused their efforts on certain techniques: methods for quantitative analysis of compound nerve and muscle action potentials in nerve conduction studies, quantitative studies of neuromuscular transmission disorders, and EMG studies of central motor disorders. The report consists of three main sections. The first section reviewed quantitative methods for traditional diagnostic EMG. Many such methods automate the measurements that previously were done by hand. They were developed to increase speed and accuracy of EMG used for diagnosis of neuromuscular disorders. The second section focused on new EMG techniques and special applications. This included such topics as EMG of ocular muscles, laryngeal muscles, and sphincter muscles as well as studies of aging, respiration, and muscle fatigue. The third section dealt with instrumentation and standardisation of equipment, particularly to interface with digital computers. The committee noted that, in this very rapidly developing area, any guidelines would need to change. There will be a meeting in Göteborg, Sweden, in 1982 to provide significant interaction between scientists, their engineering colleagues and local engineers. There will be practical demonstrations. The goal is to define methods of quantification of EMG so that practical information can be obtained.

The Committee on EEG Instrumentation Standards had submitted reports to previous International Congresses. Some were included in the 1983 *Recommendations* book. The committee continued in 1981–1985 and consisted of

H.W. Shipton (Chair), R. Cooper, G. Dumermuth, K. Ikeda, A.M. lvanitsky, S. Métral, P. Rappelsberger, P. Seaba, and L.H. Van der Tweel. The Committee felt that it could not effectively standardize auxiliary apparatus such as visual stimulators and evoked potential equipment. International standards of such equipment are desirable. The committee recommends a working group be appointed to consider these techniques. The International electro-technical commission (IEC) is developing standards for electro-technical equipment which governments can use to make judgements about equipment orders, etc. These have proven to be in many instances stricter than the standards used by individual countries. Dr. Barlow has been a member of working group 62D that deals with electro-medical equipment. These include recommendations about EEG equipment. Dr. Barlow suggested that the Federation should be represented on the working group.

The Executive Committee appointed P. Seaba from Iowa City (an engineer with considerable EEG experience) as the Federation liaison to the Organisation Internationale de Métrologie Légale (OIML), an organization established by treaty among several countries including USA, USSR and France. That organisation is evaluating the Measuring Instruments Used in the Field of Public Health. P. Seaba explained to them the differences between EEG and ECG and the group's draft recommendations have been accordingly amended. Initially the OIML had assumed that EEG instrumentation could be treated as a type of ECG. P. Seaba submitted to OIML the relevant Federation standards. As a result the OIML Secretariat invited the IFSECN to become a Collaborating Organization. The Federation, through its liaison, participated in drafting a standard for electroencephalographs. The Secretariat subsequently sent the resulting draft to collaborating countries for review and comment. In 1985 the draft standard for electroencephalographs was submitted to the International Committee of Legal Metrology (CIML). Eventually these technical standards for electroencephalographs became law in the many nations who were treaty signatories. The group subsequently considered standards for EMG equipment.

A Committee on Terminology in Paediatric EEG was charged with extending the previously published EEG Glossary to include more terms relevant for premature and neonatal patients. The existing glossary was short on terms used in those patients. The committee, chaired by C. Lombroso, continued to work on this project through the end of the Fiscal Period, and continued into the next. Eventually these terms would be included in an updated *Glossary of Terms Commonly Used by Clinical Electroencephalographers.*

5. Archives

In the preceding Fiscal Period, Otto Magnus (Chairman of the Committee on Standards of Clinical Practice of EEG and EMG) suggested that all the past documents published or filed relating to the history of the Federation should be collected and catalogued and archived preferably in London. This initial version of the archives could be the collection recently assembled by W. Cobb in preparation for his book *Wave Length: A History of the IFSECN.* Dr. Cobb reported the possibility to house the archives at the National Hospital at Queens Square without cost. That facility had no formal archivist. The Royal College of Physicians in Regent Park offered space to the EEG Society for their archives and the Federation might rent a portion of that space. A part-time archivist there might arrange and catalogue the Federation's materials in 1–2 years. The Montreal Neurological Institute was also considered. There was general agreement that the so far collected books, papers, photographs, etc. should not be thrown away, but no decision was made as to how they should be managed. The primary source material used for W. Cobb's book was eventually kept by one of the subsequent Executive Committee members. When contacted 25 years later, the material was considered lost. This points to the need for the Federation to maintain a better archive for its primary source materials.

6. New policies

The change of the title of the Federation has been already discussed during previous Fiscal Periods because the EEG had an unrealistic priority. Titles like "Federation of Clinical and Experimental Neurophysiology" (Dutch Society) or "International Federation for Clinical Neurophysiology" (S.L. Visser) were rejected in Kyoto in 1981; also the proposal of "World Federation of EEG and Clinical Neurophysiology" (J. Desmedt) was not accepted. No action was taken until the next Fiscal Period.

The Executive Committee rescinded the previous policy of allowing the other editor to participate in the Executive Committee meetings; only the Editor-in-Chief would attend the Executive Committee meeting. The other editor could come only by invitation.

General principles of meeting support were reiterated and extended, based in part on prior Executive Committee decisions from 1971. Based on three classes of support for meetings, the Executive Committee agreed on the following language and rules:

1. "Organized by IFSECN in conjunction with [host society]". This category pertains only to the quadrennial EEG and EMG congresses. Extensive financial support is provided and underwriting the costs is implied.
2. "Sponsored by the IFSECN". This category pertains to meetings organized by others. A financial contribution to such a meeting will be a loan, which will be repaid first against any profits.
3. "Under the auspices of IFSECN". This category pertains to meetings organized by others without financial obligation by IFSECN.

The Executive Committee rescinded the previous policy of allowing the other editor to attend the Executive Committee meetings, and now only the Editor-in-Chief would attend the Executive Committee meeting. The other editor could come only by invitation.

The International Organisation of Societies for Electrophysiological Technology (OSET) wants to be involved in the IFSECN congresses. The Executive Committee agreed to strongly support involvement of technicians, in general ways, especially in respect to the congresses. OSET was inaugurated in 1977. The first contact between technologists and IFSECN was established during the Advanced Course, organized by Otto Magnus and Helmuth Petsche in Salzburg, Austria in 1965. At the VIII IFSECN Congress in Marseilles, 1973, the technologists organized their own programme with great success. Since then OSET held its meetings every 4 years, 1979 in Guildford (UK) and 1983 in Winnipeg (Canada). There was no provision for formal participation of the OSET in the London IFSECN congress in 1985.

The Executive Committee discussed the issue of two Member Societies of one country. In 1978 or earlier there apparently was a Bye-Law change that two societies could be brought in from the same country. The executive committee should discuss with the societies the possibility of their amalgamation. If impossible, a second society is admissible provided that its main sphere of interest differs from that of the first. No more than two national societies from any country can simultaneously be members of the Federation.

7. Finances

Income of the Federation increased more than expected during these 4 years. The journal royalties now account for one-third to one-half of the annual income. Both royalties and dues payments are now much greater than expected when the Fiscal Period budget was proposed 4 years earlier. The General Assembly in 1981 had accepted the proposal of the Treasurer to increase the annual dues from US $3 to $4 for each member of the Member Society (there had not been an increase for 8 years). The repayment from the X ICEEGCN in Kyoto, 1981, also was greater than was foreseen.

Expenses of the Federation have also been greater than anticipated, due to increases in cost of living and transportation. Executive Committee expenses have increased modestly. The increase in expenditures was greater at the Editorial Offices, in part due to the increased throughput of manuscripts, publication of two books, and the initiation of the new evoked potential series. Travel and expenses for committee meetings tripled, corresponding to a greater use of committees for drafting standards and reports. The subsidies to the International Congresses also increased substantially, with some being loans and other expenses being grants. Overall, income nearly matched expenses with a net deficit of US $20,979 over 4 years in a total budget of US $900,000.

8. Gift committee

The Federation donated three sets of the *Handbook of Electroencephalography and Clinical Neurophysiology* to institutions in Turkey, People's Republic of China, and Thailand. Requests for donations of books and journal subscriptions were coordinated through the Gifts Committee. That committee was composed of R. Naquet (Chair), J.S. Chopra, G. Gonçalves e Silva, G. Rabending, and J. Stevens.

9. Permanent executive office

In 1983 the Executive Committee considered establishment of a permanent executive office with a professional executive secretary and/or treasurer. The growing workload, numerous detailed responsibilities, and need for continuity were cited as reasons. The executive office concept was discussed at this point but no clear action was taken. This concept would continue in discussion for the next two decades, leading eventually to the establishment of such an office.

The office of secretary transitioned smoothly to Vancouver after the 12 years in Omaha under the stewardship of Robert Ellingson. Morton Low, as the new Federation Secretary, worked closely with Dr. Ellingson in his new role as President so as to preserve excellent continuity of functions.

10. Rules committee

As described in the Statutes, the Rules Committee constantly reviewed the Statutes and Bye-Laws and made any necessary recommendations for the amendments. That committee also resolves unclear issues in applying Federation rules and reviews the proposal for new national society members.

10.1. A history of the Statutes and Bye-Laws 1947–1985

The statutes have been forever a work in progress. The original constitution was accepted at the II International Congress in Paris in 1949 and was published in the EEG Journal in 1951. Minor amendments were made in 1953 and major changes were made at the V International Congress in Rome in 1961. At that time an EMG Commission initiated and Bye-Laws modifiable by the Council, rather than the General Assembly, were introduced. These new rules were published in the EEG Journal in 1962, Vol. 14. Further major revisions took place at the VI International Congress in Vienna, 1965, at which time the Executive Committee was enlarged by the addition of a Member-at-Large. The Rules Committee was changed from an *ad hoc* committee to standing committee. Bye-Laws for the conduct of the General Assembly and Council were promulgated and published in the EEG Journal in 1965–1966, Vols. 19 and 20. Minor changes to the Constitution again were made in 1969 and 1973, published in the EEG Journal 1970 and 1974, Vols. 28 and 37. Following some small changes in 1977 the Constitution was last published at full version in the EEG Journal in 1979, Vol. 45, pp. 151–171. Those Statutes and Bye-Laws together with one change was made at the X International Congress in Kyoto in 1981, published in the 1983 *Practice Recommendations* book.

10.2. French registration and regulations

In this 1981–1985 Fiscal Period, the Rules Committee was composed of S.L. Visser (The Netherlands, Chairman), Haime Bogacz (Uruguay), William Kennedy (USA), Jerzy Majkowski (Poland), and Yasuo Shimazono (Japan).

There were continuing problems with the French legal registration. New French regulations require societies to meet for election of officers and register the elections with the local district within 3 months. For this purpose, new 1981 IFSECN registration documents were filed to indicate that Executive Committee officers were elected in June at an Executive Committee meeting in London as opposed to March 1981 in Kyoto, even though they were elected in stages over the preceding 18 months. New French regulations also require that all societies registered in France must have at least one French national on the Executive Committee, possibly as Treasurer. An attorney would be needed for consultation, since this would be incompatible with IFSECN standard procedures, possibly requiring a move of the Federation to a different site for registration or incorporation. Such discussions and consultations continued on and off in succeeding Executive Committees for the next two decades, ending eventually in the move to incorporate in Canada.

10.3. Balancing representation by geography and discipline

Membership of the Federation's Executive Committee should be representative and balanced concerning geographical and disciplinary aspects. Several steps were taken toward more democratic management. It was noted that as the Federation has grown, the rules have not necessarily followed. Rules Committee member H. Bogacz proposed that the Executive Committee should have two Members-at-Large, instead of just one, so as to promote broader representation. The Executive Committee favoured this and added three conditions to favour broad representation and turnover. The General Assembly in 1985 adopted the following new rules: First, the Members-at-Large should serve only one term. Second, the nomination and election systems should be held in three stages: first the President; second the Secretary, Treasurer and EMG Commissioner; and last the two Members-at-Large. Third the two Members-at-Large must come from societies as yet unrepresented in the new Executive Committee. One Member-at-Large must be from each of the two recognized disciplines, EEG and EMG. A special election was held after the Congress in 1985 to fill the newly created second Member-at-Large position.

The general discussion about broad geographic representation has continued over decades, to try to expand representation to be as wide as possible without making the election process too cumbersome. The Nominations Committee was charged with trying to reach the best possible broad geographic balance and to restrict nominations that do not fulfil that goal.

10.4. Turnover in Executive Committee membership

The Executive Committee suggested encouraging turnover among the Members-at-Large to encourage greater representation over time. The Rules Committee suggested that other Executive Committee members also should serve only one term in the same office. Up to that time, officers could be re-elected many times. For example, Robert Ellingson as

Secretary and Max Dondey as Treasurer each were elected three times to the same office. The eventual agreement was that the Editor-in-Chief, Secretary, and Treasurer could serve two terms because of the importance and complexity of the work in those offices. The 1985 General Assembly endorsed the expansion of the Executive Committee to two members-at-large who may not be re-elected to the same position. They also restricted the Secretary and Treasurer to re-election only once.

10.5. Multinational member societies

The Federation is composed of national societies. In two cases, multinational societies have been members: the Latin American and the Australasian Societies. The Australasian Society once represented Australia, New Zealand, Indonesia, and the Philippines. In this term, a section of the Australian Neurological Society has replaced the Australasian Society. The Executive Committee accepted this change. The Federation encouraged New Zealand and other Asian countries' individual national societies to apply for membership. Eventually those other nations' clinical neurophysiologists did form national societies, which then joined the Federation as member societies.

The Latin American Society had discontinued paying dues for more than a decade and apparently had become inactive as a society. As a result of persistent failure to pay dues, and as specified in the Bye-Laws, the previous Executive Committee voted in 1978 that the Latin American Society was no longer in good standing and its participation would be suspended because of non-dues payment. In addition, several national societies from Latin America joined the Federation, raising an issue of double representation.

In 1985, when the Latin American Society still had not rectified the dues payment even after considerable attempts to contact for a decade, the Executive Committee voted to recommend expulsion of the Latin American Society. When this matter was discussed at the 1985 General Assembly, Latin American neurophysiologist A. Mosovich reviewed the history of that society and its many achievements in promoting the development of clinical neurophysiology in the southern hemisphere. He acknowledged that the Society had indeed ceased to exist. President Robert Ellingson acknowledged those important roles played by the Latin American Society, the great contributions of individuals from Latin America to the field, and noted that the procedure for removal of a society from Federation membership is prescribed by Statute, and these rules had been followed with no intention of animosity. It was left to future Executive Committees to identify ways for Latin American clinical neurophysiologists to participate in the Federation, even for those in countries without a national society. This eventually led to the development of the Latin American IFCN Chapters a decade later.

10.6. Proportional representation in the General Assembly

The West German Society suggested that representation in the General Assembly should correspond to the number of regular members of each society. Over time, some societies have grown very large, whereas other remained quite small. Until this point, each society was allowed three representatives in the General Assembly. The proposal was that each society would have one, two or three representatives in the General Assembly in addition to their one Delegate, depending on the number of dues-paying members. The cut-off numbers were 100 and 400. Furthermore, other individuals had voting rights in the General Assembly. These were curtailed. After considerable debate, the rules' changes were approved to:

1. Eliminate the honorary presidents who are the past presidents of the Federation from voting rights in the General Assembly.

2. Eliminate members of the special commissions from voting rights during the General Assembly.
3. Eliminate members of the OCIC from voting rights in the General Assembly.
4. Reduce the representation of smaller societies.
5. Reduce the overall size of the General Assembly.

To keep the General Assembly involved as much as possible in the ongoing business of the Federation, suggestions were made to allow for meetings of that body at the EMG congresses as well as their regularly scheduled meetings at the quadrennial EEG congresses. No definitive decision was made. The General Assembly did agree that they could vote or conduct other business by mail whenever pressing issues made that desirable.

11. International congresses

The Executive Committee discussed whether to print congress announcements both in French and English. Another suggestion was to print a French summary. The second Kyoto announcement had been completely bilingual. For the then upcoming London ICEEGCN, at least the translation of essential sections of the announcement into French was required.

11.1. Seventh International Congress of EMG

The Seventh International Congress of EMG was held in Munich on October 9–13, 1983. The precedent 6 EMG Congresses had taken place in Pavia (1961), Copenhagen (1963), Glasgow (1967), Brussels (1971), Rochester, MN (1976), and Stockholm (1979). The Congress in Munich was organized by the Local Organizing Committee, which included A. Struppler (Convener), former Chairman of the EMG Commission, J. Dudel (Secretary), and H. Heintel (Treasurer) with the active participation of the German society as host. Representatives of the Federation in the Organizing Committee of International Congresses were R. Ellingson (President), M. Dondey (Treasurer), J. Desmedt (Chairman of EMG Commission). The venue was the Technical University. Travel fellowships of US $200 each were awarded to 40 attendees, mostly young investigators nominated by their national societies.

The EMG Congress was attended by 620 active members and its program included 5 symposia, workshop discussions, oral communications and poster presentations. The scientific level of the Congress was excellent and highly praised. The social program was outstanding with a welcome reception in the Antiquarium, an illustrious hall of fame in the Residential Palace of the former Wittelsbach Dynasty, an excursion to Andechs Monastery for an organ concert and a subsequent Bavarian rustic meal, and a Congress Banquette in the Hotel Bayerischer Hof.

The congress was a financial success. The EMG Commission, composed of J.E. Desmedt (Chair), H. Shimazu and Erik Stålberg during this Fiscal Period, brought forward a request by the German Society that some of the EMG Congress profits be used to support a symposium on motor control held in Germany in April 1985. This symposium was held in part to honour Professor A. Struppler, convener of the EMG Congress, who was nearing retirement. The symposium was attended by 70 scientists and included in-depth discussions of current issues in motor control.

The Executive Committee discussed Federation support of additional meetings. It was agreed that support could be given to individual meetings when approved by the Executive Committee, but these actions should not be taken as precedent. Decisions about disposition of surplus funds from congresses must be made on the individual merit of each case.

11.2. XI International Congress of EEG and Clinical Neurophysiology

The XI ICEEGCN was held in London in August 1985. The meeting took place on the week immediately prior to the World Congress of Neurology in Hamburg. The Organizing Committee for the EEG Society of the United Kingdom consisted of A.M. Halliday, S. Butler, and R. Paul. Sir Bryan Matthews served as the Honorary President. The general organization was in the hands of a professional company. The first announcement cover page is reprinted in Appendix 11, Fig. 1.

The meeting site, the Barbican Centre, is a part of the historic City of London and close to St. Paul's Cathedral. Opened just 3 years earlier, this centre was built as a cultural focus for the area. It serves the community as a hub for theatre, symphony concerts and ballet and is close by many popular sites. The Barbican as a host site presented an interesting three-dimensional maze of rooms and corridors and provided many areas where meeting's participants could sit and visit. The congress was opened by Sir Andrew Huxley, O.M., President of the Royal Society. At the opening ceremony, Sir Bryan Matthews spoke about the early days of EEG and his work in collaboration with Lord Adrian to reproduce Berger's work on the human alpha rhythm. The host society displayed several historical pieces of equipment including early EEG machines and original equipment used by Dawson to record evoked potentials in the 1940s. A course of educational activity also was organized for the International Organization for Societies of EEG Technologists (OSET).

Fellowship grants were increased both in number and in amount to US $300. The meeting was a scientific and educational success. Financial issues developed due to unexpected additional charges by the congress site, which took until the next Fiscal Period to eventually resolve.

Each registrant to the meeting received a complementary copy of W. Cobb's book *Wave Length, A History of the IFSECN.* That book is reprinted with minor editing for the first half of this book. Congress social events were organized to visit the Houses of Parliament, Westminster Abbey, Windsor, and other sites around London. The congress was held immediately before the opening of the World Congress of Neurology and International Leagues Against Epilepsy meetings in nearby Hamburg, Federal Republic of Germany (FRG).

The 1985 General Assembly discussed the location for the next International Congress of EEG and Clinical Neurophysiology. Three countries submitted bids: Brazil, the Federal Republic of Germany, and India. The General Assembly held an extended discussion about the advantages and disadvantages of coordinating the IFSECN Congress with the next World Congress of Neurology, as had been the custom for the previous several Congresses. The World Congress of Neurology had bids from Brazil, India and three other countries, and the choice of sites will be made one week after this IFSECN General Assembly meeting. The General Assembly then voted to empower the Executive Committee to set on the location of the next Congress taking into consideration the World Congress of Neurology site. In a non-binding vote, the General Assembly favoured Brazil if other factors were not taken into consideration.

12. Nominations Committee

The Nominations Committee was composed of Robert Naquet (Chair), Teruo Okuma, J. Radermecker, and José Vásquez del Mercado. Nominations were held in three stages between May 1983 and summer 1984. The committee first held the election for President, followed by a second round for election of the Secretary, Treasurer, and Chairman of the EMG Commission. Finally, a third round was held for the one Executive Committee Member-at-large and two additional Members of the EMG Commission.

The Nominations Committee was charged with selecting the nominees for the ballot with the largest number of nominations from societies while adhering to the principles of broad geographic representation. The process was discussed at the 1985 General Assembly, where the expressed sentiment was that the names of all persons who receive nominations, and who accept to stand, should appear on the election ballot. If needed, a runoff could be held among those with the largest number votes if no candidate received a majority in the initial balloting.

When these elections were held, the 1985 General Assembly had not yet met. It was at that 1985 meeting that the General Assembly established a second Member-at-large position. An election for that new position was held at the beginning of the next Fiscal Period.

The Executive Committee of the Fiscal Period 1985–1989 consisted of:

President	John E. Desmedt (Belgium)
Past President	Robert J. Ellingson (USA)
Secretary	Bram Ongerboer de Visser (The Netherlands)
Treasurer	Manuel Meyer (Switzerland)
Chairman of the EMG Commission	Stéphane Métral (France)
Member-at-Large EEG	Juhn Wada (Canada)
Member-at-Large EMG	Roberto Low (Brazil)
Editor-in-Chief	Hans van Duijn (The Netherlands)

Wave Length and Action Potentials: History of the IFCN
(Supplements to Clinical Neurophysiology, Vol. 61)
By: M.R. Nuwer and C.H. Lücking

Chapter 11

1985–1990

President: John E. Desmedt

This Fiscal Period lasted officially 4.5 years until January 1990 in order to take advantage of the summer in the southern hemisphere, where the XII International Congress was held in Rio de Janeiro, Brazil. The year 1987 was the 40th anniversary of the formative Federation meeting in 1947. Furthermore, the year 1989 was the 60th anniversary of the publication of H. Berger's first report on recording the human EEG and the 40th anniversary of the Federation.

Recognizing that anniversaries are opportunities to celebrate the past but also to look toward the future, this Fiscal Period marked the time when the Federation changed its name to the International Federation of Clinical Neurophysiology (IFCN). This was accomplished officially at the 1990 General Assembly meeting.

The Executive Committee was led by John E. Desmedt (President), who had served the Federation previously as Chairman of the EMG Commission from 1977 to 1985. Robert J. Ellingson (Past President) brought continuity to the Executive Committee based on his 20 years of service, including three terms as Federation Secretary. Bram Ongerboer de Visser (Secretary), Manuel Meyer (Treasurer), Stéphane Métral (Chairman of the EMG Commission), Juhn Wada (Member-at-Large) and Hans van Duijn (Editor-in-Chief) completed the initial Executive Committee membership. A picture is in Appendix 11, Fig. 2. Roberto Low (Member-at-Large EMG) joined the Executive Committee soon after the beginning of the Fiscal Period, when he won the special election for the newly created second Member-at-Large position. Dr. Low's election marked the first Executive Committee member from South America (Brazil). That validated the rational for increasing the number of Member-at-Large positions, which was accomplished to bring better diversity of representation to the Federation's Executive Committee.

The Federation affiliated with the World Federation of Neurology (WFN) in the special capacity of *WFN Charter Member.* The action to join the WFN in this capacity was well received and unanimous acclamation of the WFN Council, in September 1987 in New Delhi. The Federation expects this partnership more effectively to promote clinical neurophysiology together with clinical neurology.

1. The Journal

In early 1987, Editor-in-Chief Hans van Duijn and Editor Mary A.B. Brazier both asked to be relieved of their duties for personal reasons. The Executive Committee offered them both deep feelings of gratitude for their devotion and commitment to the Journal over many years.

Molly Brazier had been active in international affairs since 1947 when she helped establish the Federation at the first International Congress in London. She took part in organizing the International Congresses in Boston, 1953, and Vienna, 1965. She subsequently served as Treasurer 1953–1957, Secretary 1957–1961, President 1961–1965 and Past President 1965–1969. She was also involved with the Journal from the beginning in

1949 when she assisted Robert Schwab in setting up a business office at Massachusetts General Hospital for the Journal that had been newly founded by Herbert Jasper. She was Editor of the Journal from 1972 to 1987, served as Editor-in-Chief from 1972 to 1984. She authored and edited several books. She has a long list of publications. Hans van Duijn has been a basic scientist and clinician. As Chairman of the publication committee for the 1977 International Congress in Amsterdam he became active in the Federation. He was Editor of the journal from 1979 until 1987, was Editor-in-Chief from 1984 to 1987.

This left the need to appoint two new Editors on short notice. President J. Desmedt acted as interim editor for the Eastern hemisphere and Past-President R. Ellingson for the Western hemisphere until new permanent editors could be appointed and arranged to assume those editorial responsibilities. The Executive Committee considered this unprecedented situation as an opportunity to reshape editorial policies and further enhance the EEG Journal's status as the leader among clinical neurophysiology publications. Timothy Pedley (USA) was appointed as Western hemisphere Editor, but resigned after several months due to differences about the role of the Federation Executive Committee and President in the affairs of the journal. He was succeeded by Gastone Celesia (USA). François Mauguière (France) was appointed as Editor for the European Office. Continuing discussions were held about their respective roles, the position of one only as Editor-in-Chief, and the role of the Federation Executive Committee in the affairs of the journal. Until this time, only one Editor at a time held the position of Editor-in-Chief. At some points in the previous few years, the two Editors were each entitled to one-half of a vote in the Executive Committee. After considering the options, the Executive Committee recommended that both Editors be given the title Editor-in-Chief, and each be allowed a full vote in the Executive Committee. The related amendment of the Bye-Laws was approved by the 1990 Council in Rio de Janeiro. F. Mauguière and G. Celesia reaffirmed that the Editors-in-Chief will have independence from the Executive Committee in all the scientific issues and editorial content. The role of the Executive Committee was to appoint editors and the editorial board, to set some business arrangements of the Journal, and to oversee other Federation publications such as the Supplement series of books and the Handbook.

The volume of submitted manuscripts continued to climb. The volume in this 4-year Fiscal Period was 30% higher than in 1981–1985, and about 60% higher than in 1977–1981. The American office continued to receive about 20% more manuscripts than the European office. In 1988–1989, 45% of the manuscripts received pertained to evoked potentials. About 15% were about EEG, 10% EMG, 10% motor control, 8% sleep, 5% animal basic physiology, and only 2% were about MEG. About 36% were clinical reports, 33% concerned human physiological studies, and 26% were technical or normative data studies. The editors encouraged submission for other studies of neurophysiology such as fMRI. The large portion of submissions on evoked potentials justified the earlier decision to create a separate volume with six issues per year for evoked potential and event-related potential studies. Since all of the evoked potential manuscripts could not be included in this sub-specialized volume, most of the short communications, case reports and normative data studies remained in the EEG volumes of the Journal. The two editorial offices routinely made use of reviewers from the other region. The acceptance rate ranged between 40% and 50%.

New reviewers were added to enlarge the base of the reviewing process and as new technologies were developed. A survey was mailed in 1989 to all reviewers, requesting feedback to the editor. The feedback was overwhelmingly positive and many suggestions were adopted to improve manuscript flow while maintaining quality standards. The editors spent a considerable effort to keep the review turn-around time and the overall publication lag time to as short as possible. The journal also started a new section on Controversies in Clinical Neurophysiology.

2. Practice guidelines and other committee reports

The Executive Committee considered publishing an updated edition of *Recommendations for the Practice of Clinical Neurophysiology* (Elsevier 1983). But according to Elsevier, one such update every 4 years would not be financially feasible. As an alternative, some Guidelines Committee and other Federation reports may be published in the journal as they appeared or were accepted by the Federation.

Several committees were appointed during this Fiscal Period to produce reports on specific methodologies in clinical neurophysiology in order to pursue the task of updating the Recommendations book. These were accepted at the 1990 Rio de Janeiro General Assembly and eventually were published in the Journal between 1990 and 1994:

- Report of IFCN committee on clinical relevance of kindling. Kindling: basic mechanisms and clinical validity. M. Sato, R.J. Racine and D.C. McIntyre.
- Report of IFCN committee on basic mechanisms. Basic mechanisms of cerebral rhythmic activities. M. Steriade, P. Gloor, R.R. Llinás, F.H. Lopes da Silva and M.M. Mesulam.
- Neuromonitoring during surgery. Report of an IFCN committee. M.R. Nuwer, J. Daube, C. Fischer, J. Schramm and C.D. Yingling.
- Recommended standards for electroretinograms and visual evoked potentials. Report of an IFCN committee. G.G. Celesia, I. Bodis-Wollner, G.G.E. Chatrian, G.F.A. Harding, S. Sokol and H. Spekreijse.
- Long-term monitoring for epilepsy. Report of an IFCN committee. J. Engel, Jr., J. Burchfiel, J. Ebersole, J. Gates, J. Gotman, R. Homan, J. Ives, D. King, J. Lieb, S. Sato and R. Wilkus.
- Human reflexes and late responses. Report of an IFCN committee. J. Kimura, J. Daube, D. Burke, M. Hallett, G. Cruccu, B.W. Ongerboer de Visser, N. Yanagisawa, M. Shimamura and J. Rothwell.
- Central EMG and tests of motor control. Report of an IFCN committee. M. Hallett, A. Berardelli, P. Delwaide, H.J. Freund, J. Kimura, C.H. Lücking, J.C. Rothwell, B.T. Shahani and N. Yanagisawa.
- IFCN guidelines for topographic and frequency analysis of EEGs and EPs. Report of an IFCN committee. M.R. Nuwer, D. Lehmann, F.H. Lopes da Silva, S. Matsuoka, W. Sutherling and J.F. Vibert.
- IFCN recommended standards for short latency somatosensory evoked potentials. Report of an IFCN committee. M.R. Nuwer, M. Aminoff, J. Desmedt, A.A. Eisen, D. Goodin, S. Matsuoka, F. Mauguière, H. Shibasaki, W. Sutherling and J.F. Vibert.
- IFCN recommended standards for brain-stem auditory evoked potentials. Report of an IFCN committee. M.R. Nuwer, M. Aminoff, D. Goodin, S. Matsuoka, F. Mauguière, A. Starr and J.F. Vibert.
- IFCN recommended standards for long latency auditory event-related potentials. Report of an IFCN committee. D. Goodin, J. Desmedt, K. Maurer and M.R. Nuwer.
- Non-invasive electrical and magnetic stimulation of the brain, spinal cord and roots: basic principles and procedures for routine clinical application. Report of an IFCN committee. P.M. Rossini, A.T. Barker, A. Berardelli, M.D. Caramia, G. Caruso, R.Q. Cracco, M.R. Dimitrijevic, M. Hallett, Y. Katayama, C.H. Lücking, A.L. Maertens de Noordhout, C.D. Marsden, N.M.F. Murray, J.C. Rothwell, M. Swash and C. Tomberg.

3. New member societies

During this Fiscal Period the Federation accepted seven new member societies: Chinese Society of EMG and Clinical Neurophysiology, Valle State Society of Clinical Neurophysiology (Colombia), Dominican Society of EEG and

Clinical Neurophysiology, Indonesian Society for Clinical Neurophysiology, Philippine Society of Clinical Neurophysiology, Portuguese Association of EEG and Clinical Neurophysiology, Thailand Section of Clinical Neurophysiology. That resulted in 48 the total of Member Societies of the Federation.

Xiao-Fu Tang, Delegate from the People's Republic of China, reported about the one China issue. Her government and society were happy to see Taiwanese physicians at a Bangkok regional Federation symposium. The use of the Taiwanese flag, used there in a social event along with other national flags of registrants, caused political difficulty for her Society. X.-F. Tang described that the Chinese Society position is that there is only one China, and she requested that the Federation avoid compromising that position in its activities. She would be happy to have us refer to the Taiwanese physicians as coming from Taiwan, China. The Executive Committee expressed regrets that this is a problem in China. The Federation's position is that it does not take political positions.

4. Secretary

Communication is important but a difficult task for keeping a worldwide body organized. Federation Secretary B. Ongerboer de Visser maintained contact through correspondence with the Member Societies, keeping them informed about Federation activities. He prepared and circulated meeting minutes for the Executive Committee, Organizing Committees of the International Congresses, Council, and General Assembly. The General Assembly asked that the regular communications to each Delegate include the Executive Committee minutes. Every month the Secretary prepared the "Yellow Pages" journal section with the Federation news. These include the announcements and preparation of the International Congresses. It also included member societies' news, announcements for national or regional meetings, events, or conferences as submitted by member societies. The Secretary provided help to third parties asking for information about persons, methods, or equipment manufacturers. Contact was maintained with the Council for International Organization of Medical Sciences (CIOMS) in Geneva.

5. Finances

Treasurer Manuel Meyer watched over Federation spending carefully during the 4 years of this Fiscal Period. Total income for the entire Fiscal Period was US $848,618 and grew by 40% in 4 years. The main sources of income are the Elsevier Royalties and editorial support (US $534,107), member society dues (US $125,137) and the interest on investments (US $89,906). Congress income decreased because of the lack of profit and loan repayment from the 1985 Congress. The loans to the 8th EMG Congress in 1987 were completely repaid. The Rio de Janeiro Congress was expected to break even partially because funding was kept in more stable currencies in North America and Europe. Total expenses for the Fiscal Period were US $668,652 and increased by about 6% over 4 years. Increases were due primarily to costs of living, transportation, and additional activities for the Federation, the Executive Committee and Editorial offices. Total assets in December 1989 were valued at US $458,773, a substantial increase over the US $278,807 in August 1985. The previous policy of keeping Federation funds in many places was replaced by a plan to keep the funds in one place in Switzerland. Funds were moved to Crédit Suisse in Zurich. Investments increased in value in 4 years from US $90,595 to US $381,732.

The financial problem facing the Executive Committee during this term pertained to the Barbican Centre, site of the 1985 London Congress. The contract for which was more complex than originally expected. Many extra charges were unexpected. Auditors were hired to advise the Federation and the (British) EEG Society on settling the matter of the additional charges. After long and delicate negotiations with the Barbican Centre, Congress Convener A.M. Halliday achieved a suitable settlement. The Federation loan to the Congress was not repaid and the Federation covered an additional US $50,000 of expenses.

6. Rules committee

The Rules Committee consisting of William R. Kennedy (Chairman), David Burke, Gilson E. Gonçalves e Silva, Carl H. Lücking, and Paolo Rossini dealt with several amendments of Federation's rules raised during this Fiscal Period.

7. Federation name change

An amendment of the name "International Federation of Societies for Electroencephalography and Clinical Neurophysiology" was proposed by the Executive Committee and endorsed by the Council through a mail ballot in June 1987. At the Rio de Janeiro Congress, the Council and General Assembly considered the issue again and approved the amendment by consensus. The major purpose of the name change was to recognize that the Federation represents a broad collection of knowledge about investigating physiology and disease of the nervous system and muscles through various methods of testing, especially through electrodiagnostic methods. Over the past 40 years, the Federation's focus had expanded well beyond EEG itself. At the 1990 General Assembly in Rio de Janeiro, the vote in favour of changing the name of the Federation to IFCN was unanimous. There were no abstentions. This name change was received as a forward step, looking to the future of what this organization represents now and in decades to come.

Consideration was raised about the name of the journal, "Electroencephalography and Clinical Neurophysiology". The journal's name was well established and widely referred to, and it was important to preserve the high impact of the journal, which could be disrupted by a name change. For that reason, the journal's name was not changed at this time.

8. EMG congress name

A further discussion concerned the question whether the name of the EMG Congress should include "Clinical Neurophysiology" or whether EEG and EMG Congress should be known simply as "International Congress of Clinical Neurophysiology". The Executive Committee proposed and the Council in Rio de Janeiro approved an amendment to the Bye-Law on Other International Meetings stating: "In addition to the International Congress of EEG and Clinical Neurophysiology, the Federation organizes *an International Congress of Electromyography and may organize or sponsor other interim meetings on any topic related to clinical neurophysiology."* Future Rules Committees were encouraged to study and report back on further name changes for the congresses.

9. Two Editors-in-Chief

The Executive Committee recommended that the Federation allow for two individuals to hold simultaneously the title *Editor-in-Chief.* The Executive Committee carefully studied the problem of balancing the status of the editors who are in charge of the Western and European offices, respectively. Until 1988, the two editors had been invited to the meetings of the Executive Committee, but only one had a vote in conformity with the Federation Statutes. In early 1988, the Executive Committee agreed provisionally to grant to each editor the name of "Editor-in-Chief" and to give each of them a half vote (which amounted to having them share the one vote provided for an Editor by the Statutes). Federation President requested that the General Assembly grant a full vote to each Editor-in-Chief. This would require a change in Statutes. The Rules Committee noted that this would increase the number of Executive Committee members who had not been elected by the Council. The General Assembly voted with more than a two-thirds majority to change the Statutes and Bye-Laws as follows: "The Federation is administered by an Executive Committee composed of the President, the immediate Past President, the Secretary and the Treasurer of the Federation, the Editors-in-Chief of the EEG Journal,..." In addition, a change was made to the Journal Bye-Law, "The Editorial Staff may consist of *two Editors-in-Chief*, a Managing Editor, ...". The Rules Committee was asked to report back at the next meeting on problems this may cause in the balance between EEG and EMG members on the Executive Committee.

10. Geographic representation

Geographic diversity was desired for broad geographic representation as a goal of Federation rulemaking. The two Members-at-Large must represent geographical regions not already elected to the Executive Committee. A question arose as to whether the geographical exclusion should include or exclude the Past President's location. An amendment of the Bye-Law "Committees, The Nomination Committee" had been submitted by the Executive Committee to the Council of Rio as follows: "The Nomination Committee should ensure that Members-at-Large are chosen from geographical areas not already represented in the Executive Committee by members elected in the same fiscal period". This amendment restricts the areas represented by the current President, the Treasurer and the Secretary, but not the area represented by the Past President who was elected in the previous fiscal period. This was approved by consensus.

In the years since, the meaning of this amendment changed. When adopted, it was meant that the Member-at-Large must be from broadly defined geographic regions different from the previously chosen Executive Committee members. At the time of adopting the amendment, it was understood that example geographic regions were Western Europe, Eastern Europe, Asia, North America, Latin America, Africa and Australia.

As the years passed, this meaning was lost. The rule came to mean the Member-at-Large could not be from the same nation. Twenty years later, the original intent resurfaced in further proposed rule clarifications to ensure broad representation by defining a region to be the societies in a Chapter.

11. EMG commission

The 1985 General Assembly in London requested a special committee to examine the role and purpose of the EMG Commission and how best to ensure a fair balanced in representation of both EEG and EMG in executive operations. Based on the committee's conclusions, the Council in Rio de Janeiro voted to disband the EMG Commission. The EMG Commission was formed at the First International EMG Congress in 1961 and continued its work for three decades. Its chairmen were successively: Fritz Buchthal (1961), Edward H. Lambert (1965), Fritz Buchthal (1969), Albrecht Struppler (1973), John E. Desmedt (1977 and 1981), and Stéphane Métral (1985).

In years leading up to this and from this point on, EMG has been recognized as a core discipline of the Federation.

Nominations rules called for fair representation of the EEG and EMG disciplines in future Executive Committee composition.

12. Regional meetings

The Federation sponsored symposia besides its traditional International Congresses. This fulfilled the educational missions for the IFSECN and served to foster the vocational development among young physicians. During this Fiscal Period, the Federation sponsored several regional meetings. These included:

- Regional Symposium of Clinical Neurophysiology in Bangkok, Thailand, February 1987.
- Regional Symposium of Clinical Neurophysiology in Bali, Indonesia, September 1987, jointly with the Asian and Oceanian Congress of Neurology.
- Regional Symposium of Clinical Neurophysiology in Beijing, People's Republic of China, June 1989.

Each symposium and educational workshop served to support and promote a newly affiliated Federation member society. These symposia also served to enhance the impact of our discipline in the host and neighbouring countries by providing intensive teaching and updating in practical methodologies for young clinical neurophysiologists. Many young neurophysiologists were supported by a Federation fellowship. Work with local authorities led to new positions and laboratories for EEG and EMG. These showed the value of regional meetings toward achieving the mission of the Federation.

13. International congresses

13.1. VIII International Congress of Electromyography (ICEMG)

The EMG Congress was held in Sorrento, Italy, on May 24–29, 1987 at the invitation of the Italian Society of EEG and EMG which hosted the congress. The Organizing Committee consisted of the local organizers: Giuseppe Caruso (Convener), Paolo Rossini (Secretary), and Antonio Arrigo (Treasurer), and members of the Federation Executive Committee: John E. Desmedt, Robert J. Ellingson, Bram Ongerboer de Visser, Manuel Meyer, Stéphane Métral. Over 800 physicians and scientists attended. The education and scientific programmes were well received. The programme included 16 symposia, 8 didactic lectures, many demonstrations and workshops, and 32 poster sessions designed with active discussions lead by a chairperson. The social programme was outstanding and highly praised.

13.2. XII International Congress of EEG and Clinical Neurophysiology

The EEG Congress was held in Rio de Janeiro in January 14–19, 1990, summer time in the southern hemisphere. The choice of Brazil as host country for the major quadrennial Congress was a demonstration of support for clinical neurophysiology in Latin America. The Federation by this time had seven member societies in this region. This was taken as a step toward reaching out to be more receptive to the special problems that may be challenging our colleagues in different parts of the world. The Brazilian Society of Clinical Neurophysiology served as the host society. Its Organizing Committee representatives were Gilson E. Gonçalves e Silva (Convener), Roberto Low (Secretary), and João A.M. Nóbrega (Treasurer). Organizing representatives from the Federation, John E. Desmedt, Robert J. Ellingson, Bram Ongerboer de Visser, Manuel Meyer, and Stéphane Métral who worked tirelessly with the local society representatives to organize an excellent scientific and social event. Honorary Presidents of the Congress were: José G. Camargo Lima (Brazil), Henri Gastaut (France), Pierre Gloor (Canada), Edward H. Lambert (USA), and Yasuo Shimazono (Japan).

The venue of the Congress was Hotel Nacional Rio Convention Centre. The programme included 17 didactic lectures, 19 symposia, videotape sessions, and free communications presented in eight poster sessions. About 900 active physicians and scientists participated. The organizers faced several obstacles. The Brazilian government does not allow importation of equipment so the number of vendors was fewer than usual. Because of Brazilian hyperinflation, the congress financial transactions were handled through Zurich and New York. Despite the wide fluctuations in value of the crusado currency, the Congress was able to balance its budget.

New rules were implemented for bidding on the next International Congress. Invitations for hosting the International Congress must be sent to the Executive Committee at least 2 months ahead of the General Assembly meeting. This would allow for some time to consider the details. Proposals for hosting the next International Congress in 1993 were received from Canada–USA, Germany, Hungary, and India. Vancouver was approved by a majority of 47 votes.

14. General assembly report of the president

As a part of his report on the Rio de Janeiro General Assembly, the President presented his perception of the quiet, but significant, evolution of the challenges that the Federation has had to meet.

> "We will all agree that the Federation should maintain a prevalent position in enhancing the significance of the studies of brain and muscle functions through electrical recordings. While electroencephalography was of premier concern since the first decade of the Federation, electromyography strongly developed from the 1960s and has now established its position in our traditions. For example, both EEG and EMG are now well represented in the Executive Committee (thus removing the need for an "EMG Commission"), and their cooperation enhances the impact efficiency of our ventures.
>
> Recently, electrophysiological monitoring in surgery or sleep, evoked potentials, transcranial magnetic stimulation and brain mapping have been pushed forward. In addition, other methodologies such as CT, PET, SPECT and MRI are providing new imaging resources which become popular in clinical neurology and might pretend to substitute altogether for brain electricity studies in diagnostic applications.
>
> I am sure you will share my feeling that these recent challenges of sophisticated anatomical diagnostic tools should be taken seriously and that they should be properly responded to. It is time for us to reassess all the areas of our discipline and to actively promote our best updated electrophysiological methodologies throughout the world. Fellowship programmes and regional workshops appear to me to deserve special concern."

The complete President's report and the full Proceedings of the General Assembly are published in *Electroencephalography and Clinical Neurophysiology,* 1993, 87: 67–75.

15. Honours and awards

Honorary Fellows of the Federation elected during this term included Fritz Buchthal (Copenhagen), Pierre Gloor (Montreal), Edward H. Lambert (Minneapolis), Antoine Rémond (Paris), and Yasuo Shimazono (Tokyo). This was approved unanimously by the 1990 General Assembly.

Three honorary lectures were created and named after major pioneers of clinical neurophysiology in plenary sessions. The intention was to have these named honorary lectures at each future quadrennial congress. Major international figures in clinical neurophysiology were invited to give these honorary lectures.

The name of Hans Berger who established electroencephalography with his major paper of 1929 was an obvious choice for one lecture's name. The Rio de Janeiro Congress marked the 60th anniversary of Berger's publication. Jerome (Pete) Engel of Los Angeles delivered the First Berger Lecture on functional explorations of the epileptic brain and their therapeutic implications.

Eric Kugelberg was chosen as a name for the second lectureship, because of his work as a founding father of electromyography and on the basic classical framework for the diagnosis of neuropathic and myopathic disorders and human reflexes. Robert Porter of Victoria, Australia, delivered the First Kugelberg Lecture on brain mechanisms of voluntary motor commands.

The Third Lecture was named after Lord Adrian of Cambridge to celebrate his essential contribution to neurophysiology in animals and in humans, and as a reminder that our discipline is deeply rooted in the basic neurosciences. Fernando Lopes da Silva of Amsterdam presented the First Adrian Lecture on neural mechanisms underlying brain waves.

Another initiative introduced at the General Assembly were the Young Investigator Awards. Elsevier Science Publishers funded these awards of US $3500 for each of two. They were awarded to honour young authors submitting an excellent original manuscript to the journal *EEG and Clinical Neurophysiology*. The Executive Committee accepted this proposal and established a procedure for the designation of the laureates. The name Cobb Award would be given to the author of a manuscript submitted to the European journal office and the name Brazier Award for the Western Hemisphere office. The manuscripts would go through the standard journal review procedure. The primary author must be a person under the age of 40 years. The awards will be given during each quadrennial Congress.

16. Nomination committee

The Nomination Committee for this term was composed of Robert J. Ellingson (Chairman, USA), D.J. Brimani (Iran), Ray Cooper (UK), and Karl Hainaut (Belgium). In 1985, shortly after the 1985 General Assembly authorized a second member-at-large position, a special election was held. Procedures for this election followed the wishes as expressed by the General Assembly. All nominations received from Delegates would be placed on the first ballot as long as they were eligible for the position and agreed to serve if elected. Only nominees from geographical areas not yet represented in the Executive Committee were considered eligible: Africa, Asia, Australia, Latin America, and Eastern Europe. If no candidate were to receive a majority on the first ballot, the two with the greatest votes would be in a runoff ballot. Eleven persons were nominated. Roberto Low of Brazil won that election with the majority on the first round of voting. He served in that Executive Committee role during most of these 4 years.

Near the end of the third year, the election cycle was initiated for the next term for President, Secretary, Treasurer and two Members-at-Large. Additional constraints were applied. No one who had previously held an office was eligible for re-election to that office, except that the Secretary and Treasurer may be elected to a second term. If the Treasurer was an EMGer, the Secretary must have been an EEGer, or vice versa. The two Members-at-Large must have come from geographic regions other than those already represented by the other elected officers. One Member-at-Large must have been an EEGer and the other an EMGer. The election process had become complex.

To comply with the above restrictions, the election was held in three stages. Voting was one vote per member society. The first round elected a President and a Treasurer. Six people were nominated for President; one declined to run. Four were nominated for Treasurer; two declined to run. Election ballots were sent out on December 15, 1988. Jun Kimura of Japan received a majority of 27 votes for the office of President, Manuel Meyer of Switzerland a majority of 33 votes for the office of Treasurer; both were declared as elected without a runoff. The second round elected a Secretary. Eight people were nominated; two were excluded by rule and two declined to run. Nomination ballots were sent out on February 28, 1989. Barry R. Tharp of the United States received a majority of 20 votes and was declared elected. The third round elected two Members-at-Large, one each for EEG and EMG disciplines. To this point in the election process, unrepresented geographical areas were Africa, Australasia, the Far East, the Near East, Latin America, and Eastern Europe. This represented the original sense of the geographical diversity rule. Six persons were nominated for EEG Member-at-Large and four for EMG Member-at-Large; all accepted to run. No candidate for either office received a majority of votes in the initial ballot. A runoff listed the top two candidates for each office. In the runoff, the vote for the EMG Member-at-Large position was tied. Under Statute VIII.2 in force at that time, the President of the Federation had the deciding vote, which he cast for Jagjit S. Chopra of India. Jerzy Majkowski of Poland received a majority of 19 votes for the EEG Member-at-Large position and was declared elected.

The Executive Committee for the 1990–1993 Fiscal Period was composed of:

President	Jun Kimura (Japan)
Past President	John E. Desmedt (Belgium)
Secretary	Barry Tharp (USA)
Treasurer	Manuel Meyer (Switzerland)
Member-at-Large EMG	Jagjit Chopra (India)
Member-at-Large EEG	Jerzy Majkowsky (Poland)
Editors-in-Chief	François Mauguière (France)
	Gastone G. Celesia (USA)

Wave Length and Action Potentials: History of the IFCN
(Supplements to Clinical Neurophysiology, Vol. 61)
By: M.R. Nuwer and C.H. Lücking

Chapter 12

1990–1993

President: Jun Kimura

The Executive Committee in this term consisted of Jun Kimura (President), John E. Desmedt (Past President), Barry Tharp (Secretary), Manuel Meyer (Treasurer), Jagjit Chopra and Jerzy Majkowsky (Members-at-Large), François Mauguière and Gastone G. Celesia (Editors-in-Chief). Seven Executive Committee meetings were held during this fiscal period.

This was the first term under the new name International Federation of Clinical Neurophysiology and the first since decades without an EMG Commission. Both of the two Editors-in-Chief were full voting members of the Executive Committee. The movement toward greater numbers of regional meetings and regional presence continued, foreshadowing the eventual move toward Chapters. Rules continued to evolve to promote turnover among the Executive Committee members.

The previous IFCN 1990 General Assembly in Rio de Janeiro directed the Executive Committee to consider the holding Council and General Assembly meetings every 2 years at the occasion of both the International Congress of EEG and Clinical Neurophysiology and the International Congress of EMG. The General Assembly had established new rules for the Executive Committee. Each Editor-in-Chief has one full vote. The Agenda for Council and General Assembly was to be sent to the Delegates at least 1 month prior to their meetings. Executive Committee meeting minutes were to be distributed to the Council members after approval by the Executive Committee, so as to keep Delegates informed of Executive Committee activity.

The new name *International Federation of Clinical Neurophysiology* (IFCN) replaced the original name *International Federation of Societies of EEG and Clinical Neurophysiology* (IFSECN) at the beginning of this Fiscal Period at the 1990 General Assembly in Rio de Janeiro. The new name acknowledged the equal importance of EEG and EMG, as proposed by former president John Desmedt and others. The change reflects a unity to clinical electrophysiology as a discipline. Reflecting this spirit, the main quadrennial convention dealt with an increasing number of EMG materials. The scope of the midterm convention, previously known as the EMG Congress, likewise gradually was enlarged into a broader representation of techniques and applications. This trend in fact had already been noticeable at the 1987 EMG Congress in Sorrento and continued at the 1992 EMG Congress in Jerusalem.

The name of the journal *Electroencephalography and Clinical Neurophysiology* remained unchanged because of the well established name as well as the great importance of preserving the high impact factor of the Journal. That remained the status of the journal name until the end of that decade.

Under the Chairmanship of John Desmedt, 17 books have been sent to nine countries. These have consisted primarily of *Handbook of EEG and Clinical Neurophysiology* (Revised Series): *Volume 3, Evoked Potentials* (T.W. Picton, Editor). A Gift Committee has been established to provide books to institutions which do not have funds and not for personal libraries.

In view of the challenge by the new imaging techniques (CT, MRI, SPECT, PET), all areas of clinical neurophysiology have to be actively promoted. Therefore, fellowship programmes and regional workshops were widely promoted.

The proposed budget for this Fiscal Period by the previous Treasurer was not accepted by the General Assembly in Rio de Janeiro. The new Executive Committee was instructed to develop a new budget and communicate it to each Delegate within 2 months.

1. Journal

The IFCN was fortunate to have two excellent Editors-in-Chief during these 4 years, Gastone G. Celesia for the Western Hemisphere office and François Mauguière for the European office. They maintained the high scientific and academic reputation of the journal. The journal expanded from 18 to 24 issues annually. Six issues each year were dedicated to a separate annual volume subtitled *EMG and Motor Control*. This was similar to the action 4 years earlier to add a six-issue volume named *Evoked Potentials*. Both separate volumes were published in parallel with the main journal, which had 12 issues and two volumes. Therefore, the journal reached four volumes and 24 issues each year.

The journal continued to experience an increasing number of submissions. Overall the submissions had been increasing at about 10% per year. The increase had been mainly in the European office. The number of manuscripts received at the two offices was approximately the same, at about 240 per year, whereas for several decades the Western Hemisphere office had had the larger volume. To put that number in context, this journal's manuscript volume in 1980 was about 240 for both editorial offices combined, so that the change represented a doubling of the submitted manuscript volume over a dozen years. The volume of submissions to the European office had increased by 50% over the previous 5 years. The acceptance rate dropped to about 45% in the early 1990s from 60% a decade earlier. These numbers showed how the journal gained popularity and remained highly competitive over the years. To keep the acceptance rate from dropping too low, the journal enlarged by adding pages, issues and volumes. While some viewed that acceptance rate as rather low, the selectivity of this journal improved its academic standing in Europe. At this point, it had achieved the status as the first choice when authors submit manuscripts in the field of Clinical Neurophysiology.

This favourable situation as a highly regarded, selective journal resulted in a need to increase the total number of pages printed per year. By increasing size, the journal was able to keep the backlog at Elsevier's publication desk to a minimal duration. This helped the turn-around time, which was also regarded as very desirable to keep low for a journal. Manuscripts were submitted to three reviewers by mail including at least one reviewer from the opposite geographic region, which entailed a degree of turn-around time delay. The mean delay between reception of manuscripts and the mailing of the first answer to authors had dropped to less than 2 months. For accepted manuscripts, the time from first submission to eventual transmission to the publisher was kept to only 4.5 months — about one-half the overall turn-around time achieved 4 years earlier. These were considered good by the standards of the day in the era before routine electronic communications.

As far as the types of studies published, from 1988 to 1992 the evoked and event-related potential manuscripts gradually decreased from 65% to 50% of manuscripts published. During that same interval, EEG remained around 20% of published manuscripts, and sleep was 10%. If one excluded technical reports, those two fields actually dropped during this period. Many technical papers were about new techniques in computerized EEG and mathematical models of EEG activity. Those technical EEG reports represented nearly 40% of the EEG submissions.

The launching of the *EMG and Motor Control* subtitle explained most of the positive trend in submissions. For the European office the EMG and topics of reflexes had grown to represent 25% of manuscripts in 1992 in comparison with only 15% of submissions in 1988. The Western hemisphere office saw a smaller rate of manuscripts of EMG and reflexes. If one included all EMG, reflexes, and motor control and motor evoked potential manuscripts, the sum came to be close to one-third of submissions.

The submission rate of evoked potential reports remained stable from 1988 to 1992. The different types of evoked potentials evolved over those years. The routine somatosensory, brainstem auditory and visual evoked potential reports were steadily decreasing. Magnetic evoked field reports had been increasing, especially for the auditory magnetic evoked field papers. Event-related potentials grew to 30% in 1992 from 12% in 1988. Most of these reports concerned studies in normal subjects.

Submission pressure was high in this field and it is a matter of editorial policy to decide whether the acceptance rate should be increased. Most of the papers with no direct relevance to human studies were not given priorities, consistent with an editorial policy to promote clinical studies. This goal was only partly achieved in this time period, with clinical studies increasing during the 1988–1990 period. But this positive trend reversed beginning in 1990. In the early 1990s the percentage of studies conducted in normal subjects began increasing due to the growing number of event-related studies in normal subjects, often describing techniques which were not applicable or validated in patients.

Among clinical disease topics, epilepsy had the most reports, which were about 15% of the overall clinical reports. Sleep disorders, focal CNS lesions, movement disorders and neuropathies each represented about 10% of clinical studies published. Peripheral nervous system diseases clearly increased from previous time periods, a change that was related to the very successful launching of the *EMG & Motor Control* volume in Europe. Similarly epidemiologic trends explained the increase of papers devoted to dementia and AIDS. The gradual drop in portion of papers on epilepsy and sleep was probably related to the competition with other journals such as *Epilepsia* and *Sleep*.

The countries of origin remained widely diverse. In the Western editorial office the increase in manuscripts from Japan was notable. Japanese submissions rose to nearly 30% of the manuscripts received in that office.

The two editorial offices used nearly 600 colleagues to review manuscripts during these 4 years. Most reviewers were not on the list of official consulting editors. The consulting editors were appointed for a term of 3 years, and choosing the names for the formal editorial panel was very difficult. In order to recognize those who have accepted the task of reviewing many manuscripts, sometimes for many years, required dropping other names from this list.

Reviewers who provide excellent editorial services to the journal through the burden of reviewing papers ought to eventually see their name on the front page of the journal. This difficult task of changing names on the editorial panel raised many questions especially from those whose names were removed. The editors expressed a wish that those whose names had been dropped would understand the need to do so.

Two awards have been established for young investigators. The Brazier and Cobb Awards, sponsored by Elsevier, were awarded to the best manuscript submitted to the journal in the field of Clinical Neurophysiology in Europe and in the Western Hemisphere, respectively, at the time of the quadrennial International Congress.

The journal had achieved the recognition of citations in Biological Abstracts (BIOSIS), Chemical Abstracts, Index Medicus, Medline, Current Contents Life Science, Current Contents Clinical Medicine, Excerpta Medica (EMBASE), PASCAL M/CNRS, RIS/Reference Update, and Current Awareness in Biological Sciences (CABS). The journal had achieved and maintained the highest scientific impact factor of any journal in field of Clinical Neurophysiology.

2. New member societies

By the end of the previous Fiscal Period the Federation had 47 member societies. There were questions raised about new countries applying to the Federation. The situation of a united Germany presented no problem as the two countries had agreed upon amalgamation and formed one organization. Several other countries applied to the Federation for membership: Cuba, Malaysia, Turkey, Czech Republic, Slovak Republic. The Czech and Slovak applications were favourably reviewed after they were able to notify the Executive Committee in writing that the Czechoslovakian Society of Neurophysiology no longer existed. Turkey was notified that there was already one society recognized in their country and that a second society can apply only if its area of neurophysiologic specialization or membership differs from the other society. In the end the previous Turkish society was found to have dissolved and the new one was recognized as its successor. The Cuban application was slowed by lack of documentation. Questions were raised about the status of the Malaysian society as a formal society or section on Clinical Neurophysiology, since it appeared to be a Neurological Society itself applying for membership. A need for better guidelines for member society admission to the IFCN was noted.

Members-at-Large Jagjit Chopra from India and Jerzy Majkowski from Poland were particularly helpful in resolving various regional problems. Along this line, the Federation remained deeply interested in the activities of the West European Association for Clinical Neurophysiology and the Association of Central and East European Societies for Clinical Neurophysiology. Those autonomous regional organizations nominated François Mauguière and Jerzy Majkowski as secretaries of their respective Liaison Committees, which was very convenient in that both served at that time on the IFCN Executive Committee. These regional organizations were precursors to the eventual European Chapter that became an integral part of the IFCN.

3. Finances

Under the efficient and reliable work of the Treasurer Manuel Meyer the Federation's total income in this 4-year Fiscal Period grew to US $890,000, or 7.5% more than during the previous 4 years. The annual income reached a stable plateau, and it was not predicted to change significantly in the coming few years. Income is based on four sources: Elsevier royalties, member societies' dues, interest on investments, and repayment of loans to congresses.

Total expenses had increased considerably since the previous 4-year Fiscal Period. Support to international congresses increased 23% to US $311,974 in the form of fellowships, grants, loans and contributions to organizations. Loans to the Rio de Janeiro and Jerusalem Congresses were repaid in full. Costs of living and transportation together increased 12% for both the European and American editorial offices and for the Executive Committee functions. A contributing factor to increased Executive Committee costs was the successful broad geographically composition of Executive Committee members, a policy good for the Federation but which increased air travel costs.

The account's balance over the 4-year Fiscal Period shows an overall gain of US $86,592. Part of the gain overall was due to favourable currency exchange rate changes. Total assets had increased to US $545,366 by the end of this 4-year Fiscal Period.

Financially, the IFCN was in good financial condition, certainly far better than during darker financial days in the 1970s. For an international scientific organization this situation was excellent. The accounting was reviewed and approved by Otto Sprecher in Zurich, an outside auditor retained by the Federation for this purpose.

4. Secretary

Federation Secretary Barry R. Tharp communicated on a regular basis with the Delegates and member societies and responded to all inquiries of the Federation. The Secretary organized the business meetings of the Council and the General Assembly. His duties included keeping the minutes for the meetings of the Executive Committee, Editorial Board, Congress Organizing Committee, Council and General Assembly, and distributing minutes to the Council Delegates. The secretarial office prepared 22 issues of the Federation's Yellow Pages information section camera ready for publication in the EEG Journal, listing notices of meetings and information about Member Society and Federation activities. The Secretary organized the presentations of societies seeking to host the next International Congresses both for the EEG and EMG series. He kept the Federation Statutes and Bye-laws updated with assistance from former EMG Commissioner Stéphane Métral of France who prepared the French version.

At the Secretarial Report at the Vancouver Congress, Barry Tharp made some suggestions that arose from his experience during his Secretariat. His proposals concerned the accountability and transparency of the Treasurer's activity, the election process of the Federation's officers, the number of votes in relation to the size of the Member Societies, and the geographical distribution of the Executive Committee members. These items were discussed at the Vancouver General Assembly and the subsequent new Executive and Rules Committees, leading to a series of amendments to the Statutes and Bye-Laws.

5. Rules committee

Several sets of rule changes were discussed and approved during this 4-year Fiscal Period. The rule changes were initiated by the Executive and Rules Committees and by the General Assembly. The Rules Committee carefully considered the proposals in relation to the existing statutes and Bye-Laws. The Executive Committee approved the changes and forwarded it on the agenda of the Council and General Assembly of the Vancouver Congress.

The Rules Committee members in this term were Marc Nuwer (USA, Chairman), Jasper Daube (USA), Carl H. Lücking (Germany), Teresa Sagalés (Spain), Minoru Shimokochi (Japan).

Rule changes below show new text as **bold** and removed text in strike-through.

5.1. Conflict between the Statutes and Bye-Laws concerning two Editors-in-Chief

A Statute change was needed to allow for two Editors-in-Chief. At the Rio de Janeiro IFCN meeting, Bye-Laws were amended to allow two Editors-in-Chief instead of just one. The Rules Committee was charged with drafting Statute changes to refer to the Editors-in-Chief in the plural number. The following rule changes were approved.

> *Statute VI.1.* The Federation is administered by an Executive Committee composed of the President, the immediate Past President, the Secretary and the Treasurer of the Federation, ~~the Editor~~ **the two Editors** in Chief of the EEG Journal, ~~or his deputy,~~ the ~~Chairman~~ **Chairmen** of Special Commissions and two additional members-at-large.

Bye-Laws: Executive Committee

1. (Stat. VI.1) The representatives of the EEG Journal are normally the Editors-in-Chief. If ~~this post~~ **these posts** should be ~~in abeyance~~ **vacant**, one of the other Editors, nominated by the Executive Committee, shall represent the Journal.

5.2. Potential lack of turnover on the Executive Committee

At the time of quadrennial elections, as few as two new persons might be seated on the new eight members of the Executive Committee. Encouraging greater turnover seems appropriate. Currently contributing to the lack of turnover is a rule that the Secretary and Treasurer both may be re-elected once. The Rules Committee suggested preventing simultaneous re-election of both the Secretary and Treasurer. One easy way to do so is to allow the Secretary to serve only one term. The following rule changes were approved.

> *Statute VII. 3.* The President, Secretary, and Treasurer of the Federation, the members of Special Commissions and the Members-at-Large of the Executive Committee are elected by the Council from the nominees of the nomination committee. Their term of office is the Fiscal Period. The President, **Secretary**, Chairman of Special Committees and Members-at-Large may serve only one term in office. The ~~Secretary and the~~ Treasurer ~~are~~ is eligible for re-election once only.

5.3. Term of office for Editor-in-Chief

The unelected status of the two Editors-in-Chief contributed to lack of Executive Committee turnover, more so once the number of Editors-in-Chief was increased from one to two. In addition, there was no clear term of office for the Editors-in-Chief. Suggested solutions included specifying a term of office for each Editor-in-Chief, or allowing each new Executive Committee to re-appoint each Editor-in-Chief. The total tenure of an Editor-in-Chief could also be limited, for example, to 8 years maximum. This would have been consistent with the practice for some other journals. The current Statutes do give the Executive Committee the power to set Bye-Laws to govern the appointment of the EEG Journal Editorial Staff. A new rule was proposed and approved:

> *Statute VII. 4.* The Editorial Staff of the EEG Journal is appointed, **reappointed, or removed** by the Executive Committee. **Each Editor-in-Chief's term of office is 8 years. An Editor-in-Chief cannot be reappointed. An Editor-in-Chief cannot vote on his or her own tenure or termination of appointment and should not be present when these are discussed and put to a vote. The Executive Committee may establish policies and procedures for removal from office of Editors-in-Chief or other members of the Editorial Staff**.

5.4. Organization of a congress

There had been no Bye-Laws section about the Organization Committee of the International Congress (OCIC) panels and their work. Guidelines helped each new OCIC to standardize some aspects of each congress. These were prompted by organizational and financial problems encountered in some past congresses. A new Bye-Law about organizing a congress was adopted:

5.4.1. Bye-Laws — Organization of a congress

1. **The OCIC, constituted as indicated in Statute XII, shall have responsibility to organize all aspects of the International Congress. A budget shall be created consistent with standard accounting practices and appropriate fiscal assumptions. Responsibility for any net financial deficit of the congress shall be decided explicitly at least 2 years prior to the congress. Fiscally responsible organizations shall be presented with accounting reports and budget estimates at least twice each year through the time of the congress.**
2. **The OCIC will set aside program time for three honorary lectures, named the Berger, Adrian and Kugelberg Lectures. The OCIC will invite distinguished speakers to present these lectures.**
3. **The OCIC will budget to set aside as uncommitted funds 15% of the congress registration fee from all active members of constituent societies excluding junior members. If the congress runs a budget deficit, these uncommitted funds will be used to cover the deficit. If uncommitted funds still remain or if the congress has a net profit, these uncommitted funds will be transferred to the IFCN to defray costs of a fellowship program to help young physicians attend congresses.**

5.5. Journal Bye-Law changes

At several points Bye-Laws on the *Journal* needed clarification. These were developed following the rules adopted in Rio de Janeiro in 1990 appointing both Editors-in-Chief to the Federation Executive Committee. The rules adopted in Vancouver specify that the Executive Committee constitutes the Board overseeing the Journal's business aspects. That Editorial Board advised the Editors-in-Chief on matters of general policy but leaves the day-to-day, scientific, and editorial responsibilities for the journal entirely to the Editors-in-Chief or to the publishers. Consulting Editor appointments must be based on merit and service. This was meant to discourage purely honorary or courtesy appointments. The Editors-in-Chief are in the best position to nominate Consulting Editors because they are familiar with current Consulting Editors' and ad hoc reviewers' timeliness and content of reviews. The following amendments were adopted:

5.5.1. Bye-Laws, Journal

1. The Executive Committee ~~and the present Editors of the Journal~~ constitute**s** the Editorial Board of the Journal.
2. The Editorial Board appoints the Editors, assign to them their functions and defines their relationship. It appoints the Consulting Editors **from nominees submitted by the Editors-in-Chief based upon scientific merit and willingness to serve. Except for the Editors-in-Chief,** all these appointments may be for an indefinite period. **All these appointments** may be subject to review at any time and shall not be terminated by the end of the Fiscal Period.
3. The Editorial Board advises the Editors-**in-Chief** on matters of general policy and arbitrates on matters referred to it by the Editors-**in-Chief**, but leaves the day to day conduct of, and responsibility for, the Journal entirely to the Editors-**in-Chief** in conjunction with the publishers.

6. Ceremonial gavel

On the occasion of the OCIC meeting in Kyoto, July 1993, John Desmedt (Past President) and Carl Lücking (President elect) strolled through Kyoto to be looking for a "symbol of power" for the IFCN President (Appendix 11, Fig. 3). In a small antique shop near Kiyomizu Temple they found something resembling the most a sceptre or a gavel. They were told that this wooden piece was called "Nyoi-bo" which contains some magic power (Appendix 11, Fig. 4). At a later time, Hiroshi Shibasaki found out the legend of Nyoi-bo: it was used by an ape warrior called Songoku when he helped a Chinese priest called Sanzo-Hoshi going all the way from China to India to obtain the Buddhist Bible. During the journey the monkey was able to accomplish, by using the Nyoi-bo, all kinds of miracles to protect the priest. This is all based on a novel called Saiyuhki written in ancient China. Thus Noyi-bo is not exactly the same as either a sceptre or a gavel but it may be more or less like a magic bar with which one can do anything what one likes to do.

The Nyoi-bo was handed over to the President Jun Kimura during the OCIC session in Kyoto. The intention was that this instrument will serve for that point forward as the ceremonial gavel to be handed from president to the next president. Given its tradition, it also serves as a sign of hope that the president and the Federation will achieve its goal during each term. At the General Assembly in Vancouver, September 1993, it was presented for the first time as a ceremonial gavel to the incoming Federation President Carl Lücking with an expressed hope that the Nyoi-bo brings the new Executive Committee team success in the coming 4 years in what they wish to accomplish for the cause of IFCN.

Each succeeding President has received the Nyoi-bo from the outgoing President at the end of the quadrennial General Assembly as a ceremonial token of their authority in office and wish for good fortune throughout their term of office.

7. Regional meetings

The IFCN granted fellowships and support not only for the International Congresses but also for certain regional meetings. In the days before formal Chapter Congresses, these served the

Federation's goal of bringing education and science to the clinical neurophysiology audience where it was needed. It also served to advance the practice of the field in these areas, and to give support to newly established member societies.

The procedure for selecting the recipients of fellowships was similar to International Congresses. Each Member Society was asked to submit, with a priority ranking, a list of candidates (less than 40 years old and having a paper submitted to the Congress) with a brief CV. The final choice for regional meetings was made with due consideration of all factors involved by the Liaison Officers appointed by the IFCN (François Mauguière or Jerzy Majkowski). Initially 20 fellowships of US $400 each were provided. Since the 1992 European Congress in Lisbon, the number of fellowships was increased to 30 at US $400 each. These were granted to promote Clinical Neurophysiology in Europe as well as to effect cooperation between national and regional societies and the IFCN. Comparable efforts have been done by IFCN through Fellowship programs in conjunction with regional meetings outside of Europe such as the Bangkok, Bali, and Beijing Regional Symposia of the preceding Fiscal Period.

In general, fellowships would be considered for regional meetings involving more than one country. As the IFCN support should be available for future congresses, the Executive Committee discussed in 1991 some type of financial remuneration from the congresses and decided that congresses which want their meeting to be held under the auspices of IFCN pay US $1000 or 10% of the profits, whichever is larger, to the IFCN. If requested, IFCN would provide a US $10,000 loan to the Organizing Committee of a regional meeting that would be reimbursed if a meeting profit was attained.

7.1. V. European Congress of Clinical Neurophysiology (ECCN)

The V ECCN was organized under the auspices of all the European National Societies of Clinical Neurophysiology and held under the Presidency of Stéphane Métral in Paris, France, on September 9–12, 1990. The site was the Centre International de Conférences in the Cité des Sciences et de l'Industrie de la Vilette. IFCN provided 20 fellowships granted to young investigators. A Liaison Committee, whose Secretary was François Mauguière, brought together the delegates of each of the Western European societies for clinical neurophysiology. This was established and met during the Congress to discuss several issues. Jerzy Majkowski had been invited as an observer to represent the Eastern European Societies for CN. The Liaison Committee decided to hold ECCN every 2 years in even years to avoid the uneven years used by IFCN congresses. The next ECCN was scheduled for Lisbon, Portugal in September 1992.

7.2. XV. Congress of Eastern European Societies for Clinical Neurophysiology

The East-Central Association of European Societies organized this Congress. The Secretary for that association was Jerzy Majkowski. The Bulgarian Society organized this congress, which was held in Varna, Bulgaria, in October 1991. Twenty fellowships were granted by IFCN to young investigators. This was part of a series of such Congresses held in the Eastern Europe.

7.3. VI. European Congress on Clinical Neurophysiology (ECCN)

The VI ECCN was held in Lisbon, Portugal, in September 19–22, 1992, and followed by the "First Advanced Course on CN" from September 23 to 24. The Congress was organized under the auspices of the IFCN and promoted by the Portuguese Association of EEG and Clinical Neurophysiology. F. Lopes da Silva, who was born in Lisbon, was appointed Honorary President and gave the Egaz Moniz Lecture on basic mechanisms of epilepsy from neuronal membranes to neural networks. The Scientific Committee consisted of delegates of nearly all National Societies of East and Western Europe. The Advanced course was chaired by F. Mauguière and A. Martins da Silva. It was an excellent meeting on the scientific level and remarkable for the social events with a Welcome Reception at the Castel S. Jorge from the VIII century and the Farewell Party at a farm north of Lisbon, in the bull breeding area of Ribatejo. The IFCN provided 30 fellowship grants at US $400 each to allow young investigators to attend and present their scientific reports.

7.4. 2nd Bangkok Symposium on Clinical Neurophysiology

The 2nd Bangkok Symposium was organized in March 1993. IFCN provided 20 fellowships of US $400 each to help young physicians in the Asian region to attend. The meeting was organized by the Thailand society and involved many clinical neurophysiologists from Asian countries. This was another step toward bringing the Asian societies together in what eventually became an IFCN Chapter.

7.5. XVI. Congress of Eastern European Societies for Clinical Neurophysiology

The East-Central Association of European Societies and the Polish Society of Clinical Neurophysiology organized this XVI Congress of Eastern European Societies for Clinical Neurophysiology. The meeting was held in Poland on June 3–5, 1993. Initially no fellowships were required for this meeting. But as the Executive Committee had decided to support this meeting as any other regional meeting, seven fellowships of US $400 were provided retroactively to young scientists who had attended the meeting.

In the previous year, the Eastern and Central European clinical neurophysiologists and delegates of their societies attended the ECCN in Portugal. The political need had disappeared for two parallel clinical neurophysiology meetings. Soon after this Congress, the Eastern–Central Congress series was disbanded. Thereafter all European clinical neurophysiologists attended the ECCN series together.

8. International congresses

8.1. IX. International Congress of EMG and Clinical Neurophysiology, Jerusalem 1992

This Jerusalem Congress was among the most challenging to prepare. World politics deteriorated shortly before the scheduled Jerusalem Congress dates of June 1991. Tensions in the Near East worsened and in February and March 1991 war broke out in Kuwait and Iraq. Israel found itself under air attack. Once the ground war started, the war was apparently over quickly. A truce was declared, but public opinion still was concerned about war or further provocative actions against Israel. On many occasions, the OCIC considered and reconsidered its options. In that OCIC, IFCN Executive Committee members J. Kimura, J.E. Desmedt, B. Tharp, and M. Meyer represented the Federation and A. Gilai, P. Solzi and M. Rabey represented the Israel Society of Clinical Neurophysiology. The discussions remained always congenial, but this OCIC found it difficult to make final decisions. Some members insisted on holding the meeting in June as scheduled in Jerusalem, whereas the IFCN representatives preferred to cancel the Congress out right without taking a calculated risk. Majority votes were deeply split. Council Delegates were polled, and again there was no clear consensus. The best choices seemed be either cancellation or postponement. In the end, President J. Kimura recommended to postpone the meeting to a time substantially later than the originally planned dates. The rest of the OCIC agreed to this compromise.

When the Congress eventually took place in the following year in 1992 the organizers welcomed over 500 physicians and scientists as well as guests from all corners of the world. This attendance was much more than originally anticipated. The Federation provided 42 fellowships at US $600 each to support the attendance of young investigators. Despite a smaller number of participation than the typical EMG Congress, the meeting had remarkably strong scientific and social programs. The major items included the second Honorary Kugelberg Lecture delivered by Arthur K. Asbury on "Polyneuropathies at the Millennium" and the second Honorary Adrian Lecture delivered by John Newsom-Davis on "New Concepts in Neuromuscular Disorders". The registrants at the Congress provided excellent feedback about high scientific quality of the meeting. The Congress was accompanied by a satellite symposium on Magnetic Stimulation, organized by Kerry Mills (UK) just after the main congress itself.

Financially, the Jerusalem Congress's financial operations were well in control and the organization was able to repay the Federation's loans. Under the particularly difficult circumstance in the shadow of a war, and in fact under any circumstances, the Congress was considered a great success.

8.2. XIII. International Congress of EEG and Clinical Neurophysiology, Vancouver, BC, September 1993

This EEG Congress was held in Vancouver, British Columbia, Canada, from August 30 through September 5, 1993. It was held under the auspices of three host societies, the Canadian Society of Clinical Neurophysiologists, American Association of Electrodiagnostic Medicine, and American Electroencephalographic Society. The OCIC included IFCN members Jun Kimura (President), John Desmedt (Past President), Barry Tharp (Secretary), Manuel Meyer (Treasurer), and from the host societies Juhn Wada (Convener), Andrew Eisen (Secretary), Mark Hallett (Treasurer). See Appendix 11, Figs. 5 and 6. The OCIC hired a professional congress organizer firm, Venue West. The Congress was held just before the World Congress of Neurology in the same Vancouver Convention Hall. That site was located on the harbour with striking views of the inlet, Lyons Gate Bridge, and surrounding mountains.

Andrew Eisen, who lived in Vancouver, handled much of the difficult and often controversial issues with finesse. The effect of a depressed worldwide economy may have hurt attendance. A number of IFCN member societies were unable to send representatives because of the cost, the economy, and the distance to Vancouver. The IFCN provided 100 fellowships for young investigators. In all, 969 delegates registered for the meeting.

The congress site was the Vancouver Trade and Convention Centre. Honorary Presidents were Edward Lambert, Herbert Jasper, Peter Kellaway, Irena Hausmanova-Petrusewicz (see Appendix 11, Figs. 8 and 9). The scientific programme included 15 Plenary Sessions, 16 Hands-on Workshops, 12 Video Demonstrations, 60 Poster-Sessions of nearly 600 posters. The program was highlighted by three well received special contributions: the third Adrian Lecture was presented by John Desmedt (Belgium) on "Somatic Sensation and Its Disorders: Evoked Potential Evidence". Edward Lambert (USA) was selected to give the third Kugelberg Lecture on "Disorders of Neuromuscular Junction". Pierre Gloor (Canada) presented the third Honorary Lecture, the Berger Lecture, on the question, "Is Berger's Dream Coming True?" Abstracts of the plenary sessions, video presentations, and posters were published in a supplement of *Electroencephalography and Clinical Neurophysiology*, Number 2, August 1993.

The Opening Ceremony took place at the historic, beautifully restored Orpheum Theatre. The audience had been most eagerly awaiting the President. But Jun Kimura's flight from Japan was badly delayed so that a limousine was sent to pick him and his wife Junko up at the airport. He came straight to the "Opening" in a T-shirt and jeans! (See Appendix 11, Figs.5 and 6.) He led the audience in remarking in amusement about that attire and the need to be a patent traveller.

The highlight of the social program was the "British Columbia Night", an exciting entertainment event that offered Canadian West Coast showmanship and hospitality (see Appendix 11, Fig. 7). In a ladies' competition of hitting nails into a wooden plate, Merula Lücking, wife of the new IFCN President, was the winner and declared as "Miss Nail" and awarded a carved squirrel.

Despite the worldwide economic problems, IFCN was very fortunate to have a very successful congress both from scientific and social points of view. The Congress employed a professional congress organizer firm, Venue West. That relationship with a professional organization to help with the organizational details proved very positive. The experience of professionals in congress organizing was very helpful and this provided a way to accommodate the great amount of time and effort necessary to mind the details and budget. That firm, Venue West, would come back into the history of the IFCN later when they also assumed the role of executive administrative office for the IFCN in late 2006. The later administrative office choice was influenced by the positive experience with the firm helping to run this congress. This experience also encouraged a desire that future congresses should also use an experienced professional congress organizer firm to help with management details.

8.3. Vancouver General Assembly Report of the President

In his report Jun Kimura noted that he was the first President from Asia and the first President of the Federation under its new name *International Federation of Clinical Neurophysiology* that had been in use since the 1990 Rio de Janeiro General Assembly. The new name acknowledged the equal importance of EEG and EMG and unified clinical electrophysiology without clear division into multiple disciplines. The President underlined difficulties as well as success in organizing the IFCN Congresses of Jerusalem and Vancouver. He also acknowledged the responsible, dedicated work carried out by retiring Executive Committee officers, Barry Tharp, Manuel Meyer, Jagjit Chopra, and Jerzy Majkowski. He especially mentioned the contribution of John Desmedt, outgoing Past President, who served with distinction during this and previous fiscal periods, initially as the Chairman of the EMG Commission and later as President. He is one of the very few to have accomplished so much in improving the status of clinical neurophysiology in general and the image of the International Federation in particular. The President then continued:

> "These have been exciting four years with some unexpected problems, which we have jointly overcome and some pleasant surprises that we have enjoyed together. The system, which I witnessed over the past four years, worked very well. It was empirical and eminently efficient, providing perhaps the most practical way the Executive Committee could manage to serve its purpose. In this rapidly evolving world, however, it seems necessary to modify our operation to adapt to the emerging new expectations. We need to clarify our objectives and encourage active participation from all member societies, large or small, with different needs and problems to reflect their vision, their insight and their ideals. The Federation is a very delicate instrument with contributions from many national societies, having different priorities and preferences in regard to science in political systems. Thus, in the operation of the organization, nothing should be taken as granted. For example, those of us who speak English as their mother tongue or use it almost as the first language, as I do, must recognize how disadvantaged many delegates are who speak other languages. We must overcome national and individual differences in the interest of unity which is imperative if we are to succeed in strengthening the status of clinical neurophysiology as the unique discipline bridging the basic science and clinical medicine. We live in changing times, and the Federation is no exception."

At the end of the General Assembly the President handed the new Ceremonial Gavel, the Nyoi-bo, to the new President Carl Lücking wishing him and the new Executive Committee that the Nyoi-bo would bring the new team what they wish to accomplish for the cause of IFCN.

8.4. Vancouver General Assembly Report of the Secretary

In addition to the rule changes brought to the floor by the Rules Committee, Federation outgoing Secretary Barry Tharp presented to the General Assembly two groups of suggestions for new or future rules. The first suggestions sought to improve financial accountability. These included:

1. The Treasurer should prepare detailed accounting of costs. This should be available to the Executive Committee and to any member society requesting it.
   (a) This should include expenses for each person for each Executive Committee and Congress Organizing Committee meeting. Persons should provide receipts for their expenses.
   (b) This should include all expenses incurred by Executive Committee members outside of regular meetings, that is, to run Federation business in their offices.
2. The Executive Committee must approve of disbursements in excess of US $300.

Dr. Tharp also brought to the General Assembly suggestions for improvements in the process of electing Executive Committee members. These included:

1. The Executive Committee should monitor the election process. The Nominating Committee chairman should report to the Executive Committee about which societies voted and efforts to contact societies who failed to submit a ballot. No late ballots should be counted. Only written ballots should be accepted. Nominees must agree to have their name on the ballot. Campaigning by the Nominating Committee members is against Federation rules and Delegates should report to the Executive Committee any violations. Campaigning includes any contact with a Delegate for the purpose of influencing a vote.
2. If no candidate receives a majority, a run-off election should be held of the top two or three candidates.
3. The Federation should allow societies to cast the same number of votes in elections as the society they were entitled to in the General Assembly.
4. Additional geographical restrictions should be developed. If the president was from one region, for example Europe, the secretary and the treasurer should be from other regions.
5. No one should serve more than 8 years on the Executive Committee, as chairperson of a commission, or as editor of the journal. This would allow a healthy turnover of leadership.

To follow up on those suggestions, the General Assembly members brought forth several motions that were debated and accepted in near-unanimous votes. These Vancouver General Assembly resolutions were:

1. A more detailed and complete accounting of all expenses of the Federation should be provided to every delegate at least 3 months prior to every IFCN Congress. All records of expenditures should be open to delegate inspection upon request.
2. The Executive Committee should develop specific rules for justification of expenditures. The General Assembly rejects the budget presented at this meeting. A detailed budget for the next 2 years must be prepared immediately by the new Executive Committee and be made available to each Delegate within 2 months. In the future, the detailed Federation Fiscal Period budget proposal must be made available to the Delegates at least 3 months prior to each IFCN Congress.
3. The Rules Committee develops amendments to the Statutes that societies have as many votes in the Executive Committee elections be as they do for votes in the General Assembly. Votes would be allotted on the basis of the size of the society.
4. The Rules Committee re-evaluates the entire voting process of the Federation with respect to the issues raised in the Secretary's report and make specific recommendations for changes in the official voting rules and

regulations within the next 6 months. Furthermore, these recommended changes should be distributed to all delegates as soon as they are completed and that General Assembly vote by mail 3 months later. The issues of concern included, but were not limited to, weighing of votes by the size of societies, balancing the geographic and disciplinary considerations, that electioneering is not acceptable and that this point should be disseminated with information sent with the ballot, the relationship of Executive Committee to the Nominating Committee be reviewed and clarified, and whether Executive Committee members could vote in General Elections.

5. Council and General Assembly meetings will be held in 2 years at the Kyoto International EMG and Clinical Neurophysiology Congress.
6. The Rules Committee is instructed to develop a statute that no individual can serve on Executive Committee for more than 12 years, except that this should not preclude the Editor or any other appropriate individual from becoming President of the Federation.
7. The General Assembly in Kyoto should decide the venue of the subsequent EMG Congress.

8.5. Site of the next IFCN Congress in 1997

Ten member societies presented invitations to host the next Congress that was scheduled for 1997. Many had booths in the Congress area during the duration of the congress to encourage support for their city's bid and to allow delegates and others to ask questions about the bids and cities. This encouraged a great deal of discussion during the Congress about the choice for the next site. The General Assembly meeting was held toward the end of the overall Congress session, leading to a great deal of suspense over which national society and city would win the balloting. The invitations, presented in alphabetical order along with their presenters, included Argentina (M. Turner), Australia (R. Mackenzie), Austria (H. Lechner), Chile (N. Chiofalo), Germany (H.J. Heinze), Hungary (I. Szirmai), India (J. Chopra), Israel (A. Gilai), Italy (G. Comi) and Thailand (P. Boongird). After several rounds of secret ballots, the list was reduced to Australia and Italy. The final secret ballot tally was Italy 39 and Australia 38, which was recounted several times to assure that the total was reported correctly. The next International Congress was therefore set for Florence, Italy in 1997. The winning delegation expressed a great deal of spontaneous enthusiasm in the General Assembly meeting and wished everyone a great welcome in advance to attend the 1997 Congress.

9. Nomination Committee

The Nomination Committee in this term was composed of J.E. Desmedt (Belgium, Chairman), Nelly Chiofalo (Chile), Pierre Guiheneuc (France), and Nobuo Yanagisawa (Japan). The committee conducted the 1993 elections for President, Secretary, Treasurer and two Members-at-Large. As decided by the 1985 London General Assembly, all persons nominated by Delegates were listed on the election ballot if they accepted to run. The nominees were required to be an individual member of a Federation Member Society. Only the Secretary and Treasurer could be re-elected for a second term. In this case, the Treasurer was in his second term, and therefore he was ineligible for re-election.

No geographical restrictions were applied to nominees for the two Members-at-Large positions. Allowed nominees were from geographical areas not yet represented on the new Executive Committee officers. The definition of geographical zones to be excluded was defined until after having carrying out elections for the new President, Treasurer and Secretary.

Bye-Laws require disciplinary balance between nominees. The nominees for Secretary must be of the opposite EEG or EMG discipline than that of the just-elected Treasurer. The two Members-at-Large had to be from opposite disciplines. This latter was implemented by having two positions, one for an EEG Member-at-Large and one for an EMG Member-at-Large.

The election was held in three stages. A majority was required to win a position, and otherwise a run-off round was scheduled. The correspondence about the election process and the ballots were sent by mail to the 55 members of the IFCN Council, that is the Delegates of the 47 affiliated societies and the eight members of the current IFCN Executive Committee.

In the first round of balloting, eight persons were nominated for the President position, two of whom declined to run. Three persons were nominated for the Treasurer position. Forty-eight ballots were returned so that the absolute majority was 25. Carl Lücking received a clear majority for President and Paul Despland for Treasurer without requiring a run-off. In the second round of balloting, seven persons were nominated Secretary, among whom one declined to run. Forty-eight ballots were returned so that the absolute majority was 25. Giuseppe Caruso received a clear majority on the first ballot.

In the third election round, the geographic restrictions were used. Since the three recently elected officers were from European countries (Germany, Switzerland, and Italy), it was simple to define the "as yet unrepresented geographical areas" by merely excluding nominees from Europe for Member-at-Large positions. One person was nominated for EEG Member-at-Large and two for EMG Members-at-Large. All accepted to run. Fifty-two ballots were returned so that a majority required 27. Marc Nuwer (USA) received unanimous votes for EEG Member-at-Large, and Xiao-Fu Tang (China) received a clear majority for EMG Member-at-Large.

The identity of the person signing ballots on behalf of any affiliated society was ascertained throughout. Postal addresses were checked and updated. The number of ballots returned was greater than in the 1989 election (48 instead of 45 for the President–Treasurer election; 48 instead of 33 for the Secretary election; 52 instead of 37 for the Members-at-Large election). Several members of the Nomination Committee recounted the ballots.

The Executive Committee for the next term also will include Past-President Jun Kimura and Editors-in-Chief François Mauguière and Gastone G. Celesia. The Executive Committee for the 1993–1997 Fiscal Period will consist of:

President	Carl H. Lücking	EMG	Region 2	Germany
Past President	Jun Kimura	EMG	Region 1	Japan
Secretary	Giuseppe Caruso	EMG	Region 2	Italy
Treasurer	Paul A. Despland	EEG	Region 2	Switzerland
Member-at-Large	Marc Nuwer	EEG	Region 1	USA
Member-at-Large	Xiao-Fu Tang	EMG	Region 2	China
Editor-in-Chief	Gastone G. Celesia	EEG	Region 1	USA
Editor-in-Chief	François Mauguière	EEG	Region 2	France

Wave Length and Action Potentials: History of the IFCN
(Supplements to Clinical Neurophysiology, Vol. 61)
By: M.R. Nuwer and C.H. Lücking

Chapter 13

1993–1997

President: Carl Lücking

In this term, the Executive Committee (ExCo) consisted of Carl Lücking (President), Jun Kimura (Past President), Giuseppe Caruso (Secretary), Paul Despland (Treasurer), Xiao-Fu Tang and Marc Nuwer (Members-at-Large), and Gastone Celesia and François Mauguière (Editors-in-Chief). The initial and primary activities were to implement the urgent motions made by the General Assembly at the Vancouver XIII ICEEGCN in 1993. These included transparency of the fiscal policy, detailed budgeting, re-evaluation of the Federation voting process, and eligibility and time limitation for ExCo membership.

1. New policies

At the first ExCo meeting in Vancouver in 1993, the President declared to follow a fully democratic policy taking account of the views of the ExCo and IFCN members without pursuing personal interest. The Committee decided to increase the openness and accountability as well as the efficiency of the organizational structure of IFCN (Table 13.1). The Delegates should be informed on a regular basis about the decisions of the ExCo, the development of new rules, and the budget and spending situation. The minutes of ExCo meetings should be distributed as they are to the Delegates and regularly published as report in the Yellow Pages of the journal. In addition, the Statutes of IFCN, minutes of the General Assembly and reports of the President, Secretary, Treasurer, Editors-in-Chief, and the Nomination Committee will be published in the Journal.

The requests of the Vancouver General Assembly were accomplished in the 2 years of this Fiscal Period. Regarding financial issues, the IFCN budget was submitted for approval to national Delegates ahead of each General Assembly. All expenses were registered in an accounting book that was made available for inspection by the Delegates. Two Delegates were chosen by Council as auditors to examine the accounting books in detail, give advice, help to decide on future expenses, and report back to Council independently of the ExCo. A goal was established to set aside an amount of US $1 million that would allow the IFCN to continue to function using the interest without touching the capital. This would cushion the Federation in case of a financial disaster at an International Congress. Guidelines for the ExCo members' expenses were developed.

New rules elaborated the voting process, eligibility of officers, and geographical balance (Statutes and Bye-Laws). It is unacceptable for Nominating Committee members to contacting Delegates to campaign for particular candidates in ExCo elections. The nomination should reflect the view of the member societies.

Each year some member societies, especially from Eastern Europe and the Middle East, do not pay their annual dues. The ExCo decided not to propose to expel these societies, which would have been allowed according to the Statutes. Those societies would remain as inactive

TABLE 13.1

INTERNATIONAL FEDERATION OF CLINICAL NEUROPHYSIOLOGY POLICY FOR EXECUTIVE COMMITTEE (ExCo) EXPENSES AND ACCOUNTING

1. Office expenses

1.1. *ExCo officers*: Officers of the IFCN are entitled to reasonable reimbursement for secretarial and transcription services as well as the costs of telephones, faxing, copying and mailing. For the Treasurer, reimbursement includes the costs of auditing, accounting and other external financial services. Officers do not receive personal stipends. Each officer should be allotted a set annual budgeted allocation for these services and should be expected to provide the IFCN with appropriate accounting for disbursement of these funds at the end of each year. Suggested 1994–1995 annual budget allotments are:

President	US $10,000
Past President	US $ 3,000
Secretary	US $10,000
Treasurer	US $ 7,000

1.2. *Editors-in-Chief*: Editors-in-Chief receive reimbursement for the costs of secretarial and transcription services, phones, faxing, copying and mailing. Costs of travel related to the Journal and ExCo also come from this allotment, including costs of travel to meetings with Elsevier. There is no additional allotment for the cost of holding meetings with the consulting editors. The 1994–1997 annual recommended allotment for each Editor-in-Chief is:

Editor-in-Chief, each	US $30,000

1.3. *ExCo Members-at-Large* may be reimbursed for specific expenses incurred on behalf of ExCo and IFCN in carrying out their respective duties. Members-at-Large are not entitled to an automatic allocation at the start of each annual budget year, but rather would be reimbursed upon presentation of receipts and suitable documentation when expenses have been authorized by ExCo.

1.4. *Officers or Editors-in-Chief* who leave office during a budget year will receive a suitably prorated portion of the annual office payment. Any overpayment will be returned to the IFCN.

2. Meeting expenditures

2.1. *ExCo members* are entitled to reimbursement for the direct costs of travel to ExCo meetings, OCIC Meetings and IFCN Congresses. Travel expenses for Editors-in-Chief have to come out of their annual office expense.

2.2. *Airfare* is reimbursed at coach class except for intercontinental flights, which are reimbursed at business class. Travellers are asked to obtain the best value for airfare. Extra hotel nights may be authorized by the IFCN Treasurer in order to qualify for minimum stay requirements, but only if the total IFCN cost is less for the longer stay compared with the shorter stay. Train travel is also permitted. Before authorizing extra hotel nights to obtain a lower overall IFCN cost, the Treasurer must receive a detailed breakdown of the projected costs for both the shorter and the longer stay. Members must try to obtain the best prices for travel.

2.3. *Additional ground transportation* by taxi, or equivalent, is reimbursable. Request for reimbursement for taxi fare of US $25, or more, should be accompanied by a receipt.

2.4. *Hotel costs* for room, tax and costs for meals are reimbursable up to an amount considered usual and customary for business travel at that location. ExCo members arriving after an intercontinental flight may arrive 1 day early to adjust to time changes. Additional costs of an accompanying spouse are not reimbursable. When it is needed as a room for committee meetings, the IFCN President may arrange for a suite.

2.5. *The costs of hotel incidentals* and entertainment are not reimbursable. IFCN will reimburse the costs of a speaker phone or conference calls placed during ExCo meetings itself. The cost of one brief telephone call or one fax are reimbursable once per day, for example to reconfirm travel reservations.

2.6. *For an ExCo or ICOC meeting* occurring at an international, national, or regional meeting, reimbursement is limited to the transportation and other costs for the day(s) of the ExCo meeting (cf. Sections 2.1–2.5). Registration fees for a meeting are not reimbursed by IFCN.

3. Accounting

3.1. Members are expected to submit copies of receipts along with a summary of expenses. The IFCN Treasurer will keep these on file until 1 year after the close of the IFCN Fiscal Period. Items less than US $25 do not need to be accompanied by a receipt, but must be identified regarding the nature, date and purpose of the expense.
3.2. Annual payments for office expenditures for officers and Editors-in-Chief can be made at the beginning of each budget year in amounts specified above in Sections 1.1 and 1.2. Each officer and Editor-in-Chief must submit suitable accounting at the end of each year, identifying in detail the manner in which these funds were spent.
3.3. IFCN does not reimburse for items which are not identified, such as "miscellaneous" or "other" items not further identified.
3.4. Accounting for IFCN ExCo expenses must be carried out in a manner consistent with standard business practices with suitable receipts amenable to auditing and appropriate justifications for each expenditure.
3.5. The IFCN Treasurer is charged with assuring that all accounting and expenditures are conducted in a manner consistent with the IFCN policies and standard business practices.
3.6. An accounting report should be prepared annually by the Treasurer for presentation to ExCo. This accounting report should be mailed to IFCN Delegates. The report should break down categories of expenses into their details.
3.7. An audit of the IFCN accounting and funds should be conducted at least once every 4-year Fiscal Period (cf. IFCN Statute XV, Section 7).

4. Other policies

4.1. The ExCo needs to establish the time period for the 12-month budget years of IFCN. When a 4-year Fiscal Period is significantly longer or shorter than 48 months, suitable adjustments need to be made in the duration of the annual budget year. In the cases of shortened or lengthened budget years, suitable adjustments must be made in the annual amounts allocated to IFCN officers and Editors-in-Chief.
4.2. Although travel expenses are usually reimbursed subsequent to travel or at the conclusion of the ExCo meeting, the Treasurer may make suitable arrangements to pay in advance the cost of travel for ExCo members who require such assistance.
4.3. The Treasurer is authorized to directly pay the hotel for the costs of rooms and meals associated with ExCo Meetings. The costs of telephones, incidentals or entertainment, or additional costs of an accompanying spouse, which are not reimbursable by IFCN, may be: (A) paid directly to the hotel by the member incurring these expenses; or (B) by arrangement with the Treasurer. These costs may be deducted from the amount reimbursed for the member's airfare and other travel expenses.
4.4. The cost of currency exchange, fund transfers, check collections from a foreign bank or applicable taxes may be reimbursed to members at the discretion of the Treasurer and upon presentation of receipts or other suitable documentation.
4.5. The IFCN President is responsible for authorizing routine expenses and reimbursement to the Treasurer, whereas the Treasurer is charged with authorizing routine expenditures to all other ExCo members.

---

members without voting rights, and their members still would be able to receive fellowships and other advantages. The fellowship stipends were fixed at US $600, and authorized for 100 applicants for the International Congresses and 60 for each regional congress.

To foster clinical neurophysiology worldwide, the Members-at-large took over the special task to identify developing countries in which clinical neurophysiology could be established or supported by offering fellowships, books and journals, and invitations to IFCN congresses. The same issue will be pursued by the President in close contact with the Non-governmental Organizations (NGOs) concerned with the prevention and treatment of neurological disorders of the WHO in Geneva. A campaign of the President and Elsevier to gain support from various industrial companies to finance subscription of the EEG Journal for financially weak countries was not successful.

In August 1996, the President sent a letter to all Delegates to inform them about several achievements within the Federation. These included: efforts to establish associations of regional member societies of Asia, Latin America, and Europe in order to found Chapters of the IFCN; financial support and fellowships of US $1000 for young scientists for regional meetings and International Congresses; active participation of ExCo members in regional meetings by organizing the ExCo meeting at the same place; campaign to obtain sponsors from the industrial sector in order to provide the EEG Journal to societies and members who can afford a subscription by their own means; plan to open a home page for the IFCN in the World Wide Web; invitation of the Delegates to send any matters of concern or suggestions which would be discussed by the ExCo and put on the agenda of the Council Meeting or General Assembly beforehand.

2. New member societies

The ExCo decided that a society must number at least three members. To apply for IFCN membership a minimum of 10 members is required. After the reunification of Germany in 1989 the two German societies merged into one. The dissolution of Yugoslavia since 1991 led to independent societies in Slovenia, Croatia and in the Federal Republic of Yugoslavia (Serbia, Montenegro, Vojvodina). Czechoslovakia in 1992 was separated into Czech Republic and Slovakia, each with its own society. In addition to the society of People's Rep. of China, a second Chinese society was established in Taiwan. This was in accordance with IFCN rules which allow the existence of several societies in one country (like in Belgium or USA). Further societies were established in South Korea and Cuba, and they applied for membership. The society in Turkey had become inactive, but in this Fiscal Period it re-emerged and re-activated its membership. The society in India changed from a section of the Neurological Society of India into a section of the Indian Academy of Neurology. The Malaysian Society of Neurosciences investigated application for IFCN membership, although that was not finished until a later Fiscal Period. South Africa withdrew its membership because of the declining number of members due to physician emigration and the political situation in the country. A new society was founded in Egypt that subsequently applied for membership. Egypt would then be the only neurophysiologic society on the African continent.

The new societies, except for Egypt and Malaysia, were approved by the ExCo and the Council at Kyoto in 1995 and in Florence 1997, respectively. By the end of this Fiscal Period, the number of Member Societies had increased from 47 to 51. That number change accounted for six new Societies and two disbanded societies. To handle the politically sensitive issues of nations dividing, the ExCo adopted a policy to recognize a new nation once it was recognized and accepted by the United Nations General Assembly. In that way, the Federation would remain politically neutral and do so by deferring to that worldwide political organization to make decisions about when to recognize a nation.

3. Chapters

A new approach was undertaken to regional clinical neurophysiology organizations. This was accomplished to foster regional meetings and to pursue regional needs such as standardizing neurophysiologic training and practice. First a proposal was made by Latin American societies to establish a "Latin American Association of Clinical Neurophysiology". The European members preferred to found a "European Society of Clinical Neurophysiology" to oversee the already existing biennial European Congress of Clinical Neurophysiology.

Finally it was agreed to initiate IFCN Chapters that would include all member societies of a region. This was a major accomplishment of this

Fiscal Period. The IFCN Chapters were established in three regions: European Chapter, Latin-American Chapter, and Asian Chapter (later Asian-Oceanian Chapter).

One ExCo member serves as liaison to each Chapter. The ExCo appointed Liaison Officers for three regional areas: Marc Nuwer for Latin America, Xiao-Fu Tang for Asia, and Paolo Rossini for Europe. Several initial principles were established. The Federation would give financial support to each Chapter, for example for regional Chapter meetings. Each Chapter would choose its own ExCo. The Chapter chairman would give a regular report to the Federation ExCo. The Chapter Bye-Laws would be a part of Federation Bye-Laws, approved by the IFCN Council upon the recommendation by the Chapter's General Assembly. The Federation Rules Committee would rule on any disagreements between Chapters and the ExCo or among Chapters. Each Chapter's Treasurer would report annual expenses and income to the IFCN Treasurer along with supporting receipts and details, so that this could be included in the Federation's annual financial auditing.

By the end of this Fiscal Period, the European Chapter organizational process was fully functioning and the Asian Chapter organizational process was well advanced. European and Asian Chapter Bye-Laws were presented and approved by Council at the 1997 Florence ICEEGCN. The Latin American chapter continued its organizational stages and its Bye-Laws development.

Several factors motivated the Federation to formalize Chapters. One initial reason was to organize regional meetings. At the beginning of this 4-year fiscal period, the IFCN continued its decade long practice to support regional meetings. The ExCo recognized considerable value in such meetings. Many attendees were young physicians and scientists who did not have the financial resources to travel to the biennial International Congresses. Likewise, many senior members of regional societies were much more easily able to participate and deliver lectures at these regional meetings. Instead of making arrangements to support travel by many hundreds to the international congresses, it was financially more practical to bring excellent lectures and an international faculty to the region. Regional meetings allowed for greater involvement of the national societies in Federation activities. Meetings provided a means for some societies in a region to interact with each other more than had occurred historically. Meetings were an opportunity to approach local public officials to ask for greater resources for the national society, an opportunity that was successful on a number of occasions. Regional meetings provided a process by which additional clinical neurophysiologists from neighbouring nations could participate and discuss opportunities to establish a national society of their own. Overall, bringing some meetings to regions had achieved many goals consistent with the Federation's educational, scientific and organizational mission.

The Federation provided financial support for these regional meetings. The ExCo eventually decided to fund 60 fellowships for young physicians and scientists to attend and present at poster or platform sessions at regional meetings. Furthermore, the ExCo suggested holding its own meetings in association with these regional meetings when possible, so that ExCo members could lecture at the meetings at no cost to the meeting budget. This could reduce the substantial expense ordinarily incurred to bring international lecturers to a symposium. Requests for regional meetings would be considered individually by the ExCo, both for funding and for attendance by the ExCo.

Regional Congresses and Symposia initially arose from the joint requests of several societies in the region, and that must have represented the majority of members in that region. The IFCN ExCo reviewed each request independently. With the creation of Chapters, that responsibility devolved to the region's Chapter. IFCN Statutes require two ExCo members to participate in organizing each meeting along with the local host society and Chapter.

At the 1996 Beijing Symposium on Clinical Neurophysiology, the regional societies accepted the concept, agreed to form a chapter and elected an interim chairman, Xiao-Fu Tang of the People's Rep. of China. She currently sat on the Federation ExCo as a Member-at-Large and was a principal organizer of the 1996 symposium. In retrospect, this meeting was recognized as the First Asian Congress of Clinical Neurophysiology and the first Chapter meeting.

The Latin American Chapter took its first steps in 1995. An organization meeting was held during the Pan American Congress of Neurology in Guatemala City. During a 1-day symposium on Clinical Neurophysiology, the regional societies held a business meeting. The societies agreed in concept to form an IFCN chapter. They elected Nelly Chiofalo (Chile) as their chairperson because of her actions as the driving force behind creation of the Chapter. Enrique Delamonica (Argentina) was elected as initial Chapter secretary. They were asked to draft Bye-Laws for presentation at a next meeting, which was scheduled to be held in conjunction with the World Congress of Neurology in Buenos Aires in 1997.

In Europe, the discussion was about whether to form a free-standing society, or a Federation of European Clinical Neurophysiology Societies, or a chapter of the IFCN. At the 1996 Eighth European Congress of Clinical Neurophysiology (ECCN) in Munich, representatives from 25 European member societies debated the choices. In the end, they voted unanimously (with one abstention and no objections) to form an IFCN European Chapter. An interim group of officers was appointed: Guenther Deuschl (Germany) as Chairman pro tempore, Al De Weerd (The Netherlands) as Secretary–Treasurer pro tempore, along with additional Special Committee members Anders Fuglsang-Fredericksen (Denmark), Jean-Marie Guérit (Belgium) and Aurora Constantinovici (Romania). They were asked to develop Bye-Laws and address other organizational issues. They reported back to the societies at the Florence 1997 International Congress of EEG and Clinical Neurophysiology. Actions taken there are covered in the next chapter of this book.

In the meanwhile, the European societies continued their discussion of recognizing Clinical Neurophysiology as a specialty in European Community. J.A. Jarrett (UK) had opened discussion of this at the Lisbon ECCN. This was considered an important area for Chapter action, although there remained no consensus about what action to take.

4. Regional meetings

Regional meetings supported during this 4-year term included the European Congresses of Clinical Neurophysiology in Budapest in July 1994 and in Munich in October 1996. In the Far East, the Asian Symposium on Clinical Neurophysiology was held in Beijing in September 1996. In Latin America, the Basic and Advanced Courses and Workshops in Clinical Neurophysiology were organized in conjunction with the IX Pan-American Congress of Neurology in Guatemala in October 1995.

4.1. VII European Congress of Clinical Neurophysiology

European Congresses of (Electroencephalography and) Clinical Neurophysiology have been organized by one of the Western European Societies since 1976. The early congresses were held in Venice (1976), Salzburg (1979), Basel (1983), Amsterdam (1988), Paris (1990), and Lisbon (1992). Parallel congresses of Central East Europe were held until 1993.

The IFCN ExCo worked with François Mauguière. He both served as Federation Editor-in-Chief and was involved with organization of the European meetings. He was instrumental in presenting a plan for the European meetings to be held within the framework of the Federation and its activities. The Federation agreed to provide fellowships for young physicians and scientists to attend the European meetings. Fellowships were preferentially assigned to Eastern European societies for the Budapest Congress in order to facilitate attendance. Sixty grants of US $600 each were awarded to persons nominated by their national society. The fellowship process restricted the grants to persons below 35 years of age, who have paid their congress registration fees and actually attended the meeting, and who presented at poster or platform sessions as first author.

The VII European Congress of Clinical Neurophysiology was held in Budapest, Hungary, July 3–7, 1994. The congress venue was the Budapest Marriot and Atrium Hyatt Hotel. The organizing committee consisted of: József Czopf (President and Convener), Robert Galambos (Honorary President), and several members of the Hungarian Society; the Scientific Committee included representatives of the European societies and IFCN. The excellent programme covering all aspects of clinical neurophysiology contained 6 Plenary Lectures, 16 Scientific Sessions, 6 Free Communication Sessions, 2 Symposia, and 2 Poster Sessions with 6 different topics each. A full-day Advanced Course was organized on July 8. The social programme included the welcome party at the Duna Palace, a traditional Hungarian dinner in the garden of a restaurant in the Buda hills, a banquet and an evening pleasure boat trip on the river Danube. Nearly 400 neurophysiologists were registered for the meeting, mainly from 29 European countries but also from USA, Canada and Russia.

4.2. Asian Symposium of Clinical Neurophysiology (ASCN '96)

During the fiscal period 1985–1990 under the presidency of John Desmedt, clinical neurophysiology societies in South East Asia had organized regional symposia with intensive practical workshops in Bangkok (February 1987), Bali (September 1987), and Beijing (June 1989). The Second Bangkok Symposium on Clinical Neurophysiology was held in March 1993 at the initiative of the Society of Thailand. Following these meetings John Desmedt suggested building up a South East Asia Liaison Committee (SEALC) for Clinical Neurophysiology. This would assemble the Delegates of the IFCN member societies of this area in order to promote Clinical Neurophysiology in Asia and to organize regional symposia. At that time this committee would consist of the Delegates to IFCN of China, India, Indonesia, Iran, Japan, Philippines, Thailand, and possibly Australia.

At the start of this Fiscal Period in 1993, Member-at-Large Xiao-Fu Tang of the People's Rep. of China (Appendix 11, Fig. 10) requested support for a regional conference in the South and East Asia region. This followed the successful format of previous Asian regional meetings in Beijing, Bali, and Bangkok. At the subsequent ExCo meeting, X.-F. Tang reported that Delegates from India, Thailand, China, Japan, Indonesia, and the Philippines had agreed to a South and East Asia Conference.

Tentatively this was set for autumn 1996. To assist in organizational details, X.-F. Tang requested that J. Desmedt and J. Kimura serve as consultants to the organizers. The US $43,500 budget was spent for organizational costs plus 40 grants to young Asian physicians. By July 1994, plans were laid to hold this meeting in Beijing, China. Registration fee would need to be low, given the economic situation for physicians in China. The process of awards fellowships was revised. Instead of the figures appropriate for meetings in Europe or America, the meeting and travel costs were made more modest for young physicians from the host country. That allowed for more fellowships to be awarded at a reduced amount for each: instead of 30 fellowship awards at US $600 each, US $300 each for Chinese physicians and 15 at US $600 for physicians from other regional nations.

The Asian Symposium of Clinical Neurophysiology (ASCN '96) was held in Beijing, September 23–25, 1996. The congress site was the Beijing International Hotel. The Symposium was organized under the auspices of the IFCN, Chinese Society of Neurology, Chinese Medical Association, Chinese Society of EMG and

Clinical Neurophysiology, and Chinese Society of EEG and Epilepsy. The Organization Committee consisted of: Xiao-Fu Tang (President and Convener), Prasert Boongird, Nubuo Yanagisawa, Jos Utama (Vice Presidents), De-Xuan Kang (Secretary), Ding-Guo Shen (Treasurer). Honorary Presidents were: John E. Desmedt, Jun Kimura, Carl H. Lücking, Xin-De Wang, Xiao-Da Zhou. The programme included four sessions of a total of 15 Special Lectures, many delivered by IFCN Officers, and four Platform Sessions with totalling 40 presentations. The meeting was accompanied by a welcome reception and a farewell banquet in a wonderful, Chinese customary atmosphere.

4.3. Basic and advanced courses and workshops in clinical neurophysiology, Guatemala, 1995

In 1994 Nelly Chiofalo (Chile) and neurophysiologists from other countries of Central and South America discussed with the President the situation of clinical neurophysiology in their countries. In the past, the Latin American Society had regularly organized meetings on clinical neurophysiology. But in recent years those meetings were discontinued, the society dissipated, and lost its seat in the Federation General Assembly. In many Latin American countries clinical neurophysiologists do not have their own society, but are incorporated in the neurological society. At present, only the neurophysiologic societies of Argentina, Brazil, Chile, Dominican Republic, Mexico, and Uruguay are member societies of the IFCN. In some other countries first steps are being made to build a society for Clinical Neurophysiology. Although there were opportunities for the national societies in Latin America to work with each other on topics and issues of mutual interest, a local organizing committee is lacking. Regional Federation meetings in Latin America would be helpful and consistent with the Federation's mission; a regional organization could facilitate such meetings. The Central and South American representatives expressed their wish to form a new Latin America Society. The IFCN, besides having contact with the individual Federation member societies, could have contacts within countries without their own society of clinical neurophysiology. In general those countries have too few clinical neurophysiologists to establish their own society and apply for IFCN membership. Some other countries have sufficient clinical neurophysiologists to form their own clinical neurophysiology society, but they prefer not to do so because of their close ties with neurology.

The ExCo agreed to these ideas and needs and asked Nelly Chiofalo to call for a regional meeting for the purpose of organizing a Latin American Society as an IFCN Chapter. This meeting would include as many as possible IFCN Delegates from this region. Enrique Delamonica (Argentina) assisted Dr Chiofalo to organize the ensuing meeting, "Curso Básico y Avanzado en Neurofisiologia Clinica and Talleres de Trabajo en Neurofisiologia Clinica", which was organized in conjunction with the IX Pan-American Congress of Neurology in Guatemala in October 1995 (Appendix 11, Fig. 11). IFCN co-sponsored the meeting. The President Carl Lücking, Member-at-Large Marc Nuwer and Editor-in-Chief Gastone Celesia represented the IFCN at this meeting. The President delivered an opening address to the assembled representatives.

4.4. VIII European Congress of Clinical Neurophysiology, Munich (Germany), 1996

Two years after the European Congress in Budapest, the VIII European Congress of Clinical Neurophysiology was held in Munich in October 9–12, 1996. The Congress site was the Plenary Hall of the Technical University of Munich. The Local Organizing Committee consisted of: B. Conrad (Convener), C. Bischoff (Secretary), S. Quasthoff (Treasurer), and the International Advisory Board with representatives from the 23 European Societies (Appendix 11, Fig. 12).

The final programme welcome address by C.H. Lücking (IFCN President), R. Korinthenberg

(President of the German Society of CN), B. Conrad (Convener), and C. Bischoff (Secretary) noted:

> *"We are pleased to welcome you to the 8th European Congress of Clinical Neurophysiology which was organised under the auspices of the International Federation of Clinical Neurophysiology and the German Society of Clinical Neurophysiology.*
>
> *The meeting is intended to bring together both scientists and practising physicians and covers the latest clinical and research developments in the field of clinical neurophysiology. It will highlight various neurophysiological methods used for the diagnosis and monitoring of affections of the central and peripheral nervous system. Particular emphasis is put on recently developed methods as well as on advances achieved through a combination of neurophysiological and imaging techniques. Nine invited lectures will focus on different neurophysiological techniques as well as on disorders that can be monitored or diagnosed using clinical neurophysiological methods. In addition, in 8 workshops a large number of invited international experts will give an overview about current concepts regarding intra-operative and intensive care monitoring, nerve excitability, magnetoencephalography, neurophysiology of cognition, motor control, pre-surgical epilepsy evaluation, clinical neurophysiology in psychiatry, and neuroimaging. Throughout the conference 60 free communications and about 400 posters will provide intensive coverage of the 'state of the art' of clinical neurophysiology. The congress will be followed by advanced courses of clinical neurophysiology designed to give a critical review of well-established and innovative neurophysiologic techniques.*
>
> *The social programme commences with a welcome reception in the famous art gallery* Neue Pinakothek. *A Bavarian evening has been planned to give you an impression of the local traditions. An outstanding sightseeing programme has been arranged to give accompanying persons an opportunity to explore Munich, the beautiful capital of Bavaria, with its cultural treasures and magnificent Alps and lakes."*

During the Opening Ceremony an Honorary Lecture was given by Wolfgang Singer, Frankfurt (Germany) on temporal coherence as a coding principle in the cerebral cortex. About 800 neurophysiologists attended the congress. Thirty fellowships of US $600 were granted by the IFCN for young fellows from 16 European countries. The abstracts of the Morning Sessions, Poster Sessions, and Workshops were published in a special issue of the EEG Journal, October 1996. Overall, this was considered an exciting scientific meeting that was well organized in a wonderful atmosphere and in a splendid place.

5. The journal *Electroencephalography and Clinical Neurophysiology*

At the beginning of the Fiscal Period the journal *Electroencephalography and Clinical Neurophysiology* was divided into three separate sections: the main set of issues without a subtitle, a section subtitled *Evoked Potentials*, and another section subtitled *Electromyography and Motor Control*. In 1994 a new cover of the Journal went into effect. An electronic version of the EEG Journal became available in 1996.

The two Editors-in-Chief managed an increasing number of manuscripts submitted during these 4 years. Quality of the articles continued its trend of improvement, as did the formally measured journal impact factor (1.872 in 1993 and 2.400 in 1997). Review Articles were introduced to add another dimension to the usefulness and acceptance of the journal. The distribution of the journal was noted to be limited especially in the economically weak countries. To address this, the ExCo unsuccessfully looked for companies to sponsor journal subscriptions to economically disadvantaged areas. Therefore the ExCo initiated direct gifts of subscriptions to societies or medical centres in economically weak areas. For this purpose the Delegates were addressed to identify key institutions that would make the journal accessible for all the neurophysiologists of the city or area.

The total number of subscribers was in decline. It dropped from 2363 in the early 1990s, to 2262 in 1993, and to 1896 in 1995. The ExCo discussed this with Elsevier representatives. The drop was mainly among individual subscribers. Institutional subscriptions dropped much less. Reasons included the proliferation of journals, availability through academic libraries, and constrains on expenses at departments and laboratories. Actions considered were deeper reductions in individual subscription prices and greater incentives for individuals to maintain their subscriptions. Discussions continued beyond this Fiscal Period.

The ExCo serves as the Editorial Board for the journal. The minutes and meetings are kept separate from the ExCo meeting and minutes. The ExCo, in its role as the Editorial Board, makes decision making about finances, contracts, and other business matters of the journal and other Federation publications. The Editors-in-Chief remain in control of the scientific and content issues of the journal. The Supplements are included in the subscription of the journal. Upon the recommendations of the Editors-in-Chief, Consulting Editors, Book Editors, and Associate Editors are appointed by the ExCo. The ExCo also appoints each Editor-in-Chief. During this 4-year term, the appointment of Western office Editor-in-Chief Gastone Celesia was reaffirmed. Upon the announced intention to resign of European Editor-in-Chief François Mauguière in 1995, an international search was initiated. The ExCo evaluated applications from Geoff Barrett (UK), Jerzy Majkowski (Poland), Milos Matoušek (Sweden), and Paolo Rossini (Italy). The ExCo appointed Paolo Rossini as the new European office Editor-in-Chief effective in 1995.

When Gastone Celesia announced that he would retire at the end of 1999 the ExCo discussed for the first time to return to the previous policy of a single Editor-in-Chief. This was not decided at the time, but continued as a topic for discussion into the next Fiscal period and for the next ExCo.

William Cobb (UK), a past Editor-in-Chief and Federation President, had decided to discontinue his work on language correction for the Journal that he had done for many years. He did so to improve the English of the manuscripts coming from non-English-speaking countries for publication. He was succeeded by Geoff Barrett who served well in that language editing role during this Fiscal Period.

In 1996, the 50th anniversary of the Federation and the Journal was discussed. While it was without any doubt that the Federation was born in 1949, the year of the birthday of the Journal was less certain. Finally the birthday was scheduled for 1999 according to the quotation of William Cobb in a letter from September 1996: "The [Journal's] conception was certainly in 1947 but gestation was rather long and delivery of the first number was not until February 1949".

6. Practice guidelines

A Subcommittee on Monitoring in Coma submitted an initial report to the Council and General Assembly at the IFCN Congress held in London 1985. The committee included B. Bergamasco, A. Bricolo, G.-E. Chatrian (Chairman), J.D. Frost, and P. Prior. In 1993 and 1995 this Committee updated the report which was approved by the ExCo and published in the EEG Journal in 1996.

Practice and safety of repetitive transcranial stimulation (rTMS) was a new growing area of interest. A committee was formed to report on this technique. As the rTMS appears destined for use in different disciplines, many outside of clinical neurophysiology, the IFCN felt obliged to create this committee to promulgate standards of techniques and guidelines for indications of this method. The committee was composed of M. Hallett (Chair) A. Pascual-Leone, E. Wassermann, P. Rossini, W. Paulus, C. Epstein, J. Rothwell, C. Tassinari, R.H. Belmaker, H.A. Sackheim, L. Ladegoard, and equipment vendor representatives J. Cadwell, and R. Jalinous. The committee continued its work beyond the end of this Fiscal Period.

As digital methods replace analogue ones, another process was undertaken to give guidance to digital techniques and equipment. A committee was constituted composed of Member-at-Large Marc R. Nuwer (Chair), with committee members G. Comi, R. Emerson, A. Fuglsang-Frederiksen, J.-M. Guérit, H. Hinrichs, A. Ikeda, F.J.C. Lucas, and P. Rappelsberger. The committee was charged to work with manufacturers and users to develop a report for digital equipment when used in clinical settings. The committee sought advice from the Delegates in order to establish the minimum standards for conducting digital EEG and digital neurophysiologic studies. Standards were drafted, circulated and underwent a series of revisions. Open meetings were held to involve manufacturers and any interested persons. These were held at the Kyoto International Congress and at two regional meetings. An eventual consensus was reached, endorsed by the Council at the Florence Congress, and published in the journal.

Concern was raised about commercial firms making claims that their equipment meets the IFCN Digital EEG Standards. The concern was that such a claim may be incorrect, and the Federation should have some control over the use of its name. A process was developed so that vendors could seek IFCN review before using the Federation's name in commercial advertisements, particularly when they make claims that their equipment meets Federation standards. The ExCo wanted to prevent claims of compliance for equipment that is actually not in compliance. On the other hand, the IFCN does not endorse products, nor does it wish to be viewed as such. The concern focused on how vendors could use the IFCN name to say that they comply. They could not use the IFCN logo. The size of font announcing that it meets IFCN digital EEG standards should be informational, not a large advertising banner using the IFCN name. The advertisement must state that the IFCN does not endorse the product. The process would go through the IFCN secretary office. Further concerns were raised about a hold harmless process in case equipment caused damages or injuries. The IFCN may need insurance in case commercial firms are disagreeable about the IFCN withholding its authorization from them. However, given the French registration of the organization, standard insurance could not be found, and not even ordinary directors' and officers' insurance could be found. Eventually this took two directions. First the published document stated that no commercial advertisements could use the IFCN name to claim compliance unless the IFCN agrees. At the same time, no process was developed to give such an authorization. This led in the next Fiscal Period to questions about liability insurance, which led to inquiries about the legal status of the Federation and the need for an Executive Secretariat and permanent address in order to obtain insurance.

7. Finances

At the request of the Vancouver General Assembly for transparency of fiscal policy the ExCo kept a detailed budget for each year. An independent auditor was appointed. In January 1994 ExCo approved a Policy Document for expenditures to ExCo members in accordance with the business practices used by US universities for reimbursement for travel expenses. The policy was endorsed and accepted as enduring Federation policy by the 1995 Kyoto General Assembly (see Table 13.1).

7.1. Budgets and gains

For the first 2 years (1994 and 1995) the total income of US $475,000 was from member society dues, Elsevier royalties, repayment from congresses, and investment interest. This was balanced by the total expenses of the same period for Editors-in-Chief and ExCo member office expenses, ExCo meetings and travel expenditures, OCIC meetings and travel expenses, International Congress and Chapter meeting subsides, support for congress fellowships, along with payment for banking, currency exchange, legal and accounting expenses. For the first time the budget was voted on by postal ballot: 18 out of 24 responses of the delegates were in favour, 4 against, 2 were in abstention.

At the 1995 Kyoto General Assembly, Treasurer Paul Despland's budget report was approved. The IFCN assets had increased from

US $545,365 in 1993 to nearly US $880,864 in 1995. The profit was mainly through careful spending policies and favourable exchange rate changes. Robert Miller (USA) proposed a motion, "The Executive Committee is charged with developing a long-range financial plan, to be completed before the Florence meeting, in view of our large reserves, to include a re-evaluation of dues structure, fellowships, funding, and the allocation of votes to each society". Michael Aminoff (USA) congratulated the Treasurer on the favourable fiscal report and extensive details provided for review, and seconded Dr. Miller's motion that was unanimously approved. This motion was in keeping with the action already underway by the ExCo over the previous 2 years. The Treasurer agreed to modify the budget accordingly when the reserves reached US $1 million.

By the time of the 1997 Florence General Assembly 2 years later, Treasurer Paul Despland was able to report a favourable 4-year Fiscal Period report and propose to do the same in the next 4 years' budget. At the end of each year, Mr. Alain Maillard, the external financial advisor audited all the accounting books and the receipts from each ExCo member. Receipts were kept for all expenses over US $10. The liquid funds, as well as the investments, had been transferred from Crédit Suisse Zürich to the Union Bank of Switzerland in Lausanne. The Union Bank of Switzerland regularly made suggestions for reinvestments when necessary. The essential objective of the investments is to keep safe the Federation assets and derive a reasonable income without any speculation. It has to be noticed that our income is mostly based on the royalties from Elsevier. These royalties were paid in Dutch guilders, which explains why most Federation investments were expressed in this currency. International currency conversion rates adversely affected the total assets in the years 1995–1997, because the income and assets are in Dutch guilders whereas the accounting books are kept in US dollars.

7.2. Comparison between 1993 and 1997 assets

Due to increased income and expense controls during these 4 years, the Federation's assets rose to US $865,138, which was almost 60% more than at the beginning of the Fiscal Period. A special reserve account was created of US $48,000 from favourable financial results in the years 1994 and 1995. This reserve was set aside as a buffer against depreciation of currency rates in the near future. On the other hand, favourable exchange rates could provide appreciable marked profits in the following year. The balance sheet showed a Fiscal Period profit of US $319,772, and improvement over the previous Fiscal Period profit of US $86,592.

7.3. Budget for 1997–1999

The Treasurer presented a budget for the next 2 years. Paul Despland was re-elected as Treasurer for the next Fiscal Period, so that he would continue to watch over this next budget too. The Treasurer proposed the motion: "The budget for the next two years should be similar to the budget of previous years." The motion was approved with one abstention. The General Assembly asked that future budgets be presented with all detail shown down to levels below US $10,000, and as much additional detail as possible below that level, that is, down to less than US $2000 wherever possible. This level of detail should be made available both for the Council and General Assembly. The budget presented was renewed for 2 years.

The ExCo was charged with developing a long-range financial plan to be completed before 1999. This plan would include an evaluation of dues structure and fellowship funding. As an endowment strategy, a long-range planning may involve deposit into a non-profit foundation or other accounting processes to isolate the assets from the ordinary operating funds of the IFCN. It would be used for educational purposes. That proposal was approved unanimously. The

Treasurer proposed to set aside a US $500,000 for this purpose. A Long-Range Financial Planning Task Force was established that included Andrew Eisen (Canada), Kjeld Andersen (Norway), François Mauguière (France) and Robert Miller (USA). The Task Force was charged with developing a plan regarding societies' dues and spending on fellowships. The Task Force was asked to report back at the 1999 Prague meeting. It was discussed that a membership dues reduction would be advantageous for large societies, but not to small societies who have difficulties in paying even small dues amounts thus risking to lose their IFCN membership.

Some societies asked to have their dues waived for reasons of financial difficulty. The ExCo did not agree to those requests. Instead the ExCo indicated that non-paying societies would lose voting rights, but they would retain all other privileges including the right to have fellowship funding for their young members.

7.4. Fellowships

The ExCo in 1996 noted that the Federation provides a much greater number of fellowships compared with other international federations. The ExCo reduced the number of International Congresses fellowships from 100 to 70 and increased the amount awarded from US $600 to US $1000. Fellowships for members of the host society that organizes the congress were reduced to US $500. Thirty fellowships would be awarded for regional meetings; also in this case fellowships for the host society will he halved. The fellowships were awarded on the condition that the scientific work will be first submitted to the EEG Journal like all the work presented at IFCN congresses.

Fellowships were given to individuals not to their societies. Individual candidates from non-dues-paying societies remain eligible to receive fellowships. To make sure that information about fellowships reaches young candidates, the ExCo discussed the possibility to send information about fellowships not only to the Delegate but also directly to the members of IFCN-affiliated societies. That would reduce the time lag in between when national societies receive this information and when it reaches their members, but could result in fellowships being awarded to candidates not approved by their national society. This issue was discussed with the Delegates. Eventually, information about the fellowships was added to the Congress abstract forms.

8. Gift committee

In the past Fiscal Periods, the Gift Committee under the chairmanship of John Desmedt had provided copies of the *Handbook of Clinical Neurophysiology*. In recent years, nine copies of *Evoked Potentials* Vol. 3 of the Revised Handbook Series was donated to neurophysiologists in China, Thailand, and Poland.

The new Gift Committee consisted of: F. Lopes da Silva (The Netherlands, Chair), M. Gourie-Devi (India), Mario Medici (Uruguay), Slavcho Slavchev (Bulgaria), and Valeria Strelets (Russia). In 1994 the ExCo donated Handbook volumes when requested, provided that such requests are made by institutes or clinics and not by individuals. Due to the previous financial situation of IFCN, neither journal subscriptions nor equipment were to be granted at that time. Any request normally would be submitted by the Delegate and examined and decided by the Gift Committee. The President would then order the handbook from the publishers and send it to the recipient with an accompanying letter.

During this fiscal period, the ExCo broadened its mission by soliciting from industrial companies some donated journal subscriptions from economically disadvantaged societies and institutions. This project to find commercial sponsors failed. Subsequently, once the IFCN finances had improved, the ExCo authorized donations of journal subscriptions financed by the Federation. Delegates were asked to identify key institutions as sites for making the journal accessible to neurophysiologists.

9. Secretary's report

IFCN Secretary Giuseppe Caruso actively communicated with the member societies. A continuing task communication is to maintain updated information on the officers and number of members for each society, delegate's name and contact information for the society, its officer and its delegate. The lists needed to be kept updated even with entrance of new societies, withdrawal of another, separation of some into multiples, and joining together of another pair. Many national societies changed their executive offices, officers and delegates, and too often this news was not promptly reported to the IFCN Secretary. This caused communication problems, wasted time, and may have had adverse effects on balloting and submission of fellowship applications. The Secretary needed to work hard to keep the proper lines of communications open. Some IFCN announcements should be transmitted to members of affiliated societies, and often the easiest way is to send notices and announcements to the national societies for distribution. This sometimes ran into delays, for example if the national societies received a communiqué just after sending out their periodic newsletter. To help communicate directly to clinical neurophysiologists, the Secretary requested membership lists from each society for the purpose of some direct mailings. Unfortunately only 14 societies replied with membership lists. Communications with societies and individuals remained an active and continuing task for the Secretary.

The Secretary also had other regular chores. This included preparation of the arrangements for, agenda of, and minutes for twice annual ExCo meetings. In this term, those meetings were held in Vancouver in September 1993, Lyon in January 1994, Freiburg in April 1995, Kyoto in October 1995, San Francisco in March 1996, Beijing in September 1996, Boston in April 1997, and Florence in August 1997. During the same period six postal ballots were held of Council — practically blocking the fax and telephone lines. The newly developed IFCN ExCo Expense Policy was circulated to the Delegates. Information on the International Congresses was sent out, and invitations to bid on next congresses were organized. As a member of OCIC, the Secretary also was involved in the organization of the Kyoto and Florence Congresses. A report of the Vancouver General Assembly was submitted to and appeared in the journal.

Finally, the Secretary reorganized and standardized the style for the Yellow Pages section in the EEG Journal. The text was sent monthly to Elsevier for monthly publication as the Yellow Pages in a form camera ready for publication. Where possible, in all correspondence to delegates and secretaries of member societies, they were encouraged to use the Yellow Pages to advertise their activities.

ExCo minutes were sent to Delegates after the ExCo approved the minutes. A brief synopsis of each meeting was published in the journal Yellow Pages. This was done to facilitate good communication with and improved participation by the societies in ongoing Federation activities.

Given the amount of correspondence and organization required in the Secretary office, the General Assembly in Kyoto suggested for the first time to consider an executive director or a permanent Secretariat to take over much of the routine work, improve the quality and continuity of information flow, and serve as a possible source of continuity when the Secretary position changes hands.

10. IFCN Statutes and Bye-Laws amendments

At the beginning of this Fiscal Period the Vancouver 1993 General Assembly instructed the ExCo to amend several parts of the IFCN Statutes and Bye-Laws. The Rules Committee, consisting of Mark Hallett (USA, Chair), G. Barrett (UK), Jan Daniel Gieu (France 1993–1995), François Mauguière (France 1995–1997), Hans-Christian Hopf (Germany), and Motohiro Kato (Japan), was charged with developing draft wording and reviewing the justification of the amendments to implement the General Assembly's motions.

The first amendments concerning the role of Council and the eligibility of the ExCo members have been approved by the Council and finally submitted to the General Assembly in Kyoto in 1995.

10.1. Executive Committee voting by societies

The Vancouver General Assembly's requested to change the format of voting for the ExCo members. The previous system gave one vote for each society. The new methods would be like the General Assembly voting with 2, 3, or 4 voted for each society depending on the society's number. However, the ExCo members themselves would be ineligible in this voting, even though they do have voting rights in ordinary General Assembly voting. The Rules Committee drafted the following rule changes. In this and following rules text, the new inserted text is shown in **bold** and the deleted text in strike-through. This set of rules changes were adopted at the Kyoto General Assembly with five abstentions and no vote against.

10.2. Statutes

VI, 2

The Council is composed of the ExCo together with one delegate from each of the Member Societies. It votes on the proposals submitted to it by the ExCo, on applications for membership of the Federation and ~~on the proposals of the Nomination Committee for the officers of the Federation and the members of Special Commissions, and~~ on any other business appearing on the Agenda.

X

On recommendations of the ExCo, with the approval of the Council, the General Assembly may set up Special Commissions, each to represent a special branch of Neurophysiology. Each Special Commission shall be composed of three members, one of whom shall be designated Chairman; they will be proposed by the Nomination Committee and elected by the **member societies similarly to the members of the ExCo** ~~Council~~. The Chairman will be a member of the ExCo and will advise it of the interests of his speciality. The members will be members of the General Assembly. The President may delegate tasks, such as the organization of specialized meetings, to the appropriate Special Commissions.

XI, 2

This Committee shall invite nominations from the members of the Council, who may each consult with his parent Society if he/she so wishes for the offices of President, Secretary and Treasurer of the Federation, the Members-at-Large of the ExCo, and those of the Chairman and the two members of each Special Commission to hold office for the following fiscal period. Having ascertained the willingness of the candidates to serve, the Chairman of the Nomination Committee shall submit their names to the postal vote of the **member societies** ~~Council~~, and inform the Secretary of the result of the ballot. **Each society has the number of votes to which it is entitled in the General Assembly. The ballot is to be sent to the delegate of the society who will be responsible for returning the ballot by the specified date. The vote may be split among the different candidates.**

10.3. Executive Committee turnover

The Vancouver General Assembly expressed concern about individuals serving on the ExCo for an extended period, sometimes serving in various roles over time. In the not too distant past some ExCo members had served continuously for 20 years. The General Assembly asked for a rule to mandate turnover in ExCo membership. Specifically, the motion was that no one should serve more than 12 years, except in the case of a president who could take office after having served 8 years. In the latter case, the president's eventual term would total 16 years. To implement that, the Rules Committee proposed the following rule:

VII, 3

The President, Secretary, and Treasurer of the Federation, the members of Special Commissions and the Members-at-Large of the ExCo are elected by the member societies Council from the nominees of the Nomination Committee. Their term of office is the Fiscal Period. The President, Secretary, Chairmen of Special Commissions and Members-at-Large may serve only one term in office. The Treasurer is eligible for re-election once only. **No person shall serve as an elected or an appointed member of the ExCo for more than 12 years total, except that a person who has served already for 8 years would be allowed to run for President and, if elected, serve for 8 years as President and Past president.**

This was approved at the Kyoto 1995 General Assembly with four abstentions and no vote against.

10.4. Geographical and disciplinary balance among Executive Committee members

The ExCo wanted to assure both geographical and disciplinary balance among its members. For geographical purposes, the Federation already used a geographical distinction for the journal *Electroencephalography and Clinical Neurophysiology*. The journal had two Editors-in-Chief each representing a different geographical region. This could be carried over to the ExCo member elections. The disciplinary designations already in the Statutes mention only two classic designations of EEG and EMG. There was a concern that some of candidates perform both EEG and EMG, and others do neither but engage in other aspects of clinical neurophysiology.

The following rules were submitted to the 1997 Florence Congress Council. Amendments to most paragraphs were unanimously approved. The third paragraph was approved with 25 votes in favour, 3 against, and 3 abstentions.

Committees, 2

The Nomination Committee shall ensure **geographical and disciplinary balance in the ExCo** ~~that the Secretary and the Treasurer be elected the one from amongst electroencephalographers and the other from amongst electromyographers. It should also take steps to ensure that the two Members-at-Large be elected the one from amongst electroencephalographers and the other from amongst the electromyographers.~~

~~The Nomination Committee shall ensure that Members-at-Large are chosen from geographical areas not already represented on the Executive Committee.~~ **Geographical areas are (1) North and South America, Australasia and Japan, and (2) Europe, Asia (except Japan), and Africa. At the time of their nomination, nominees should be given a disciplinary designation of electroencephalographer or electromyographer by the nominating society. The designation should be justified on the basis of practice or research. The Nominating Committee should approve the designation. If the designation is disapproved, the decision may be appealed to the ExCo whose decision is final. The disciplinary designation cannot be changed during a voting cycle. Even if a society is not eligible to vote (Statute XI.2), it may still nominate persons for any position, and its members remain eligible for nomination.**

The President and Past-president should preferably be from different geographical regions and cannot be from the same geographical region in more than two consecutive elections. The Secretary and Treasurer should be from different geographical regions. The two Members-at-Large should be from different geographical regions and from countries different from those of the President, Past-President, Treasurer and Secretary. Concerning disciplinary balance, the members should be either four from each discipline or five from one discipline and three from the other.

Voting for members of the ExCo should occur in the following sequence: First round: President and Treasurer. Second round: Secretary. Third round: Members-at-Large. For each round, voting should be by written ballot only (post or fax is permitted) and adherence to the deadline is mandatory. To declare an election valid, ballots must

be received from at least 50% of the societies eligible to vote (by Statute XVI.2). The deadline can be extended to achieve a quorum. Extension is limited to the time when the quorum is achieved. To win an election, an absolute majority of the votes cast is required, and a run-off election between the top two candidates should be held if necessary. If a society ineligible to vote (Statute XVI.2) becomes eligible during an election, it may initiate participating in the voting when the next round of the election begins.

10.5. Electioneering by the Nominating Committee

The Vancouver General Assembly asked to prohibit members of the Nominating Committee from campaigning for one or another candidate in the election. Instead the Nominating Committee should be a neutral body set to assure a fair and organized election process. The nominations and voting should be by the societies without interference from committee members. The ExCo should oversee that the election is conducted in that manner. To implement that motion, the Rules Committee proposed the following text to append to the Nomination Committee section in the Bye-Laws.

Committees, 2

The members of the nominating committee should not promote a particular candidate for any office. The nominating committee should report to the ExCo after each step of the election process. The report must include the number of votes for each candidate.

This Bye-Law was approved unanimously at the Florence Council meeting. In addition to the Bye-Laws, the ExCo adopted an additional policy of its own that the members of the current ExCo should not campaign for any individual in the election.

10.6. Selection of time and place of a subsequent international congress

The ExCo recommended a great degree of structure in the process for selecting the next congress site. This amendment asked for more specific information from the presenters about their bids. It also limited the time for presentations, because some presenters were very extensive in marginally relevant portions of their presentation such as videotapes about their country and city in general. The Rules Committee developed the following language to address that need. This was placed among the Bye-Laws on the conduct of the General Assembly. This was approved with one abstention.

Selection of the time and place of the international congresses should be made al least 4 years in advance. Nominations may be made by any member society. Preference should be given for successive congresses of each type to be in different geographical areas. Nominations must be less than 10 min each and should include both oral and written information about the proposed organizing committee, the congress venue, the hotel arrangements and a preliminary budget. General information about the city or country of the nomination cannot exceed 5 min of the presentation time.

The final selection should be by majority vote, each member of the General Assembly casting one vote. After the first round of voting, should no nomination receive a majority, a second round should consider only those nominations receiving the four highest numbers of votes. After the second round of voting, should no nomination receive a majority, a third round should consider only those nominations receiving the two highest numbers of votes.

10.7. General Assembly voting by mail for amendments

Concern was raised that some societies have difficulty in sending representatives to General Assembly meetings. Changes in statutes might be conducted more fairly by mail so that all societies have the opportunity to vote. The Rules Committee drafted the following language. The rule was approved with one abstention.

XVIII

The present Statutes may be amended by a two-thirds vote of the General Assembly, the proposed amendments having been accepted by the Council and ~~included in the Agenda~~ **having been discussed at a meeting** of the General Assembly. **Proposed amendments must be submitted to the General Assembly by mail ballot which may be by post or fax. Each society will be entitled to the number of votes to which it is entitled in the General Assembly. The ballot will be sent to the delegate of the Society, who will be responsible for returning it by the deadline, specifying the number of votes to which that Society is entitled. Each Society will be asked to specify the names of the voting persons, and require their signatures on the ballot. Votes for a Society can be split. To declare a vote valid, ballots must be received from more than 50% of the Societies eligible to vote (by Statute XVI. 2). Adherence to the deadline is mandatory, except that the deadline can be extended to achieve a quorum. Extension is limited to the time when the quorum is achieved.**

10.8. Council and General Assembly meetings at international congresses

The Council discussed for the first time the frequency of Council and General Assembly meetings whether they should further be organized only at the ICEEGCN Congress (meeting every 4 years) or also at the IFEMGCN Congress (meeting every 2 years). At this time, the General Assembly ordinarily met only at the quadrennial ICEEGCN meeting, not at the EMG meetings. The discussion raised the further issue about the general tendency was to eliminate the words EEG and EMG from the congresses. On the whole, delegates favoured eliminating the EEG–EMG distinction and agreed to holding the Council and General Assembly meetings every 2 years. This would be effective starting in 2001. No final decision was made. This issue continued into the next Fiscal Period.

10.9. Named lectureship of the IFCN congresses

Named lectureships at congresses remained a topic of discussion during this Fiscal Period. Three Honorary Lectures in memory of Edgar Lord Adrian, Hans Berger, and Erik Kugelberg have been sponsored by the IFCN beginning at the 1990 Rio de Janeiro XII International Congress and since then regularly at the ICEEGCNs. A special lecture in honour of Fritz Buchthal was proposed by the Danish society in 1997 to be given in addition to the three honorary lectures. A honorary Buchthal lecture was held at the Florence congress, 1997. This lecture originally was to be sponsored by the instrument company Dantec. Since the ExCo required that sponsors of honorary lectures should be silent sponsors who provided an unrestricted educational grant, Dantec withdrew from sponsoring this lecture. Therefore IFCN provided the financial support for this honorary lecture at the Florence meeting.

Questions continued about whether honorary lectureships should be only named after persons who already passed away and how to avoid that the lectures are named only after European personalities. The 1997 Council recommended further study for the problem of Honorary Lectures with all their many political and cultural aspects, and keeping the Buchthal lecture temporarily while the matter was studied. The Council sent the question of a Buchthal lecture to the ExCo for a careful evaluation. The General Assembly subsequently passed a motion to send the matter back to Council with a recommendation to establish the Buchthal lectureship permanently.

11. X International Congress of EMG and Clinical Neurophysiology

The X International Congress of EMG and Clinical Neurophysiology was held in Kyoto on October 15–19, 1995. The Organization Committee of the International Congress (OCIC) consisted of three appointees from the Japanese Society, Jun Kimura (Convener), Nobuo Yanagisawa

(Secretary), and Koki Shimoji (Treasurer). Organizers from IFCN initially were Jun Kimura (President), John Desmedt (Past-President), Manuel Meyer (Treasurer), and as invited guests Carl Lücking (President Elect) and Giuseppe Caruso (Secretary Elect). Beginning in mid-1993, the IFCN was represented by Carl Lücking (President), Jun Kimura (Past-President), Giuseppe Caruso (Secretary), and Paul Despland (Treasurer). Hiroshi Shibasaki was additionally appointed for the scientific programme and Andrew Eisen as an advisor. The Program Committee represented all the Federation member societies. OCIC meetings were held three times in Kyoto (July 1993), Vancouver (September 1993), and Washington (July 1994). The budget was US $2 million, of which 1 million came from registration fees, from Japanese Society members' donations, and from the Japanese government. The second million was raised from pharmaceutical manufacturers and donors. The Local Organizing Committee did not engage a professional congress organizer because of the high costs involved. A loan of US $30,000 was provided by IFCN to cover the initial organizing costs. One hundred fellowships of US $600 each for young neurophysiologists were paid by the congress organization from congress profits. The social events were designed to be as simple and inexpensive as possible.

Nearly 40 different topics covering many disciplines including EEG and functional imaging as well as disease- and symptom-oriented clinical categories. Although this was an EMG Congresses, and that major topic was maintained in lectures and symposia, the Congress covered EEG free communications. One programme goal was to look to the future of clinical neurophysiology by having relatively young, emerging workers preferred over the already established personalities for symposia faculty.

The OCIC addressed concerns from the previous IFCN Congress in Vancouver. Too many accepted posters were not presented by the authors who did not come to the Congress. Some poster session Chairmen did not report for their walking poster sessions. The OCIC and the Programme Committee considered the problem of scientifically poor posters, but determined that some authors worked in difficult economic circumstances and were unable to attend the congress unless they presented a poster. The OCIC decided to deal with the absent poster problem by not accepting them into the programme until the presenting authors paid their congress fees.

Two prizes of US $3000 each for studies on epilepsy were awarded during the congress to authors below the age of 40 years. One prize was dedicated to Henry Gastaut (for Japan, Europe, and Asia) and the other to Herbert Jasper (for America). The aim was to increase the number of studies on epilepsy appearing in the EEG Journal.

In his greeting message in the Second Announcement, President Carl Lücking stressed the IFCN's important missions to impart a high standard of knowledge in the area of clinical neurophysiology, and to promote international cooperation. In a time in which imaging methods and molecular-biological procedures in the diagnosis of neurological diseases are becoming increasingly more important, clinical neurophysiology has needed to work constantly to define and maintain its unique status to evaluate function rather than structure. It must be shown that the different methods complement rather than mutually exclude each other. The International Congress in Kyoto accepted this challenge and aimed to present the importance, the current standards, and future direction of electromyography and clinical neurophysiology.

The venue of the Congress was the Kyoto International Conference Hall that synthesized the best of contemporary design and traditional Japanese architecture. In 1981, the X International Congress of EEG and Clinical Neurophysiology had been organized in the same Conference Hall.

For the 1995 meeting, the Honorary Presidents were John E. Desmedt, Karl-Erik Hagbarth,

Edward H. Lambert, Teruo Okuma, Yasuo Shimazono, Naoichi Tsuyama. The scientific programme included 3 Special Lectures, 9 Invited Lectures, 12 Symposia, 12 Satellite Symposia, 37 Workshops, 5 Pre-Congress Hands-on Workshops, and about 600 Free Communications as Posters. T. Tsumoto presented the honorary Berger lecture on mechanisms underlying synaptic plasticity in the neocortex. For the Adrian lecture, Stephen Waxman presented a lecture on ion channels and nerve conduction. The Kugelberg lecture was presented by K.-E. Hagbarth on muscle spindles and fusimotor system.

All participants were invited to the social events and receptions: opening ceremony and welcome reception, garden party, and closing ceremony and get-together reception without the need to pay an extra fee for entry to some social events.

The Proceedings of the Congress were published as *Recent Advances in Clinical Neurophysiology*, edited by J. Kimura and H. Shibasaki, in the International Congress Series 1101, by Excerpta Medica, Elsevier, Amsterdam, 1996. All manuscripts of Special Lectures, Invited Lectures, Symposia, Workshops, and Satellite Symposia were included.

11.1. Kyoto 1995 General Assembly report of the President

The President remembered two past Federation Presidents, Mary A.B. Brazier and Henry Gastaut, who had passed away in 1995. Marc Nuwer paid tribute to the lifetime achievements of Mary Brazier. François Mauguière did the same for Henry Gastaut. Then the General Assembly held a moment of silence in memory of the two deceased colleagues of enormous importance in the history of the Federation.

The ExCo had been hard at work at and between its four meetings during the previous 2 years. All motions from the 1993 Vancouver General Assembly were prepared for action by the Council and General Assembly in Kyoto. New amendments to the Statutes and Bye-Laws were worded and approved by the Rules Committee. A number of the new Bye-Laws were approved by the Council in Kyoto. For details, see the above section on IFCN Statutes and Bye-Laws Amendments.

The IFCN budget was approved for each fiscal year, in which specific sums for the individual areas were presented to the delegates for their perusal and comment. For details, see the section above on Finances.

In the middle of 1995 François Mauguière resigned as Editor-in-Chief for Europe, Africa and Asia after an 8-year tenure. During this time the acceptance of the EEG Journal continued to improve and the number of manuscripts increased. The Journal was divided into three sections. The excellent job Dr. Mauguière did for the Journal was especially praised.

Member societies were asked for proposals for a successor to Dr. Mauguière. Several highly qualified persons were suggested. The ExCo unanimously selected Paolo Rossini (Italy) as the new Editor-in-Chief. The main reason for this decision was Rossini's vast experience over the years as the book reviewer for the EEG Journal. At the same time, Nick Murray (UK) was appointed as the new book reviewer.

The President's numerous visits to various countries helped bring together the activities of neurophysiologists in the individual countries in preparation for the founding of new societies. Among other activities, a meeting was held with neurophysiologists in Estonia. The Estonian and Baltic clinical neurophysiologists were encouraged to form a society and apply for Federation membership.

The IFCN proposed a particular successful meeting of the Latin-American societies on the occasion of the 1995 Pan-American Congress in Guatemala. A day-long Basic and Advanced Course of Clinical Neurophysiology was organized as a satellite meeting to the Pan-American Congress of Neurology. The Clinical Neurophysiology courses were a great success as far as the participation, the quality of lectures, and the practical work were concerned. During that day, the Latin American societies held a business meeting that was the first step in founding a Latin American Chapter of the IFCN. Several Latin American countries have shown an interest in founding their own national societies and becoming member societies of the IFCN.

Contacts to the Eastern European societies were strengthened by the President's visits to Hungary, Bulgaria, and Romania. These visits identified the numerous difficulties, especially of economic nature, in this region at that time. The President recommended that these circumstances should be taken into consideration in future policy-making.

All in all, the 2 years 1993–1995 were successful in consolidating the IFCN finances, in gaining increased participation from the individual societies in IFCN decision-making, in the founding of regional chapters, and in forming new societies in various countries. Goals for the years 1995–1997 were increased attention to the subject matter of clinical neurophysiology and competition with the new imaging technology. The President encouraged that the international congresses and regional meetings provide basic and advanced courses on the new topics, and the Federation develop standards for new technology.

11.2. Kyoto 1995 General Assembly report of the Secretary

The Secretary's report, usually covering 4 years, in Kyoto covered a 2-year period because of the extra General Assembly meeting at Kyoto called by the 1993 Vancouver General Assembly. Former IFCN Secretary, Barry Tharp, was helpful for smoothing the transition in the Secretary offices and duties, and for redirecting relevant documents and material to Naples.

A first and continuing task was to communicate with the secretaries of IFCN member societies to obtain contact information on the officers of the individual societies and the number of members. The secretarial office reorganized and standardized the style of the Yellow Pages and prepared 25 issues for publication. The Secretary organized and circulated agendas for four ExCo meetings, and wrote and circulated the minutes. During those 2 years the secretarial office organized four postal ballots, practically blocking fax and telephone lines. The office circulated for comment the IFCN ExCo Expense Policy Document. The Secretary requested authorization from delegates to release or otherwise provide mailing lists of their officers. The office invited applications from member societies to organize the 1999 EMG International Congress. These 2 years also saw an abundant exchange of correspondence with the Chairman of the IFCN Rules Committee concerning mainly changes to the IFCN Statute and Bye-Laws. Where possible, in all correspondence to delegates and secretaries of member societies, the office encouraged them to use the Yellow Pages to advertise their activities.

The Secretary organized the presentations at the Kyoto Congress of those societies bidding for the 1999 ICEMGCN. Those societies were Argentina, the Czech Republic and Yugoslavia. At the time of the 1993 Vancouver Congress, the General Assembly requested that the site of the next ICEMGCN should be voted on during the Kyoto Congress. This was different from the usual process in which the ExCo chooses the EMG Congress site upon recommendations made by the EMG Commission and national societies. Kyoto was different in part because the General Assembly chose to meet during this EMG Congress, whereas it usually only met at the quadrennial International Congresses of EEG and Clinical Neurophysiology. By the time of the Kyoto Congress applications had been received from Argentina, the Czech Republic and Yugoslavia to host the next EMG Congress. Each national society presented its proposed congress venue site, proposed budget and registration fees, the names of the organizers, and information about the city and region. The result of the voting was: Argentina (Buenos Aires) 22, Czech Republic (Prague) 39, Yugoslavia (Belgrade) 3. Therefore, the next International Congress of EMG and Clinical Neurophysiology was scheduled for Prague in spring 1999.

12. XIV International Congress of EEG and Clinical Neurophysiology

12.1. 50th anniversary of the International Congresses

The XIV International Congress of EEG and Clinical Neurophysiology celebrated the 50th anniversary International Federation Congresses. It was held in Florence, August 24–29, 1997. The Organizing Committee of International Congress (OCIC) consisted of IFCN officers Carl Lücking (President), Jun Kimura (Past-President), Giuseppe Caruso (Secretary), Paul Despland (Treasurer), and the officers from Italy Roberto Zappoli (Convener), Giancarlo Comi (Secretary), and Domenico de Grandis (Treasurer). Four OCIC meetings were held: in Florence in July 1995, in Kyoto in October 1995, and in Milan and San Francisco in 1996. The budget was about US $1 million. The scientific programme included Plenary Sessions, Special Lectures, Poster Sessions, Seminars, Advanced Courses, Hand-on Workshops, Didactic Lectures, News, Video Demonstrations, and Satellite Symposia. The fellowships for young investigators were raised from US $600 to $1000. Seventy fellowships in total were provided in Florence for fellows not older than 35 years in general.

In the Second Announcement and Call for Abstracts the IFCN-President invited the world community of clinical neurophysiologists to the ancient and famous city of Florence. He emphasized that "the Congress will address all aspects of clinical neurophysiology. The structure of the Congress will be in line of the preceding meetings in offering special and didactic lectures, plenary and poster sessions, advanced courses, seminars, workshops, and satellite symposia. For the first time the presentations within the plenary sessions will be partly chosen from the abstracts. Therefore, all scientists including active young research fellows are kindly asked to submit their papers.

There is no doubt that the field of clinical neurophysiology has experienced many technical advances in the past several decades. But at the same time an increasing amount of experience has been gained in new imaging techniques and applied molecular biology. It is one of the major aims of the International Congress to demonstrate that all these methods compliment rather than mutually exclude one another. In addition, the Congress provides a unique opportunity to review the latest advances in clinical neurophysiology and also the clinical application of the electrophysiological studies. It will be demonstrated that clinical neurophysiology remains an important tool to understand and diagnose disorders of the nervous system."

The 14th ICEEGCN was held at the Pallazo dei Congressi and Centro Affari of Florence. Honorary Presidents were P. Pinelli, E. Lugaresi, C. Ajmone Marsan, T. Okuma, H. Petsche, and A.M. Halliday. The scientific programme included 4 Special Lectures, 9 Didactic Lectures, 27 Plenary Sessions, 15 Breakfast Workshops, 20 Hands-on Workshops, 886 Poster Presentations, and Satellite Symposia. There were about 1500 participants from 45 different countries. All participants were invited to attend the social events, which were an opening ceremony (Appendix 11, Figs. 13 and 14) at the Palazzo Vecchio (the 13th Century City Hall), concert in the Church of Santa Croce, banquet, and a farewell party.

The opening lecture "Mapping the human nervous system in health and disease" was given by J.C. Mazziotta. J. Kimura presented the Kugelberg Lecture on "Principles and pitfalls of nerve conduction studies". The Buchthal Lecture on "Acute and chronic demyelinating polyneuropathy" was presented by W. Trojaborg. The Congress proceedings were published as *Clinical Neurophysiology: From Receptors to Perception*, edited by G. Comi, C.H. Lücking, J. Kimura and P.M. Rossini. That book was

Vol. 50 in the *Electroencephalography and Clinical Neurophysiology Supplement* series, Elsevier, Amsterdam, 1999.

12.2. The opening address of the IFCN President at the Palazzo Vecchio

President Carl Lücking addressed the Opening Ceremony (Appendix 11, Fig. 13):

"On behalf of the IFCN I would like to welcome you to the 14th International congress of EEG and Clinical Neurophysiology. I am pleased and very grateful to see so many neurophysiologists having decided to attend this meeting. Florence is truly a wonderful place and worth visiting. But it is also the outstanding programme which is indeed very attractive. I would like to thank the members of the Scientific Committee and the local organizers, especially Professor Zappoli, the convener, and Prof. Comi, the secretary, for having organized this exciting congress.

This is the 14th International Congress of EEG and Clinical Neurophysiology. Since the first international meeting in London in 1947 under the chairmanship of Lord Adrian, every 4 years an International Congress of EEG and Clinical Neurophysiology has been organized without any exception. Therefore this year we are celebrating the 50th anniversary of the International Congresses of IFCN. This is, however, not identical with the 50th anniversary of the Federation and the EEG Journal. The Federation was founded in 1949 and the first issue of the EEG Journal appeared in the same year. We are looking forward to celebrating that anniversary in Prague in two years.

Until 1961, EEG was the main field of interest of the Federation and at that time there was considerable resistance to the idea of deliberately expanding the scope of the Federation. But when EMGers and ENGers arranged a meeting in Pavia in 1961 and planned to set up their own Federation, the IFCN gave way to an EMG Commission within the Federation and to a direct representation in the Executive Committee. Since that time, an International Congress of EMG and Clinical Neurophysiology is organized every 4 years, with a 2-year interval from the EEG Congress. The meeting in Prague in 1999 will be the 11th International Congress of EMG.

But for some time the size and the scope of both congresses have become virtually the same. And it is obviously becoming more and more anachronistic to separate neurophysiology, the IFCN Congresses, and also the IFCN officers on the basis of EEG and EMG, disregarding the fact that clinical neurophysiology comprises meanwhile several other sub-specialities. During this congress in Florence we have to discuss whether we want to continue having an International Congress virtually every 2 years or only every 4 years as it is provided in our Constitution.

When I look at the program of this congress there is no doubt in my mind that we will have an outstanding meeting. Latest advances in clinical neurophysiology as well as current clinical applications of established electrophysiological studies will be presented. Simultaneous updates of clinical disorders will provide comprehensive statements of pathogenic mechanisms and new therapies. Despite the progress and value of imaging techniques and their use for functional analyses, this congress will demonstrate that clinical neurophysiology remains essential for our ability to understand and diagnose disorders of the nervous system.

It is my pleasure now to officially declare the 14th International Congress of EEG and Clinical Neurophysiology open. And as our Constitution is bilingual I want to add: C'est un grand honneur pour moi d'ouvrir officiellement le Quatorzième Congrès d'EEG et de la Neurophysiologie Clinique."

12.3. Award presentations

The winners of these two awards were selected by the two Editors-in-Chief. The awards consisted of a Certificate and a cheque of US $3500, funded partly by IFCN and partly by Elsevier Science. The awards were named after William Cobb, who served as Editor of the EEG Journal from 1962 to 1973 and as Federation President from 1973 to 1977, and after Mary Brazier, who was Editor of the EEG Journal from 1973 to 1983 and Federation President from 1961 to 1965. During the Opening Ceremony the Cobb Award was presented to Giampiero Zanette (Italy) and the Brazier Award to Daniel Javitt (USA).

The Moruzzi Prize, sponsored by the IFCN and co-sponsored by Elsevier Science, was awarded for the first time. The award — a gold medal — is named after the great Italian neuroscientist Giuseppe Moruzzi, head of the Institute of Physiology in Pisa, who lived from 1910 until 1986. It was presented to Elio Lugaresi (Italy) for his lifetime's devotion to clinical neurophysiology.

12.4. President's report to the General Assembly

President Carl Lücking addressed the General Assembly:

"At the end of my Presidency I would like to give a short report on the main achievements of the Executive Committee during the last 4 years. Two years ago in Kyoto, I already presented an interim report as requested by the General Assembly of Vancouver.

When I assumed the Presidency I was not aware that the Federation had developed towards a difficult situation. It was not before the General Assembly in Vancouver that I realized the Federation was facing a lot of conflicts. The new Executive Committee left Vancouver with several precise requests from the General Assembly. Meanwhile all these proposals and requests have led to amendments of the Statutes and Bye-Laws that already passed the Council or will be voted on in this meeting. The Delegates are informed on a regular basis about the decisions of the Executive Committee and the financial situation.

Due to the excellent work of our Treasurer, Paul Despland, the discipline of all officers, and the important income from the EEG Journal, and despite the number of member societies, who do not pay their annual dues, the IFCN is now in the position to create a foundation as a financial backbone. The idea is to use the interest from this endowment to finance the fellowships and other kinds of support in order to foster the clinical neurophysiology. Paul Despland will provide more details in his report.

Another area of activity was devoted to get new member societies of the IFCN, especially in Eastern Europe, Asia, Latin America, and Africa. We succeeded in having Croatia, Slovakia, and Slovenia as new members from Eastern Europe, Korea and Taiwan from Asia and Cuba from Latin America. New societies have been founded in Costa Rica and Egypt, which will soon apply for membership. Egypt will then be the only African society because unfortunately South Africa has recently cancelled its membership.

There is a new approach to form subgroups of the IFCN member societies in order to organize regional meetings and to standardize neurophysiologic training. Accordingly, IFCN Chapters have been formed in Asia, Europe and Latin America. For each Chapter there is a liaison officer in the IFCN ExCo; the chairman of the Chapter will give an annual personal report to the ExCo. I am convinced that the Chapters will be able to facilitate the contact of the member societies with the ExCo and among each other.

I would like to mention the enormous and successful work of the Editors-in-Chief of our Journal. The number of submitted manuscripts has increased and the quality of the articles is continuously improving. The introduction of Review Articles to the journal will lead to a further increase of acceptance worldwide. Unfortunately, the distribution of the EEG Journal is still limited. This is especially true for the financially weak countries. Last year we started a first campaign by asking companies to be generous enough to provide a certain amount of money that would be used for the subscription to the EEG Journal being sent to the financially disadvantaged countries. Of more than 20 companies only two responded and declined such a sponsorship. Recently we have started a new approach in asking the Delegates of financially weak countries to list key institutes or hospitals where the EEG Journal could be placed in order to be available to neurophysiologists from this area. I will then ask the companies again to be willing to sponsor a limited number of subscriptions directly to these institutes. I hope that the second campaign will be more successful.

It is one of the main goals of the IFCN to foster clinical neurophysiology when, where, and how ever possible. In the past we discussed the formation of a special commission for teaching and for standardizing clinical neurophysiology. The idea was postponed for the time being because of the new Chapters which declared the training as one of their main aims. But for the special issue of repetitive transcranial magnetic stimulation (rTMS) we recently formed a Special Committee under the chairmanship of Mark Hallett. As rTMS is going to be used in different disciplines mainly outside of clinical neurophysiology, the IFCN felt obliged to create this committee that should elaborate standards of techniques and indications of this method.

Looking back on the past 4 years I personally feel that the IFCN ExCo has been successful in stabilizing and enlarging the Federation, in supporting the advances in clinical neurophysiology, and in demonstrating convincingly that clinical neurophysiology remains an indisputable instrument in neuroscience."

12.5. Decision for the 2001 congress site

The General Assembly decided on the site for the IFCN Congress in 2001. The ExCo and the Council favoured eliminating the words EEG and EMG from the title of the congresses, but no definitive decision was made yet. Argentina, Germany, and Yugoslavia presented applications to host the 2001 congress. Germany and Argentina presented last-minute applications. It was decided that bids for the next congress should be submitted at least 6 months before the General Assembly to give more time to evaluate the bids. Presentations to host the 2001 congress were presented by Dr. Medina for Buenos Aires (Argentina), Dr. Deuschl for Berlin (Germany) and Dr. Martinovic for Belgrade (Yugoslavia). Voting representatives present were 88 delegates, society officers, and ExCo members. A majority required 45 votes. In the first round of voting, no site obtained a majority: Argentina 40 votes; Germany 36 votes; Yugoslavia 7 votes. In a run-off ballot 47 were for Argentina and 36 for Germany. The General Assembly declared Argentina the organizer of the 2001 Congress.

12.6. Honorary gavel

The President ended the General Assembly meeting by thanking everyone and passed the Federation's honorary gavel, the Nyoi-Bo, to the new President Marc Nuwer, who awarded certificates to the previous ExCo members as a sign of gratitude for their service to the Federation.

13. Nominating Committee

The Nominating Committee consisted of Jun Kimura (Past-President, Chair), Aurora Constantinovici (Romania), Robert Miller (USA), Juan Santoni (Dominican Rep.). New constitutional restraints were applied for this election cycle. The two Members-at-Large should be from countries different from that of the President, Treasurer, and Secretary. The members of the Nominating Committee should not promote a particular candidate for any office. According the ExCo's own new policies, no member of the ExCo should campaign for or contact Delegates to support any candidate. The principle was that nominations and election should reflect the view of the member societies.

The ExCo for the 1997–2001 Fiscal Period will consist of:

President	Marc R. Nuwer	EEG	Region 1	USA
Past President	Carl H. Lücking	EMG	Region 2	Germany
Secretary	Hiroshi Shibasaki	EMG	Region 1	Japan
Treasurer	Paul A. Despland	EEG	Region 2	Switzerland
Member-at-Large	David Burke	EMG	Region 1	Australia
Member-at-Large	Günther Deuschl	EMG	Region 2	Germany
Editor-in-Chief	Gastone Celesia	EEG	Region 1	USA
Editor-in-Chief	Paolo Rossini	EMG	Region 2	Italy

Wave Length and Action Potentials: History of the IFCN
(Supplements to Clinical Neurophysiology, Vol. 61)
By: M.R. Nuwer and C.H. Lücking

Chapter 14

1997–2001

President: Marc R. Nuwer

The Federation celebrated Golden Anniversaries in 1999. The Prague International Congress marked the 50th anniversary of the founding of the Federation and its Journal. A group of renowned neurophysiologists had organized an international meeting in London in 1947. They discussed the "Formation of a World EEG Organization and the Foundation of an International Journal". This 1947 meeting was considered, in retrospect, as the First International Congress. Its 50th anniversary was celebrated at the 1997 Florence International Congress. Two years later in 1949, at the Second International Congress in Paris, the Federation formally was constituted and the first full set of officers was elected. In the same year the first issue of the Federation's journal, *Electroencephalography and Clinical Neurophysiology,* appeared. The year 1999 also marked the 70th anniversary of H. Berger's first publication on recording the human EEG.

Looking back from 50 years later, the Federation had come a long way. The initial proposal for a federation involved just three societies: in the UK, France and USA. By 50 years later the Federation had 55 member societies on six continents. In 1949, EEG and EMG were used at tertiary and academic medical centers, requiring PhDs to keep the equipment running. By 50 years later, clinical applications were routinely applied in hospitals and medical offices worldwide, and the techniques had expanded to include evoked and event-related potentials, magnetoencephalography, polysomnography, autonomic testing, ultrasound, functional magnetic resonance imaging, and many variations on those themes. The science of clinical neurophysiology broadened to methods too numerous to mention here. Eight Nobel prizes were awarded for scientific advancements in neurophysiology during these years. The field evolved to use terms of microseconds, nanovolts, and femtotesla. Digital methods were replacing many analogue early generation recorders.

Despite changes in techniques and science, the mission of the Federation remained as it was at the beginning. That mission can be summarized as: to discover new knowledge, teach others what has been found, integrate that into a better understanding of nervous system function, to encourage high quality medical care for diagnosing, treating, teaching, and comforting patients, and to train new physicians and scientists to meet the scientific and clinical missions of the Federation. A formal mission statement is included in the Federation Statutes.

To help celebrate this 50th anniversary, the Federation published a new Practice Guidelines book and gave copies to all registrants at the 1999 International Congress.

During this Fiscal Period, five Honorary Fellows were appointed unanimously by the General Assembly. An Honorary Fellow was someone who had rendered important services to the Federation. The Honorary Fellows appointed at this time were Past-Presidents John Desmedt (Belgium), Jun Kimura (Japan), Robert Ellingson (USA), and Robert Naquet (France), and former Editor-in-Chief Gastone Celesia (USA).

During this term, the IFCN Executive Committee (ExCo) was composed of President Marc R. Nuwer (USA), Past-President Carl H. Lücking (Germany), Treasurer Paul A. Despland (Switzerland), Secretary Hiroshi Shibasaki (Japan), Members-at-Large David Burke (Australia) and Günther Deuschl (Germany), and Editors-in-Chief Paolo M. Rossini (Italy) and Mark Hallett (USA) (Appendix 11, Fig. 16).

The Federation continued its move toward unification as a broad discipline covering more than just EEG. In 1990 the Federation changed the official name from *International Federation of Societies for Electroencephalography and Clinical Neurophysiology* (IFSECN) to *International Federation of Clinical Neurophysiology* (IFCN). Building upon that, in this term the IFCN changed the name of its journal from *Electroencephalography and Clinical Neurophysiology* to the simpler name *Clinical Neurophysiology.* The accompanying book series name was changed in the same way to *Clinical Neurophysiology Supplement Series.* Finally, the two separate series of International Congresses were combined and the name changed to *International Congresses of Clinical Neurophysiology.* In this way, the Federation recognized its evolution from its origin in the field of EEG and related techniques to its new expanded position representing a broad discipline, its science, and clinical applications as a recognized medical specialty or subspecialty.

1. Congresses and courses

1.1. Scheduling of meetings

By 1997, the Federation schedule included two separate series of worldwide congresses, three Chapter congresses, plus other sponsored local or regional meetings. One or another occurred once or two each year. In addition, other non-Federation specialty and subspecialty meetings had become more numerous. A consensus opinion was that there were too many meetings.

The two major meetings were the International Congress of EEG and Clinical Neurophysiology (ICEEGCN or the EEG meetings) and the International Congress of EMG and Clinical Neurophysiology (ICEMGCN or the EMG meetings). Each met every 4 years in an alternating pattern with 2 years between congresses. Over time the scientific, clinical and academic disciplines of EEG and EMG had become an intertwined collection of many techniques and applications beyond those first two. The distinction between the two meeting series became blurred with each containing courses, lectures, and presentations on the other topic.

The General Assembly decided to discontinue holding separately named series and combine them into one series simply named the International Congress of Clinical Neurophysiology (ICCN). The new combined series would be held every 4 years. The numerical congress identifying system would be combined. The last meeting in the EMG series would be in 2003 in San Francisco, and that meeting's official name was changed from ICEMGCN to ICCN.

The European Chapter congresses also were held at 2 year intervals. These were known as the European Congress of Clinical Neurophysiology (ECCN). The European Chapter proposed that each Chapter hold its own congress once every 4 years. These Chapter meetings could be held halfway between the quadrennial ICCNs. Together with the ICCN change, this reduced the number of Federation congresses from two per year to one on average.

The Federation also sponsored other local meetings. According to an Executive Committee decision from 1981, there are three levels of Federation meeting support. The first level is "Organized by IFCN in conjunction with [host society]". This level is for the major International and Chapter Congresses. They receive direct grants, loans, and fellowship support. The second level is "Sponsored by the IFCN". This level is for additional regional meetings sponsored by a national member society. They may receive financial support from the Federation. An example is the 1993 Bangkok Symposium on Clinical Neurophysiology. Some are held on specific subspecialty topics. The third level is "Under the auspices of IFCN". This level is for other meetings of interest in the general area of clinical neurophysiology without financial obligation by IFCN. Those meetings are usually organized by another organization.

1.2. Organizing congresses

Each ICCN is supervised by an Organizing Committee for the International Congress (OCIC). This is composed at this point by seven voting members, four from the Federation and three from the Congress's sponsoring national society. The Federation's four members are established in the Rules as the President, Past-President, Secretary and Treasurer. The national society's OCIC members are the Congress's Convener, Secretary and Treasurer. These seven organizers have overall authority for the Congress. The OCIC decides the Congress's dates, hotel sites, schedule of events, major lecturers, budget, and contracts.

Details of collecting registration fees, contracting for hotel space, organizing the exhibit hall, and arranging social events usually are contracted with a Professional Congress Organization (PCO). Each PCO is a business experienced in organizing such a medical or scientific meeting. They bring to the organizing activity the knowledge of local customs, laws, import customs regulations for exhibitors, and personal contacts to facilitate business at a local level.

Some congress details are proposed before the Congress is awarded to a particular national society, for example the city, estimated dates, and convention center. This constrained the OCIC options. To assure that congress details were set wisely from the beginning, both financially and educationally, congress proposers were asked to provide more details of their tentative plans and commitments, not just the name of the city. The Executive Committee in this term screened congress proposals before the General Assembly and asked for more details where needed.

Past congress organizing problems prompted the Executive Committee in this term to increase the details needed from proposers. In one case a PCO hesitated to provide a final financial report and return congress profits to the Federation, doing so only after an extended time. One root cause was the contract signed between the national society and PCO, and that led to greater OCIC attention to the PCO contracts. In another case, the proposed convention center closed for renovation so that the meeting needed to be moved to a hotel that had insufficient size. That prompted a request for a preliminary contract with the proposed site before presentation to the General Assembly. In another case, the PCO itself put a hold on all available hotel sites during the desired time and proposed an exorbitant fee to organize the congress in the city at the time desired. The OCIC needed to move the congress to a different time. The lesson was to have a hold on hotel or convention center space in the name of the congress and to have a tentative agreement with the PCO that includes financial details. In another case, the contracted hotel was under construction, construction was delayed. In that case, the congress moved to a different city. For one congress, a substantial cost overrun was attributed to expensive contract details with the convention center that had not been properly budgeted. Given these experiences, a two-stage process was desired. Before being awarded a congress franchise, proposers needed to be more specific about the site, PCO, and budget and have preliminary contracts for those details.

This affected the congress proposal process. National societies were invited to submit bids at least 6 months before an ICCN. Last moment bids no longer would be allowed. Proposals provided details of dates, city, site, hotels, budget, registration fee, possible social events, national society's organizers, PCO business, and preliminary contractual financial arrangements. The Executive Committee reviewed the proposals and approved for presentation those with sufficient, satisfactory detail. Bids then could be presented to the General Assembly meeting at a congress. Each bidding society was given a defined amount of time to present video and business details. Once the General Assembly awarded a bid, the OCIC still needed to review and approve the congress's business and organizational details.

This expanded bid process was used during the 1997–2001 fiscal period to prescreen the 2006 congress bids presented to the 2001 ICCN General Assembly. In addition, a similar process was used at the 1999 Prague ICEMGCN, at which the General Assembly voted on the 2003 EMG Congress sites. The latter vote broke from tradition because EMG sites previously had been chosen directly by the Executive Committee. Bringing the choice to the General Assembly was consistent with the movement to unify the congresses as ICCN meetings. In both cases, an Executive Committee member presented a review to the General Assembly of each bid's strengths and weaknesses.

1.3. Named lectureships

A decade earlier the 1990 Rio de Janeiro General Assembly had endorsed Past-President John Desmedt's proposal for three named lectures at the quadrennial EEG congresses. The 1997 congresses considered a fourth lecture named after EMG pioneer Fritz Buchthal. EMG machine manufacturer Dantec wished to sponsor this. This opened a debate about additional named lectureships. Some considered that the formal named lectureships should honor only those pioneers who were no longer alive, and Fritz Buchthal was in an active retirement — still very much alive and holding discussions at meetings with those who wished to hear his stories about development of EMG "back in the early days".

A member society survey inquired about naming the international congress lectureships. Responses of 38 member societies were divided equally on whether new lectureships could be created and named after founders who still were alive. The societies were evenly divided also about whether to aim for geographic balance in these honors. There was no clear consensus about how many named lectureships to have, with preferences ranging between 2 and 5, or whether a named lectureship should be at every congress or alternate at every other congress. Overall there was no consensus.

This discussion continued on and off for over a decade. One option for holding a half dozen named lectureships was the international congresses held every 2 years, alternating between EMG and EEG meetings. That allowed for more possible different names. That option disappeared with the unification of the congresses during this term. With only half as many opportunities, the discussion dissipated and left the previously endorsed Adrian, Berger and Kugelberg lectures.

1.4. International Congress of EMG and Clinical Neurophysiology 1999

The XI International Congress of EMG and Clinical Neurophysiology was held in Prague, Czech Republic in September 1999. The Congress had 1200 registrants, and received over 800 abstracts. Young Investigator Fellowships were awarded to 70 young physicians and scientists. A group of 160 speakers were invited to lecture at organized courses and symposia. The program included 3 Honorary Lectures, 18 Main Sessions, 18 Topical Seminars, 17 Morning meetings, 5 Free Communication Sessions, 37 Poster Sessions, 16 Teaching Courses, and a Satellite Symposium and Annual Meeting of the International Society for Transcranial Stimulation (ISTS). The social program was full of highlights with the opening ceremony and welcome party in the Concert Hall *Rudolfinum* in a splendid New-Renaissance style, a concert in *St. Nicholas*, a famous Prague Baroque church, and the farewell dinner on the Slavonic Island in the middle of the Vltava River.

The Czech Society of Clinical Neurophysiology organized the congress under the able leadership of Convener Zdenek Ambler, Secretary Soňă Nevšímalová and Treasurer Zdenek Kadanka, together with the IFCN Officers Marc R. Nuwer,

Carl H. Lücking, Hiroshi Shibasaki, and Paul A. Despland (see Appendix 11, Fig. 20). Honorary Presidents were Jun Kimura (Japan), Donald Saunders (USA), Erik Stålberg (Sweden), and Frantisek Véle (Czech Rep.). The Czech Medical Association served as the professional organizer under the executive meeting leadership of Helena Lonekova. The American Clinical Neurophysiology Society sponsored Continuing Medical Education (CME).

To celebrate the 50th anniversary of the 1949 International Congress of EEG and Clinical Neurophysiology, special 50th Anniversary Awards were made to six young investigators who delivered platform presentations at a 50th Anniversary Symposium. Over 150 applications were entered into this competition. The local organizers selected 30 semifinalists and the Executive Committee chose the winning abstracts. Each winner received a certificate, a cash award, and a free 1-year subscription to the journal Clinical Neurophysiology, all provided by the Federation's publisher, Elsevier. Award recipients were A. Brusa (Italy and UK), R. Jech (Czech Republic), V. Marchand-Pauvert (France), S. Ohara (Japan), K. Rosenkranz (Germany), and M. Valeriani (Italy).

Congress registrants were given a complementary copy of the new Federation guideline book, *Recommendations for the Practice of Clinical Neurophysiology*. This book was a compendium of older and new practice guidelines brought together under the able leadership and editing of Andrew Eisen and Guenther Deuschl.

Abstracts were published in the special issue of the journal *Clinical Neurophysiology*. This led to one of the interesting but little known stories about this meeting. The abstract books were published in Western Europe and shipped by truck to the Prague meeting. They were scheduled to arrive at the meeting hotel days before the meeting. At the border to the Czech Republic, the truck was turned back because it lacked one of the necessary paper forms for importing these books across the border. On the day before the meeting, the books were on the truck heading back to Amsterdam. Meeting organizers scrambled to intercept the truck and divert it to an airport. Proper paperwork was completed and faxed to the airport, and arrangements were made to ship the books by air to Prague. As the meeting registration opened just before the evening opening reception, the books were still en route to Prague. Organizers simply notified the registrants to pick up their abstract books the next morning at the registration desk. Overnight, the books arrived and were available in the morning. Registrants were generally unaware of this adventure. As a more general observation, congresses have these interesting issues out of sight of the meeting attendees, who may be unaware of the amount of detail and problem solving needed to accomplish a major meeting.

The Prague Congress also incurred an unanticipated change in location. The Prague Convention Center, the originally intended meeting site, was closed for renovation. With the Convention Center closed, there was no other optimal site in Prague for a meeting of our size. The Hilton, the best alternate site, was smaller than the usual venue. To use the Hilton, temporary tent structures were built in a parking lot to house exhibits and certain other meeting activities. Even with the suboptimal location, exhibit space was quickly filled and overflow space was arranged in other hotel common space.

The major honorary lectures included the Kugelberg lecture on "Neurophysiological studies of collateral reinnervation in man", delivered by Erik Stålberg (Sweden). Roger Broughton (Canada) gave the Berger Lecture on "The chronobiology of sleep/wake and of sleepiness/alertness states in normal and sleep disordered human subjects". The honorary Adrian lecture was delivered by Mark Hallett (USA), asking "Can EEG coherence help solve the binding problem"? The many symposia were collected together and published as the book, *Clinical Neurophysiology at the Beginning of the 21st Century,* Vol. 53 of the Clinical Neurophysiology

Supplement Series books, edited by Z. Ambler, S. Nevšímalová, Z. Kadanka, and P. Rossini.

Meeting jointly with other societies is a suitable way to help with the widely acknowledged problem of too many meetings. It also encourages exchange of ideas among groups who often travel to different meetings. Just prior to the congress meeting the ISTS held a satellite session on transcranial cortical stimulation science and clinical applications. The congress overlapped 1 day with the 23rd International Epilepsy Congress of the International League Against Epilepsy (ILAE) on Saturday September 11, just at the end of the ICEMGCN. The International Epilepsy Congress continued on the subsequent days. The overlapping day was a joint meeting of the two organizations. The ILAE and Federation jointly advertised the two meetings, increasing the visibility and attendance at each. The joint meeting day was on a Jewish holiday, Rosh Hashanah. Arrangements were made to open four downtown Prague synagogues for services for those who wished to attend. The Epilepsy meeting used the Hilton as a hotel but held its sessions at a temporarily renovated fairgrounds venue. Together with the ILAE and other joint and satellite meetings, over 4000 neurologists, clinical neurophysiologists, neuroscientists and others attended the collected Prague meetings. The years long good working relationships between ILAE and the Federation was enhanced by the curious coincidence that the two organizations' presidents were clinical and academic colleagues together at UCLA. Occasional organizational issues were resolved by walking 10 m down the hall to discuss the problem face to face.

1.5. International Congress of Clinical Neurophysiology 2001

The XV ICCN was held in Buenos Aires, Argentina, in May 16–20, 2001 in the Sheraton Buenos Aires Hotel and Convention Center and in the Marriott Plaza Hotel. The Federation Congress attracted 900 registrants and received over 400 abstracts, an excellent size for a Latin American congress site. Young Investigator Fellowships were awarded to 75 young physicians and scientists. The program included: Named Lectures, Advanced Courses, Basic Courses, Teaching Courses, Symposia, Workshops, Video Presentations, and Poster Sessions. A group of 130 speakers were invited to lecture at organized courses and symposia. The Sociedad Argentina de EEG y Neurofisiologia Clinica organized the congress under the able leadership of Convener Carlos Medina, Treasurer Alicia Cueto, Secretary Roberto Reisin, Roberto Sicca (Scientific Committee) together with the IFCN Officers Marc Nuwer, Carl Lücking, Hiroshi Shibasaki, and Paul Despland (Appendix 11, Fig. 19). Dr. Reisin served as the principal physician organizer. Ana Juan, a Buenos Aires professional congress organizer, was chosen eventually to serve as the business organizer for the meeting. The American Clinical Neurophysiology Society provided CME credits for the congress.

Building on the successes of the tandem Prague Congress, the meeting was planned to be joint with the International Epilepsy Congress of the ILAE and International Bureau of Epilepsy (IBE). Former IBE president Richard Holmes coordinated the joint events and budgets. The International Epilepsy Congress met in Buenos Aires May 14–18 at the same site, a 2-day overlap with the ICCN. Three additional affiliated symposia were integrated into the ICCN. These were the VII International Symposium of Spinal Cord Monitoring (ISSCM), the seventh International Evoked Potential Symposium EP7, and the International Transcranial Magnetic Stimulation.

The VII ISSCM meeting drew surgeons and anesthesiologists in addition to clinical neurophysiologists. Organizers include neurophysiologists Vedran Deletis and David Burke, and orthopedic surgeon Tetsuya Tamaki designed a 2-day meeting standard for ISSCM series meetings. The ISSCM covered the topics of intraoperative motor, somatosensory and auditory evoked potential monitoring, their known physiology and clinical applications.

The 7th International Evoked Potential Symposium (EP7) organizer, Colin Barber, designed a meeting for neurophysiologists, audiologists and other physicians on modern topics in evoked and event-related potentials. EP7 activities were held throughout the ICCN including an all-day session on 1 day.

The International Transcranial Magnetic Stimulation Symposium was organized with the help of Leo Cohen, Eric Wasserman and Martín Segura. The sessions were designed to draw additional neurophysiologists as well as psychiatrists interested in this technique. This was a meeting in the series of International Symposia of Transcranial Stimulation (ISTS). The sessions covered enhancement and depression of cortical excitability, cortical plasticity, and studies of cognitive processes. Clinical topics were the use of transcortical stimulation in epilepsy, movement disorders, and psychiatry.

Brazier and Cobb Awards were given at the Opening Ceremony. The competition was drawn from among manuscripts submitted to the journal by young investigators. The honorary lectures included the Kugelberg lecture delivered by Carl H. Lücking (Freiburg) on "The role of the basal ganglia in the control of tremor and epilepsy". The Berger lecture on "Cognition, gamma oscillations and neuronal synchrony" was given by Wolf Singer (Frankfurt). The symposia were collectively published as *Advances in Clinical Neurophysiology,* Vol. 54 in the *Clinical Neurophysiology Supplement Series*, edited by R.C. Reisin, M.R. Nuwer, M. Hallett, and C. Medina.

The General Assembly considered the 2006 ICCN site (see Appendix 11, Fig. 24). Two candidate sites submitted bids that were prescreened by the Executive Committee and judged to be suitable for presentation. The bids were for an Edinburgh Congress in September, received from the British Society for Clinical Neurophysiology, and for a Lausanne Congress in August received from the Swiss Society for Clinical Neurophysiology. Executive Committee member David Burke prepared comments on the strengths and weaknesses of the two proposals. In a close vote, Edinburgh was chosen as the site for the 2006 ICCN.

The social program was excellent with opening and closing ceremonies in the Sheraton Hotel, a welcome party in the Marriott Hotel, an Argentinian Night with an exciting dinner and tango show. Social tours were organized to view this "Paris of Latin America" with its wide avenues and parks, and to visit the famous Colón Theater Opera House. Some attendees were able to take the side trip to Iguassu Falls or tours of the semi-tropical Tigre and Paraná River delta region.

2. Publications

1999 marked the 50th Anniversary of the journal *Electroencephalography and Clinical Neurophysiology*. The journal continued to be the premier publication in clinical neurophysiology worldwide, with the best impact factor of any journal in our specialty area. Impact factor is the most common scale for measuring the quality of scientific reports published in a journal. It is related to how often the reports are cited by other publications. By 1999 the journal's impact factor was 2.86, the best of any journal in this discipline and an excellent number for any scientific publication. This level is nearly twice the impact factor achieved by the journal a decade earlier. The journal needed to choose carefully among the manuscripts submitted so as to stay within its allotted pages and to maintain high quality of published reports.

By 1999, submission acceptance rate was 50% for 500 manuscripts received. The acceptance rate was gradually dropping and submission volume continued to grow. A greater variety of manuscripts were published as the field expanded to include manuscripts dealing with the physiology of motor control and movement disorders, as well as psychophysiology, cognitive neuroscience, and event-related potentials. The traditional topic of routine EEG gradually decreased.

This term saw a change in the journals name, consolidation of its three separate titles, and initiation of electronic publishing. Topics of discussion remained how best to balance high quality while allowing sufficient pages. Color pages were increased to add quality and attractiveness.

The two Editors-in-Chief were Paolo Rossini in Europe, and Gastone Gelesia through 1999 and Mark Hallett beginning in 2000 in America. Elsevier's primary contact was manager Tatjana Fischer-Driessen of Amsterdam.

2.1. Consolidating journal sections

For over a decade, the journal was composed of three separate titles. The original journal series *Electroencephalography and Clinical Neurophysiology* was published in 12 issues annually. A section subtitled *Evoked Potentials* was published in six issues annually. A third section subtitled *Electromyography & Motor Control* also was published in six issues annually. These three sections amounted to 24 issues per year.

The Federation sought to improve problems with time to publish an accepted manuscript, a need for more pages annually, and an imbalance among the pages needed for the three sections. A solution was found in combining the issues together into 12 unified, longer issues per year. This reduced publication delay because two sections had been published only every other month. Now those manuscripts could be published a month earlier. By reducing issues the publisher reduced costs, and those cost savings could be converted into extra journal pages. This also would remove differences in acceptance rates, publication time, and pages needed among the sections.

2.2. Title change

The journal title was changed to *Clinical Neurophysiology*. The 50th anniversary was considered a good opportunity to do so. This was a time to reflect on not only our past but also the future. The journal should aim for broad set of issues in clinical neurophysiology, including consciousness, pain and emotion, cognitive neuroscience, central control of autonomic regulation, magnetoencephalography, neurosonology, and functional imaging. Whereas the discipline began with EEG, it had grown far beyond that technique and its variations. The title change recognized that evolution.

This change was consistent with other name changes. In 1990 the Federation's name was shortened from IFSECN to the IFCN. A decade later, the meetings' names were shortened from International Congress of Electroencephalography and Clinical Neurophysiology and International Congress of Electromyography and Clinical Neurophysiology to the new name International Congress of Clinical Neurophysiology. It seemed appropriate for the journal to participate in this expanded vision of the Federation. The Federation is a broad discipline of medicine and science, and this change de-emphasized a focus on one technique. Many national societies also adopted this vision and accomplished an analogous name change.

The Rules Committee reported on Statutes and Bye-Law changes needed to accomplish the journal name change. Advice was sought from the national societies. Generally this was met with enthusiasm from national societies, who recognized the historical ties to the old name but the need to move forward into the 21st Century. The only expression of concern came from the French society, who noted the proposed name's similarity to their national society's journal's name, *Neurophysiologie Clinique: Clinical Neurophysiology*, abbreviated as *Neurophysiol. Clin.* The Federation and the publisher Elsevier agreed to do whatever they could to avoid confusion.

2.3. A new cover

The name change required a cover change, at least a modest one. Other concomitant changes were considered. The new cover emphasized the two words *Clinical Neurophysiology* in a large font size. The IFCN logo appeared more as a subtle watermark rather than in bold black. A figure from a current issue article would be published on the front cover, with a subtitle referencing the manuscript from which the figure was taken. The color was changed from the previous beige to a warmer brighter color. Several color schemes were considered, and the one chosen was sun yellow with a sky blue top banner. This color scheme was carried further as the journal's branding for its other products, for example Supplement Series books, the Handbook series, the web page, and advertisements.

2.4. Editors-in-Chief

The end of 1999 marked a transition in the Editor-in-Chief for the Western region. At this time, the Federation had two Editors-in-Chief. One received manuscripts from the Eastern region, composed of Europe, Africa, and Asia (except Japan). The other received manuscripts from the Western region, composed of The Americas, Japan, and Australasia. This practice derived from the days when overseas mail delivery was slow and expensive. An expeditious way to solve the speed and cost problem had been to have two sites to which manuscripts could be sent for review, one site in Europe and another in the Western hemisphere. In the early days, the Editor-in-Chief was in one region and an Editor was in the other. The Editor-in-Chief took overall publications responsibility and attended Executive Committee meetings on behalf of the journal. Over time, this situation evolved into two persons both of whom held the title Editor-in-Chief, one for each region. Both attended Executive Committee meetings.

The Prague 1999 Congress marked the end of Gastone Celesia's term as Western region Editor-in-Chief. In January 2000 the mantle of responsibility passed to Mark Hallett, well known to the Federation for his scientific and educational work over the decades, and his then current leadership role in Clinical Neurophysiology at the US National Institutes of Health. Paolo Rossini continued to serve as the Editor-in-Chief for the journal's European office.

Before leaving his post, Gastone Celesia suggested converting back to a single Editor-in-Chief. He noted that the time of slow, expensive overseas mail was being replaced by instantaneous worldwide electronic submission and review. Paolo Rossini, the other Editor-in-Chief, agreed with this and went further. He suggested that no new European office Editor-in-Chief be appointed at the end of his term. Instead a single office would cover the Editor-in-Chief role from that time forward.

Advantages of returning to a single unified Editor-in-Chief included:

- Reduce confusion when one Editor assumes the other has taken care of an issue.
- Economies of scale.
- Motivation regarding clear leadership.
- Better position with a single voice in dealing with the publisher.
- Better staffed office with a unified budget.
- Cost saving from one fewer person attending distant Executive Committee meetings.
- Editor-in-Chief should attend OCIC meeting, preferably one person instead of two.

A disadvantage was that the Editor-in-Chief would have less contact with the other area or with subspecialty disciplines within clinical neurophysiology. This was remedied partially by appointing a half dozen Associate Editors carefully chosen so as to have at least one from each of several geographic regions and one from each of several subspecialty disciplines.

2.5. Three journal boards

The Federation Executive Committee's role for the journal was renamed the Executive Board. The role was to oversee the business side of the journal and other Federation publications. This board should not interfere with the editorial decisions of the Editor-in-Chief. The Editor-in-Chief remains operationally in charge of routine journal function. The Executive Board oversees issues such as the finances, contacts, and major issues of journal operations. The Executive Board appoints and can remove the Editor-in-Chief or any subordinate journal editors such as the Associate Editors, Consulting Editors, and Book Editor. The Editor-in-Chief brings to the Executive Board, for their advice and consent, his or her nominations for subordinate Editorial positions. This policy helped clarify the relative relationships of the board and editors, an issue that had been controversial a decade earlier.

The Board of Consulting Editors was renamed the Editorial Board. Both new board nomenclatures took effect on the journal inside cover in January 1999. Both changes cleared up ongoing confusion in the use of terms.

A new Journal Liaison Board was created. To promote the journal better within our member societies, Mark Hallett and Paolo Rossini established a board of journal representatives. This Journal Liaison Board is separate from the Editorial Board. Each Federation member society was asked to appoint one representative. Terms were limited to encourage rotation of this responsibility. The representatives are charged with reporting journal issues to their society, promoting increased individual subscriptions by society members, and reporting back to the journal Editors-in-Chief about journal-related issues from their society. In turn, each representative receives a complimentary individual subscription to the journal.

2.6. Celebrating 50 years

To celebrate the 50 years anniversary of the journal, extra events were scheduled at the 1999 Prague Congress. A celebration book was planned initially with reprinting of 25 previously published, historically significant journal articles with comments about the significance of each article. The book would be offered for sale and given out free to each registrant at the Prague Congress. Over time, the scope of the celebration book changed. In its place was substituted a new Practice Guidelines book that was already in development under the editorship of Guenther Deuschl and Andrew Eisen. A reason to change in scope was pressure of time to accomplish the initially proposed scope before the Prague congress.

Publisher Elsevier sponsored a 50th Anniversary Symposium at the Prague Congress. Elsevier provided 6 US $1000 monetary awards. These awards went to young physicians, up to 40 years of age, who made presentations at this plenary symposium. Awardees were chosen from among abstracts submitted to the meeting.

2.7. Entering the electronic era

When the name change was initiated, the manuscript volume increased. In 1998 before the name change, the publisher had received 178 accepted manuscripts. In the first 8 months of 1999 with the new name, 230 manuscripts already were accepted. The system for processing manuscripts needed improvement. Editorial time was 26 weeks for receipt, review, revision, and decision. The production time, from the arrival at Elsevier to publishing, was another 25 weeks. Consolidation of the three sections into one decreased this to 15 weeks. Electronic submission should substantially reduce editorial time and further speed production time. The publisher at this time was testing an electronic system with another of its journals *Brain Research*. The Smart Works software for electronic submission was scheduled to begin in January 2001. The review process would be done electronically by Internet. Unfortunately the system encountered operational problems and delays. When the system was implemented for *Clinical Neurophysiology*, it still needed improvement. Eventually this whole Smart Works system was replaced by the software system Editorial Manager, which continues to be used effectively to this day. Editorial and publication times became much shorter. Decision times dropped from 126 days to 42 days from manuscript arrival.

Elsevier reported its plans to publish electronically its neuroscience journals beginning around 2000. Libraries would be asked to subscribe to the electronic journal service. Concomitant major reductions in library subscriptions to print issues were expected. Physicians, scientists and students would be able to access the electronic subscriptions through their local library. Personal electronic subscriptions would also be made available. Considerable worry was expressed about the future of publishers worldwide when the web and electronic publishing replace print publishing.

At the same time, the Federation was moving into the 21st Century by establishing a website. The IFCN Secretary had established an initial website at his own university in 1998. Elsevier agreed to host and maintain a more formal site that could continue uninterrupted even when the Executive Committee membership changed. Advertisements on the website were debated, with sponsors possibly linking back to their own home pages. The IFCN Secretary would serve as the web site supervisor even when Elsevier took over hosting the site.

2.8. Journal content

Review articles were increasing in number. These were popular with the readers and were well cited. Major invited lecturers at congresses were asked to submit a review article to the journal. Review articles also were solicited from other senior leaders in their respective subspecialty fields. Each underwent standard peer review. The Editors-in-Chief aimed for one invited review article in each issue.

Editorial comment opportunities were sought when research reports were sent for review. Each reviewer was asked if editorial comments would be helpful or needed. The Editor would then assign a person to write editorial comments and may use one of the reviewers for this purpose. These editorial comments could appear at the front of the journal, separate from the article itself.

Journal page space traditionally was used to publish abstracts from member national societies' meetings. This took a progressively larger number of pages over the decades of this practice. Suggestions were considered about how abstracts would be published. The Executive Committee, in its role as the Journal Executive Board, decided to publish an annual December 13th issue to be mailed along with the 12th regular journal issue. Abstracts should be submitted no more than 6 months after a meeting. Eventually that plan was rescinded because too many abstracts were published more than a year after the meeting at which they were presented.

The abstract books for ICCN and ECCN Congresses would appear as supplemental journal issues, published at an additional cost to each congress. Congress organizers could choose whether the issue would be sent out to all subscribers or delivered only for the congress registrants. The smaller chapter congresses in Asia–Oceania and Latin America might be included in the regular issue's abstract collection, since they were smaller and more manageable.

The journal decided to accept and encourage Letters to the Editor. These would be in response to recent journal publications, not as a substitute for Brief Communications. They would appear at the end of an issue. They would appear in a smaller font size than usual journal articles and run one after another consecutively without page breaks. Letters assisted to refine areas of controversy, clarified methods and conclusions, allowed others to draw different conclusions from the data, and pointed to other publications on that topic.

Difficulty with English language use continued as a problem for submitted manuscripts. Corrections were accomplished at several stages. Reviewers occasionally contributed needed changes. It was unclear who was responsible for thoroughly vetting word use, grammar and spelling in each manuscript — the editor or the publisher. A sample of accepted manuscripts confirmed continuing problems. A quality improvement process focused on manuscripts submitted by non-English speaking authors as reviewed by English speaking MD or PhD neurophysiologists. Each reviewer was asked to indicate whether a particular manuscript needed extra attention to language editing. Elsevier decided to give the editorial offices funding for manuscript language editing before manuscripts are submitted to Elsevier.

The Yellow Pages are a section at the end of each issue that prints society news and meeting announcements. The IFCN Secretary submits them as camera-ready copy. Using smaller fonts shortened the section. The difference in pages was converted to white pages, allowing publications of slightly more manuscripts. Some announcements were judged inappropriate for our journal. Several principles for announcement inclusion were: accept any IFCN member societies announcements, accept announcements for clinical neurophysiology meetings organized by other groups, and for other meetings the IFCN Secretary judges the merit or seeks advice from other Executive Committee members.

Supplemental journal issues were optional. Abstracts of the ICCN or ECCN ordinarily were published as a supplemental journal issue. Satellite symposia to the ICCN or ECCN could publish a supplement for abstracts, or for review articles or research reports based on their symposium. Other requests for supplemental issues would be judged individually. The Editors-in-Chief would decide about these supplemental issues, or may bring them to the Executive Board for advice. The organization requesting a supplemental issue was responsible for paying the publication costs.

2.9. Reduced member subscription prices

Elsevier agreed to reduce the individual subscription price very substantially for members of Federation member societies. A new annual price for 2001 was set at US $130.00. For this price, the Federation would collect subscription payments and submit the collected list and payment to the publisher. An independent office was sought to collect those subscription fees. Bids were solicited from prospective vendors in the US and Europe. The winning bid was from a small US association executive firm. Society members were encouraged to take advantage of this reduced subscription price. In addition, the first 200 persons to sign up for this new subscription price received a copy of the recent book *Recommendations for the Practice of Clinical Neurophysiology: Guidelines of the International Federation of Clinical Neurophysiology* at no additional cost.

To encourage further these reduced subscription prices, the Executive Committee encouraged societies to sign up their entire membership for subscriptions at a price even lower than the individual prices. Contacts were pursued first in Japan, Germany and Italy, and some societies did contract for this deeply discounted package subscription relationship. The journal became an official journal for those societies.

2.10. Recommendations for the Practice of Clinical Neurophysiology: Guidelines of the International Federation of Clinical Neurophysiology

At the beginning of the term, the Executive Committee agreed to publish recent practice guidelines as a compendium book. A previous practice guidelines compendium, published in 1983, was well received at that time. Many guidelines had been developed and approved by the Federation since then.

The Executive Committee appointed Andrew Eisen (Canada) and Guenther Deuschl (Germany) as book editors. A contract with Elsevier called for the books to be ready for the 1999 Prague ICEMGCN. The Federation agreed to pay for the printing, since Elsevier was not interested in separately selling the book on the open market. It was designated as Vol. 52 in the *Electroencephalography and Clinical Neurophysiology Supplement Series* of books. Many libraries around the world had standing orders for that book series and automatically would purchase copies.

Drs. Deuschl and Eisen collected the various Federation Practice Guidelines adopted since 1981, the last year in which reports were included in the 1983 compendium. Additional documents were included to round out the collection to cover most current areas of clinical application.

The book was published on time and given free to all registrants at the Prague 50th Anniversary Congress. Additional books were given to fellows at subsequent congresses, to individuals who subscribed to the journal, and to hospitals and societies from economically disadvantaged regions.

The Federation retained the book's copyright with an explicit contract clause about translations. The Federation retained sole authority to translate the book into other languages and publish the translations with any publisher. National societies and Chapters were given the opportunity to translate the book into their language, print or publish the translation at their own expense, and to keep any proceeds from selling that book. Societies that share a language were encouraged to coordinate or agree upon these translation endeavors. The Société de Neurophysiologie Clinique de Langue Française organized and published a translation into French with participation of Belgian and Swiss neurophysiologists.

2.11. Handbook of Clinical Neurophysiology

The Executive Committee decided to publish a new Handbook series. Previously the Federation published an extended series of books in the 1970s known as the *Handbook of Electroencephalography and Clinical Neurophysiology*. This was a collection of reviews of the academic field of clinical neurophysiology. They were drafted by individuals and small working groups established by the Federation in a process dating to the 1969 San Diego ICEEGCN meeting. Former IFSECN President Antoine Rémond served as the primary series editor. A short Revised Handbook series appeared a decade later, with Antoine Rémond in an encore role as series editor.

The name of the new series was shortened to *Handbook of Clinical Neurophysiology*. This name change paralleled the movement to drop from other Federation names the technique-specific term *Electroencephalography*.

Jasper Daube (USA) and François Mauguière (France) were appointed as book series editors. Most individual volumes would focus on a particular disease and discussed the neurophysiology techniques that can be useful for diagnosis or better understanding of the pathophysiology of disease. Emphasis was on volumes on specific areas of clinical interest, for example epilepsy. This disease-oriented approach contrasted with the Practice Guideline book that is technique-oriented. The editors proposed publishing two volumes annually for 5 years. Affiliated physiological techniques can easily be included in the disease-oriented books, including techniques not covered in the Practice Guidelines book. Examples of these additional techniques were magnetoencephalography and function neuroimaging.

2.12. Supplement Series

The *Electroencephalography and Clinical Neurophysiology Supplement Series* continued to produce books, including the Congress Symposium book for the Florence 1997 Congress, the 1998 International Evoked Potential Symposium book, and the Prague 1999 Congress book. Other books published in this series were based on specific topics or other meetings. Topics were proposed ad hoc, some through the Federation and others coming from Elsevier based on the interests of specific individuals. An advantage of this series for book editors and authors is that the series already has a wide existing distribution through subscription lists to individuals and medical libraries.

The series was renamed *Clinical Neurophysiology Supplement Series* in keeping with the movement to change names of other publications and congresses. The series has no overall named editor. The Executive Committee approves new titles in the series. Individual volume editors then work directly with Elsevier to produce the book.

3. Chapters

During this Federation term, considerable progress was made to establish and organize Chapters in Europe, Asia–Oceania and Latin America. Development of regional chapters advanced several Federation goals. This continued the Chapter organizational efforts begun in the previous term by then IFCN President Carl Lücking and that Executive Committee.

3.1. Organizing chapters

Many physicians, scientists and trainees found it difficult to travel to international meetings every other year. The Executive Committee and General Assembly developed the chapters to take educational and scientific opportunities to more convenient locations. Regional chapters gave a better voice within the Federation to neurophysiologists who share common interests in their geographic region. In Latin America, the region also shared a common language among a majority of societies. In Europe, political and educational issues in clinical neurophysiology were best handled through a regional organization.

These regional organizations were best accomplished as a part of the Federation rather than as individual stand-alone organizations. In the formulation of their place in the Federation, Chapters were viewed to give them considerable discretion in their own activities. They commission and oversee their own Chapter congresses. At the same time, they need to work within the aims of the Federation in general and should not compete directly with each other, with the national societies, or with the Federation's global activities. To help keep a suitable balance, each Chapter drafted its own Bye-Laws. Those Bye-Laws are considered Federation Bye-Laws, subject to ratification by the Federation General Assembly. The Federation Rules Committee serves as the arbiter of conflicts between the Executive Committee and Chapters, and among the several Chapters. The Chapters were asked to keep the other parts of the Federation informed of their activities, congresses and other meetings through their semi-annual reports to the Executive Committee, summaries of which are included in the periodic reports to all Delegates. Chapters were encouraged to post their congresses and meetings in the journal's Yellow Pages, so individuals worldwide can know about a Chapter's meetings.

Two initiating events led to the development of Chapters. These were the needs of Latin American neurophysiologists as championed by Chilean delegate Nelly Chiofalo, and the movement in Europe for an organization to perpetuate the periodic European Clinical Neurophysiology meetings.

The old Latin American Clinical Neurophysiology Society had been removed from the Federation at the 1985 London ICEEGCN General Assembly meeting. This was based on two reasons. First, that society had not paid Federation dues for many years. Second, many members of that society were simultaneously members of a national society, giving them a kind of double vote in Federation activities. Yet, that Latin American Society had served as the only vehicle for participation for members who did not have a national society. Once the Latin American Society was excluded from the Federation, they had no home or voice — not even a clear way to communicate about upcoming congresses.

Forming a national society was not a possible option for those who had an insufficient number of neurophysiologists in their country. Belonging to another country's national society was possible for some, but not others, and seemed to be an artificial solution. Some sort of multinational organization was needed to include these neurophysiologists in some way. Yet, a multinational organization could stifle creation of new national societies.

At the same time in Europe, a process was underway to consolidate medical policies across the European Community. Neurophysiology needed a voice there to present its vision of how clinical neurophysiology should evolve in this new European organization. European clinical neurophysiologists had a European Congress series and desired an organization to perpetuate these meetings in an organized way. Both of these needs came together in a wish to form some sort of European Clinical Neurophysiology organization.

Discussions about both issues were underway during the previous Federation Fiscal Period 1993–1997. The discussions involved many individuals, and chief among whom were Federation Presidents Carl Lücking and Marc Nuwer, Chilean delegate Nelly Chiofalo, Editor-in-Chief Gastone Celesia, and former Editor-in-Chief François Mauguière. The various needs were best resolved by developing a new kind of Federation body, one establishing a body to address region needs.

3.2. Guiding principles for Chapters

Several guiding principles were defined for establishment of Chapters. The national societies in each region needed to be involved in the new bodies, so as to minimize the chances of conflict between a Chapter and its national societies. To do so, the new bodies should have a General Assembly constituting representatives from each Federation member national society in their region. Each regional body would need its own Executive Committee to organize and implement activities. Each would need funds for their operations, which could be drawn from any of several sources. Funds could come from regional congress profits, transfers from the Federation treasury, or individual profitable projects. Transfers from the Federation treasury would be at the discretion of the Federation Executive Committee. Projects could include publications of Practice Guidelines translations or other books. The regional bodies should not compete with the Federation's journal by establishing their own journals. Instead, the journal *Clinical Neurophysiology* should be recognized as the official journal of each Chapter.

The Federation has some guiding principles to which each Chapter should adhere. There is an annual audit of the income, expenses, and accounts of the Federation. The Rules Committee resolves conflicts among organizations within the Federation, and that should include the Chapters. Even if a Chapter had its own internal Rules Committee, the Federation Rules Committee should have the final say to resolve disagreements. Appeals, in the form of rules changes, still can be brought to the floor of the Federation General Assembly, the body that oversees most broadly the Federation's organization and rules.

Erik Stålberg, the founding president of the European Chapter, made further suggestions to avoid conflicts in timing between regional and global congresses. The suggestion was to reduce the ICCN meetings to once every 4 years as a unified congress, instead of every 2 years in two series of alternating EEG and EMG congresses. During the middle of the inter-congress interval, the Chapters would hold their Congresses. Major Chapter congresses would be held once every 4 years for each Chapter. That reduced the overall major Federation meetings from two to one per year on average.

Each congress should oversee the organization of other Federation meetings and activities in their region. Up until this time, the Federation occasionally funded or lent its name to the organization of smaller symposia or other meetings. Some were held in regions where additional general educational activities were desired. Others were held on specific topics, for example evoked potentials. With the establishment of Chapters, those bodies should have oversight or give approval for these secondary meetings in their region. These would be in addition to the major quadrennial Chapter congresses.

To facilitate communications, a member of the Federation Executive Committee should be included in the Chapter Executive Committee. The position was named the Liaison Officer. Ideally that Liaison Officer would be an Executive Committee member from that geographic region.

The initial Chapters considered were from Latin America and Europe. Eastern and Southern Asia region was identified as an additional area that could benefit from a Chapter to foster periodic meetings and education in the region.

3.3. Latin American Chapter

The Chapter was formally organized during this term. Bye-Laws were written and accepted by the General Assembly. The foundational work was accomplished during the previous Federation Fiscal period of 1993–1997. During that time, discussions were held on the conceptual issues. The First Latin American Congress of Clinical Neurophysiology was held as a symposium during the Pan American Congress of Neurology in Guatemala City in 1995 during the previous Fiscal Period. Chapter founder Nelly Chiofalo organized that Clinical Neurophysiology Symposium with help from Enrique Delamonica (Argentina). Representatives attended from Argentina, Brazil, Bolivia, Chile, Colombia, Cuba, Costa Rica, Dominican Republic, El Salvador, Ecuador, Guatemala, Honduras, Mexico, Panama, Peru, Puerto Rico, Uruguay and Venezuela (Appendix 11, Fig. 11). That symposium primarily was a scientific and educational program with workshops and breakout sessions. One portion of the symposium was set aside for the business meeting, at which enthusiasm was voiced for the formation of a regional organization as an IFCN Chapter. Executive Committee President Carl Lücking, Member-at-Large Marc Nuwer, and Editor-in-Chief Gastone Celesia attended on behalf of the Executive Committee. Chapter Officers were chosen and appointed to the task of drafting formal Bye-Laws. Nelly Chiofalo was chosen as Chapter Chairperson and Enrique Delamonica (Argentina) as Chapter Secretary–Treasurer. The Brazilian Society of Clinical Neurophysiology subsequently volunteered to host the Chapter's administrative office in the same site as its own society office in São Paolo. In follow-up, Dr. Chiofalo drafted Bye-Laws in Spanish. Francisco Luccas and Jose Xavier de Castro (Brazil) translated them into Portuguese.

In this 1997–2001 Federation Fiscal Period, the chapter held its Second Latin American Congress of Clinical Neurophysiology in Buenos Aires just prior to the World Congress of Neurology in September 1997. About 100 physicians attended, representing nearly all of the Federation's Latin American member societies. The Organizing Committee was President Nelly Chiofalo (Chile) and from the Argentine Society of Clinical Neurophysiology Vice-President Marcos Turner, Chairman of the Scientific Committee Enrique Delamonica, Secretary Ricardo Reisin, Treasurer Ana Maria Pardal. The site was the Sheraton Hotel and Convention Center. Most of the IFCN ExCo Members were actively involved in the program. The 2 days included 5 Scientific Sessions, 8 Poster Sessions, 2 Workshops, and 1 Symposium. At the Chapter General Assembly meeting during this Congress, draft Bye-Laws were discussed. The Chapter organized a mailing list and began periodic communication with member societies.

The chapter worked with Dr. Gustafo Pradilla and Luis Morillo (Colombia) representing the Colombian Clinical Neurophysiology Society to try to organize a 1999 Third Latin American Chapter Congress in association with the Pan American Neurology Congress in Cartagena in October 1999. This was difficult to organize and eventually support was withdrawn from this meeting. In part, this was because the site was very distant from many members. A decision was to hold initial formal Chapter congresses closer to a large number of participants so as to build more momentum for Chapter activities.

An interim Chapter symposium was held in Buenos Aires in October 2000. Both a scientific symposium and a Chapter business meeting were held at that time, organized with the help of local physicians under the leadership of Carlos Medina. The meeting was well received by the 150 registrants. The scientific topic was focused on the occipital lobe function. IFCN provided fellowships for young physicians and scientists to attend this meeting. Chapter Chairperson Nelly Chiofalo (Chile) led the business meeting. Francisco Luccas (Brazil) was elected as the Chapter Secretary–Treasurer. Olga Sanz (Argentina) was selected as a new Chapter Executive Committee Member-at-Large for terms beginning in 2000. The Federation Executive Committee appointed Member-at-Large Marc Nuwer to succeed Editor-in-Chief Gastone Celesia as Liaison Officer for the Latin American Chapter. By this point, the Chapter approved its new Bye-Laws and submitted them to the IFCN Executive and Rules Committees. The Bye-Laws were written in Spanish, Portuguese and English.

In 2001, Daniel Cibils (Uruguay) was chosen as the new Chapter President. Augusto Fernando-Guardiola (Mexico) was chosen as a new Chapter Executive Committee Member-at-Large. The greatest Chapter activity at this time was preparations to host the 2001 ICCN in Buenos Aires, which has taken much time from organizers in the Sociedad Argentina de EEG y Neurofisiologia Clinica.

Overall, this term saw the Chapter evolve from its 1995 inception to an organized set of interested and active participants representing many Latin American societies, and drawing in the interest of many clinical neurophysiologists. The preponderance of activity in these formative years was from the southern region. Meetings were at a high scientific and educational quality, well attended, and conducted mainly in Spanish and Portuguese.

3.4. European Chapter

The European Chapter grew out of a desire for an organized group to continue the ECCN meeting series and the need for a voice for Clinical Neurophysiology in the European political community. The European subsection of IFCN had been active for years in organizing meetings such as those in Paris, Lisbon, Munich, and Budapest. There was interest in organizing the European chapter of IFCN discussed at the Munich ECCN. An ad hoc committee was chosen in Munich to consider forming a Federation Chapter and drafting Bye-Laws. Guenther Deuschl (Germany) served as committee chairman. The committee included Kjeld Andersen (Norway), Aurora Constantinovici (Romania), Al De Weerd (The Netherlands), Andres Fuglsang-Frederiksen (Denmark), Jean-Marie Guérit (Belgium), and Paolo Rossini (Italy). That committee reported back to the European Chapter at the Florence 1997 International Congress, where the European delegates spent 2 days discussing the proposed European chapter statutes. These were modified, approved, and submitted to the Federation Rules and Executive Committees for approval. These committees recommended accepting the proposal and sent them to the Federation Council, which voted formally to accept this Chapter as a part of the Federation. This was the first Federation Chapter formally established in this way. Initial officers were Erik Stålberg (Sweden) as Chairman, Al De Weerd (The Netherlands) as Secretary–Treasurer, and Theresa Sagalés and Giorgio Cruccu (Italy) as Members-at-Large. At this initial election, the chairman and one member-at-large, Dr Cruccu, were elected for a term ending in 2000, and the secretary–treasurer and the other member-at-large, Dr Sagalés, were elected for terms ending in 2002. Several years later, those four all were re-elected to additional 4-year terms. In addition to those Chapter officers, Paolo Rossini (Italy) served as the IFCN Liaison Officer for the Chapter. IFCN Executive Committee member Guenther Deuschl (Germany) also continued active involvement with the Chapter.

The Chapter establishing a host-section status for Clinical Neurophysiology in the European Society of Medical Specialists, giving itself a formal voice in medical politics. The place of Clinical

Neurophysiology as a specialty on its own or as a subspecialty of Neurology was debated. A Chapter Task Force of Kjeld Andersen (Norway), Theresa Sagalés (Spain) and J.A. Jarrat (UK) evaluated the specialty status for clinical neurophysiology. Dr Andersen described how the Medical National Associations cooperate to organize and formalize medical issues and influence European medical decisions taken in the European Commission (EC). Union Européenne des Médecins Spécialistes (UEMS) organized cooperation and some uniformity among specialties. A European Union council directive determined the rules for free movement of physicians and mutual recognition of their diplomas and board certificates. UEMS issued charters organizing specialist training, quality assurance, and CME. Details are then implemented within specialist sections and boards. In 1997 the Federation European Chapter Task Force organized contacts with representatives from countries where Clinical Neurophysiology is recognized as a specialty. Nine European Federation member nations recognized Clinical Neurophysiology as a specialty. There were many similarities in training among these countries but also some differences. Further organization and uniformity were needed to comply with UEMS rules. The European Commission did not recognize Clinical Neurophysiology. Clinical Neurophysiology was offered a position as an observer in the European Board of Neurology.

The Task Force noted Directive 93/16/EEC, which organized European medical specialties. An August 1996 letter from UEMS to Dr. Andersen suggested approaching the Advisory Committee on Medical Training that includes governmental and professional representatives. He also could contact the Ministry of the Committee of Senior Officials on Public Health (CSOPH) and government representatives to recommend Clinical Neurophysiology as an independent specialty. Theresa Sagalés, writing in 1997 on behalf of the European Task Force for Clinical Neurophysiology, contacted the Secretary General of the CSOPH in Brussels. Her letter requested assistance recognizing Clinical Neurophysiology as a specialty in the revised version of the 93/16/EEC Medical Directive. Representatives from the societies in Norway, Italy, Spain, Denmark, Finland, UK, Sweden, The Netherlands and Slovenia signed the letter. Commission directive 98/63/EC in 1998 amended directive 93/16/EEC and recognized Clinical Neurophysiology as an independent specialty recognized in Denmark, Spain, Ireland, Sweden and the UK. It asked for development of training standards. The specialty was not granted a specialist section within the UEMS because it was not recognized in more than one-third of the member states. The management council instead accepted Clinical Neurophysiology as a host section.

The Chapter established several committees. One began work on unified training standards for Clinical Neurophysiology in Europe. Chapter Bye-Laws recognized *Clinical Neurophysiology* as the official journal of the European Chapter. The Chapter adopted EC-IFCN as an abbreviation standing for European Chapter of the IFCN. The Long-Term Planning Committee recommended reducing the ECCN meetings to every 4 years, a proposal subsequently taken to the Federation General Assembly by EC-IFCN President Erik Stålberg.

Turkey and Israel applied for Chapter membership during the Lyon Congress. Some discussion was held about Chapter membership of societies from countries not geographically in Europe. Turkey pointed out that a part of Turkey is in Europe including its largest city. Israel was asked why it should be recognized for membership in the European Chapter. Among the various points presented was an interesting, nonmedical, nongeographic one — that Israel participates in the European football leagues. In any case, the Chapter General Assembly voted to accept the both bids for membership.

Erik Stålberg (Sweden) was reelected as EC-IFCN Chairman. Giorgio Cruccu (Italy) was reelected as Member-at-Large of the EC-IFCN Executive Committee, both for terms lasting until 2005.

EC-IFCN funds would be raised from several sources. One is the profit from each ECCN, which will be applied to start-up funding for the next ECCN. The Chapter also asked the IFCN Treasurer for a stipend to support annual operating expenses and for ECCN fellowship stipends. The Federation Treasurer requested that the EC-IFCN Executive Committee should be the source of requests for funds. The Chapter should maintain a separate account in the IFCN Treasury. Accounting must be audited periodically as for any Federation funds.

The 9th ECCN was held in Ljubljana, Slovenia, in June 1998. It was organized by the Slovene Society of Clinical Neurophysiology under the auspices of the European Chapter of IFCN. The Organizing Committee was Janez Zidar (Convener), Tone Zaklj (Secretary), Jelka Brecelj, and David Neubauer. The International Scientific Committee consisted of delegates of the Member Societies of the Chapter. IFCN provided US $30,000 for fellowships. Clinical Neurophysiology as a distinct medical specialty has had a longstanding tradition in Slovenia. Its beginnings, with the first home-built EEG machine, date back to 1947. The Congress intended to touch on a number of different aspects of clinical neurophysiology; from the recent developments in basic neurobiological sciences to advances in practical application of neurophysiologic methods. The program included 3 Plenary Lectures, 21 Scientific Sessions, 7 Poster Sessions, and 18 Advanced Courses. The well appreciated social program started with a welcome reception, continued with an organ concert at the Cathedral and ended with a social event in the Grand Hotel Union. The Congress attracted 550 registrants from 36 countries. Abstracts were published in a supplement of the journal *Electroencephalography and Clinical Neurophysiology*. Monduzzi Editore (Bologna) published the Congress Proceedings (see Appendix 11, Figs. 17 and 18).

The 10th ECCN at the Lyon Conference Center, Lyon, France, in August 2000 attracted over 800 registrants. This excellent congress was organized by François Mauguière (Convener and Chairman of the Organizing Committee), C. Fischer (Secretary/Treasurer), and members of the Société de Neurophysiologie Clinique de Langue Française together with Officers of the EC and IFCN. Honorary President was J. Courjon. The program included an opening lecture by R. Frackowiak, closing lecture by R. Hari, tutorial lectures by J. Kimura and M. Jouvet, four Advanced Courses Sessions, eight Platform Sessions, two Topical Seminars, two Symposia, three Poster Sessions with about 300 posters in total, and two Video-EEG Sessions (see Appendix 11, Fig. 23). The social program was very well accepted with a welcome party, a City Hall reception and a gala dinner. The Federation provided US $18,000 for Young Investigator Fellowships of US $500 per person. Satellite Symposia covered two additional topics: "Functional Neuroimaging of the Epilepsies" and "Vagus Nerve Stimulation".

The EC-IFCN and Federation sponsored several local meetings during this period. Erik Stålberg organized a course on "EMG and Related Clinical Neurophysiology" in Budapest. Professor Falck of Finland and Drs. Dioszeghy and Mechler of Hungary served as faculty. The attendance was 46 and rated the educational experience very highly. The general concept seems successful. Another Electromyography course was given in Warsaw in 2001 at the Institute of Biocybernetics and Biochemical Engineering, Polish Academy of Sciences. Organizing committee chairperson Prof. Barbara Emeryk-Szajewska arranged for Profs. Stålberg and Falck and five members of the Polish Society of Clinical Neurophysiology. The 45 registrants from the throughput Poland were trained with demonstrations on normal subjects and on patients, whose EMGs displayed on one video projector and details of needle positions and other details of the demo were displayed via an extra video camera and video projector. It was very well received by the participants and considered as a success by all parties involved. The Federation also let its name be used to promote the International SFEMG course and VII Quantitation EMG Conference in Uppsala in 2001. These all were excellent educational programs. The Federation Executive Committee decided that the sponsoring of such local meetings should be under the general jurisdiction of the Chapter. Beginning around 2001, the EC-IFCN should be the group approached by those who wish to involve the Federation in local courses in Europe.

3.5. Asian–Oceanian Chapter

The Asian Chapter chose Prof. Xiao-Fu Tang (China) as its Chairperson and Prof. Nubuo Yanagisawa as Secretary at its founding. In 1997, incoming Federation Secretary Hiroshi Shibasaki replaced outgoing Member-at-Large Xiao-Fu Tang as the Executive Committee Liaison Officer for the Chapter. At the Florence 1997 ICEEGCN, the Chapter delegates met with the President Carl Lücking to discuss organization and Bye-Laws. Following that discussion, Chapter Secretary Dr. Yanagisawa circulated the draft Chapter Bye-Laws to delegates of national societies. One issue raised in reply was a move to include Australia and New Zealand in the Chapter region. Australia did have an official society, and New Zealand at this time did not. To designate the Chapter as covering this region, a better title could be the Asian–Oceanian Chapter instead of Asian Chapter. Chapter delegates supported this name change. The Bye-Laws were further revised to include some elements adopted for the other two chapters, for example regarding periodic financial report to the IFCN Treasurer.

Asia had been the site of several previous regional and local Federation meetings during the previous two decades. Organized in large part by former Federation President John Desmedt, these were held in Beijing, Bangkok, and Bali. Now that the region had a Chapter, those delegates would decide where in the region to hold Chapter congresses and other local meetings. The first of those Asian–Oceanian Chapter meetings was held in Manila in January 2000 in conjunction with the Asian–Oceanian Congress of Neurology. Convener Zenaida Bagabaldo, Secretary Marita Dantes, Treasurer Alejandro Diaz and their Philippines clinical neurophysiology colleagues, working together with IFCN Secretary Hiroshi Shibasaki, organized a very interesting and highly appreciated meeting that took place in The Heritage Hotel. IFCN ExCo held its meeting in Manila so that all members could give presentations at the Chapter congress (see Appendix 11, Figs. 21 and 22). This included seven Sessions with didactic lectures and hands-on workshops, two Sessions of Free Presentations, one Symposium, and two Poster Sessions. The Federation provided fellowship stipends of US $18,000.

At the 2000 Chapter meeting in Manila, Prasert Boongird (Thailand) was elected as the Chapter Chairman. Nobuo Yanagisawa (Japan) was reelected as the Chapter Secretary. Draft Chapter Bye-Laws were again discussed at the assembly business meeting. The Chapter established a process to consider future official Chapter and additional local meetings. The next Chapter meeting was scheduled as the Asian–Oceanian Symposium on Clinical Neurophysiology to be held in Bangkok in January 2005. By 2001, this meeting was moved to northern Thailand. So as to keep the momentum going for Chapter activities, an interim local meeting was scheduled for Bangkok in conjunction with a meeting of the Neurological Society of Thailand, March 2001.

3.6. North American region

The largest region not then covered by a Chapter was North America. The three societies in the USA and Canada were among the largest in the IFCN, one the single largest member society. In other regions the Chapters provided a way to promote Federation goals. This was lacking in North America. The Executive Committee developed a pilot project for supporting physicians and scientists from disadvantaged regions to participate in some North American Congresses. Council was consulted, and the delegates agreed with this pilot plan. The North American societies were invited to request Federation funding for travel fellowships for overseas physicians and scientists to attend their meetings, particularly for those from economically disadvantaged member nations. The American Association for Electrodiagnostic Medicine accepted this proposal and established and ran such a program for several years until the eventual formation of a formal North American Chapter in a later Fiscal Period.

3.7. African region

IFCN policy has been to foster clinical neurophysiology worldwide. In Africa there was no longer any society, since the South African society had disbanded IFCN membership in the previous Fiscal Period. Egypt started to build up an Egyptian Society of Electrodiagnostic Medicine (ESEM) and Clinical Neurophysiology. It was officially founded on the occasion of the First Alexandria International Symposium on Electrodiagnostic Medicine and Clinical Neurophysiology. That meeting was initiated and organized under the auspices of the IFCN. The symposium was held in Alexandria, Egypt on October 30–31, 1997. The Organizing Committee included Abdel-Moneim Helal (President) and Ibrahim Khalil Ibrahim (Secretary) and the IFCN Officers Carl H. Lücking, Giuseppe Caruso, and Paolo Rossini, all of whom were actively involved in the program. The meeting included three Scientific Sessions and a half-day Round Table Discussion. The new Egyptian Society eventually joined the IFCN as a member society.

4. Encouraging diversity and inclusion

A Federation goal is to encourage worldwide high quality science and education in clinical neurophysiology. There have been a number of approaches to pursuing that goal. These have included encouraging new member societies in previously unrepresented nations. The Federation also has worked with other international organizations to jointly foster mutual goals. It has provided fellowship funding support for young investigators to attend meetings. In addition, the Federation has arranged for journal subscriptions and books for major teaching institutions that otherwise were unable to afford them.

4.1. Societies and individuals

In this Fiscal Period one new member society was accepted into the Federation in 1999, the Egyptian Society of Clinical Neurophysiology. This marked the return of the Federation to the African continent, after a 5-year interval since the closing and withdrawal of the previous South African EEG Society in the previous Fiscal Period. The Executive Committee inquired of other nations whose clinical neurophysiology activities might lead to formation of further new national societies in the future.

In Latin America, the Chapter was encouraged to create mailing lists for individuals in unrepresented nations. The lists could be used to keep open lines of communications with individuals and small groups who might form the nucleus of future national societies. It also provided a practical way to let those physicians know about Chapter and other Federation activities and meetings, and to invite participation from those countries in future Federation and Chapter meetings.

4.2. Sponsorship assistance for education in disadvantaged regions

The Executive Committee desired to provide resources to teaching hospitals and medical centers in regions that are economically disadvantaged. Those areas have had difficulty obtaining resources. The IFCN is able to provide books and journal subscriptions at a discount. Book contracts for books produced under the auspices of the IFCN often have included a contract clause giving a certain number of books to the

Federation without charge. This included some contracts for the *Handbook of Clinical Neurophysiology* series, copies of *Recommendations for the Practice of Clinical Neurophysiology: Guidelines of the International Federation of Clinical Neurophysiology,* and volumes in the *Clinical Neurophysiology Supplement Series*. In addition to those free books, the Federation was able to purchase more at a discounted price.

The Past-President Carl H. Lücking was asked to oversee arrangements for these books and journal subscriptions to be distributed to worthy organizations. In this process, he solicited ideas from delegates and received spontaneous requests from institutions or professors. Some delegates from economically advanced countries were able to identify contacts they had in other countries who could benefit from these resources. Others identified opportunities in their own country where these resources would be of most value. After screening the financial reasons for needing assistance, he arranged to ship books or sign up professors at teaching hospitals to receive journal subscriptions. In each case, the recipient agreed that these resources would be placed in libraries or otherwise be made available openly to clinical neurophysiologists or others at their institution; they were not for private office shelves.

The donation of these was explicitly meant to be just that — a donation for the advantage of the local physicians and scientists. Carl Lücking assured each recipient that this in no way was meant to influence a delegate's vote in any IFCN matters. A feedback system was devised to evaluate the effectiveness of this program. The Federation desired to continue its support only to those institutions where it appeared effective that many individuals used these resources for clinical, educational, or scientific purposes.

5. Practice Committee

The new guidelines book, *Recommendations for the Practice of Clinical Neurophysiology: Guidelines of the International Federation of Clinical Neurophysiology* was published. As described in greater detail above, the book served as a single source compendium of Federation guidelines adopted and published over the previous 18 years in the journal.

5.1. Transcranial Magnetic Stimulation Committee

The Transcranial Magnetic Stimulation (TMS) Committee was reappointed with the same members as in the past Fiscal Period. The committee's focus now was on repetitive TMS, its safety and uses.

The TMS Committee includes Robert Belmaker (Israel), Charles Epstein (USA), Mark Hallett (USA), Alvaro Pascual-Leone (USA), Walter Paulus (Germany), Paolo Rossini (Italy), John Rothwell (UK), Harold Sackeim (USA), Carlo Tassinari (Italy), and Eric Wassermann (USA). It also includes as nonvoting representatives from industry John Cadwell (Cadwell Laboratories), Reza Jalinous (Magstim US), and Jorn Ladegaard (Medtronic Dantec). TMS reports were included in the 1999 Practice Recommendations book.

5.2. Digital EEG Standards Committee

In the previous Fiscal Period, the Digital EEG Standards Committee published a report on minimum technical standards for clinical digital EEG recording and review. The committee then included Marc Nuwer (USA), Giancarlo Comi (Italy), Ronald Emerson (USA), Anders Fuglsang-Frederiksen (Denmark), Jean-Michel Guérit (Belgium), Hermann Hinrichs (Germany), Akio Ikeda (Japan), Francisco Luccas (Brazil), Peter Rappelsberger (Austria). In this Fiscal Period, the Chairperson was Ronald Emerson. The IFCN developed relationships with manufacturers to encourage them to adopt the standards.

The Digital EEG Standards describe the process for claiming in advertising that the vendor's equipment meets the IFCN Digital EEG Standards. The vendor was required to ask for permission in advance. The Digital EEG Standards Committee or its designees would judge whether the hardware and software does indeed meet the standards. This raised a significant new problem, that of liability in case a vendor fails to meet standards and challenges the determination in a legal setting. To protect the Federation against those adverse actions, or any other legal adversity, it should have General Liability insurance and Directors and Officers insurance. At this time the IFCN carried no insurance. Implementing the Digital EEG Standards reviews was put on hold while the issue of insurance was reviewed. An attorney, one with experience in international legal matters, was sought to advise the Federation about the best ways to protect itself from legal actions. In turn, this raised issues about the Federation's legal status as a French nonprofit organization and French customs about insurance for such organizations, and those topics initiating a broad set of actions in the next Fiscal Period.

5.3. Medical Economics Committee

The Executive Committee in the previous Fiscal Period established an International Medical Economics Committee. The name was subsequently changed to the Professional Practice Committee. The Committee was charged with drafting a report comparing the different medical economic models and their impact on test procedures, access to testing and care, and the quality for common clinical neurophysiology techniques. The committee focused initially on several developed nations, sought methods to evaluate the different economic models, and measure influence of the economics on variations in testing procedures, access, quality, and cost. Additional issues included a central listing of available practice guidelines, development of demographic and practice surveys, and other issues about the professional practice of Clinical Neurophysiology.

Initial members were appointed representing USA, Canada, UK, and Germany. This was later expanded to include Switzerland, Japan, Italy, France, Japan and Norway. The situation encountered might differ among countries. Development or use of guidelines could be suggested based on the results.

The committee ran into substantial problems. It became clear that the economic situations were very complicated and hard to compare among the countries. The incentives for cost containment, quality, access, and procedural details varied greatly among countries. The committee members had difficulty obtaining the needed details from their own countries; much of the needed detail was not readily available in the literature or from their national medical organizations. This stood in the way of achieving the primary goals of the committee.

An observation from the committee's work was that the variations were greater than expected in many ways. The systems for medical care in different countries were difficult to compare because of the numerous confounding variables that would have to be taken into account. In the end no formal report was forthcoming beyond those observations.

6. Communications

6.1. Mail, fax and e-mail

The Executive Committee sought better ways to communicate with Delegates, among the Executive Committee members, and with the various committees. Two Fiscal Periods ago in 1989, the standard communication was airmail. During that time international faxes came into use, which were helpful to speed communications. In the last Fiscal Period starting in 1993, e-mail was adopted for Federation business. All the Executive Committee members were able to exchange e-mails, and most committee members used e-mail for their professional business. At the beginning of this Fiscal Period in 1997, about half the Delegates from national societies were using e-mail for Federation communication. The other half still replied on faxes or airmail. As e-mail use increased, Delegates were reached more often and more easily, and their advice was sought more often.

Delegates with only fax numbers, no e-mail address, were consulted somewhat less often. It was slower to reach Delegates by fax, and international fax lines were not always successful in transmissions. Delegates who only were available by airmail were consulted less often, and questions continued whether communications actually reached them.

Communications with Delegates always had been a problem for the Federation. Apart from the above issues about mail and faxes, Delegates moved their street or changed e-mail address or fax phone number, but without informing the Federation. Societies changed their Delegates without informing the Federation. Sometimes those communications to the Federation were not received. This was always a continuing struggle, especially for the Federation Secretary who was charged with keeping current the contact information for each society and its Delegate.

6.2. IFCN on-line

This term saw the start of the IFCN website. Secretary Hiroshi Shibasaki first opened this at his home institution in Kyoto. Subsequently the Federation publisher Elsevier offered to host the website and provide a technical manager. The website at the time of this printing is at http://www.ifcn.info. Chapters and many national societies also maintain websites, much of which has been made accessible as a web link through the IFCN website. The site contains information about the Federation's officers, national societies, meetings, fellowships, Executive Committee reports, and financial audits.

Elsevier also established on-line journal access during this Fiscal Period. These were available to libraries, some of which then discontinued receiving the printed hardcopy of the journal. Through the academic medical libraries, many members were able to access, read, print and save journal publications. Back issues were scanned into the publisher's on-line database, so that issues available on-line dated back to the first issue in 1949. This provided a greater access to the journal than was available to many before these changes.

Elsevier established a process for individual subscribers to access the journal on-line for those whose local medical library did not give them the needed access. Individual subscribers also were given the ability to conduct automated searches across all Elsevier journals for articles with user-defined keywords, with reports e-mailed to the user each month.

Elsevier implemented the on-line publication submission, review and management software system, Smart Works, to aid authors in tracking their accepted manuscripts through the publication process. This was eventually replaced by the Editorial Manager software system in use now.

7. Rules Committee

The Rules Committee developed new Statutes and Bye-Laws for several purposes during this fiscal Period. Rules changes included the number of Editors-in-Chief, journal name change, General Assembly mail voting, and combining the two Congress series into one. The committee also reviewed, commented upon, and approved Bye-Laws for the three Chapters. The committee included Austin Sumner (USA, Chairman), François Mauguière (France), Americo Sakamoto (Brazil), Kjeld Andersen (Norway) and Ryuji Kaji (Japan).

7.1. Combining and scheduling congresses

At the Florence 1997 ICEEGCN General Assembly, Delegates asked to combine the two separate Federation Congress series, the ICEEGCN and the ICEMGCN, more informally known as the EEG and the EMG meetings. The new series combined meetings would be held every 2 years starting in 2001. The Rules Committee was directed to develop rules renaming each congress as an ICCN instead of identifying separate EEG and EMG meetings.

At the 1999 ICEMGCN General Assembly, concern was voiced about too many meetings. The European Chapter suggested holding International Congresses and Chapter congresses each every 4 years. The Chapter Congresses would be held during the interval between the International Congresses. Business issues could be dealt between meetings by e-mail, reducing the pressure for face-to-face General Assembly meetings every 2 years. The European Chapter's motion was adopted without dissent.

The Rules Committee was directed to develop such rule changes. A choice was needed about which meeting to skip or move to convert to change the International Congresses to every 4 years. Options were skipping the 2003 or the 2005 meeting. As an added complication, the Executive Committee terms are usually 4 years long. The current Executive Committee cycles would end in 2001 and 2005. By mail ballot, a majority of Delegates favored holding the 2003 meeting. Delegates suggested shortening or extending the usual 4-year Executive Committee term once, so as to accommodate the conversion to ICCN meetings every 4 years. No congress would be held in 2005. Choices for the next Executive Committee term were from 2.5 to 6 years. Four years was excluded because the General Assembly already decided not to hold a meeting in 2005. The best choices were a Fiscal Period and Executive Committee term of 2 years 4 months, or 5 years, or 6 years. Delegates ranked the three options by mail, and 58% chose "5 years", 25% chose "2 years and 4 months", and 17% chose "6 years". The Council recommendation of "5 years" was adopted, that is holding an ICCN in 2006.

Through this action, the ICCN meetings were gradually spread out to every 4 years. ICCN 2001, 2003, 2006 and 2010 meetings were separated by 2, 3 and 4 years in that order. This had the effect of moving the ICCN meeting to even years, no longer occurring in the odd-numbered years with the World Federation of Neurology Congresses or the ILAE Congresses.

7.2. Reducing two business meetings to one

Traditionally both the Council and the General Assembly meet during each quadrennial ICEEGCN and occasionally during the ICEMGCN. At that time, Council was composed of the Delegates, one per society. The General Assembly was composed of two, three, or four representatives from each society, including the Delegates. The size of the General Assembly delegation depended on society membership size. Those two business meetings covered much the same topics with similar audiences. Discussions overlapped and usually arrived at the same conclusions. Some issues differed, for example only Council discussed Bye-Law changes whereas only the General Assembly voted on future Congress sites.

The Rules Committee was charged with evaluating combining the two business meetings. The committee recommended that the two bodies meet together as the General Assembly at Congresses. No important constitutional function was served by having a separate Council meeting. Between Congresses, Council continued to serve an important role by giving advice and consent to Executive Committee actions. The 2001 General Assembly agreed with this plan.

This was part of a series of actions that led eventually to dissolution of the Council in the next Federation term.

7.3. Journal name change

The committee introduced the rules to change the journal's name to *Clinical Neurophysiology*. Discussion centered on potential confusion with the other journals of similar names. The confusion was considered relatively modest, and examples of similar names occurred in other scientific fields. The name change was approved unanimously.

7.4. One Editor-in-Chief

The General Assembly in Florence and Prague in 1997 and 1999 discussed combining the two Editors-in-Chief positions into one. Reasons were reviewed above in the Publications section. The Rules Committee was charged with reviewing the options and making specific suggestions to the Council.

The rules did not actually mandate one way or the other. The Bye-Laws on the Journal stated: "The Editorial Staff *may* consist of two Editors-in-Chief, an Assistant Editor, two or more regional editors, a review editor, a consultant for supplements and such others as the Editorial Board may decide. At any time, these posts may be in abeyance and any two or more may be combined at the discretion of the Editorial Board [the Executive Board]. The Rules Committee opined that if the intention is to irrevocably consolidate the office of Editor-in-Chief as a single position, then it is a simple matter to amend the Statutes and Bye-Laws to strike the words, "two Editors-in-Chief" and replace it with "one". The Rules Committee suggests that maximum flexibility is desirable and that the simplest solution would be to insert the wording that the Editorial Staff may consist of one or more Editor(s)-in-Chief. Throughout the text wherever "Editors-in-Chief" was used the rules could state "Editor(s)"."

The General Assembly accepted this compromise in the rule. It left it to the journal's Executive Board, which is the Federation Executive Committee, not to replace Paolo Rossini as Editor-in-Chief when his term ended.

7.5. Editor-in-Chief on the OCIC

The Editor-in-Chief has a potentially important contribution to each ICCN's scientific program. This has been informally conducted by allowing the Editor-in-Chief to contribute suggestions during the scientific program's development. He or she is most current with the interesting new manuscript topics as well as the scientists and physicians who are involved with those studies. For those reasons, the Executive Committee asked for a rules change to appoint the Editor-in-Chief to each Organizing Committee for an International Congress (OCIC). In discussion of the matter, the General Assembly suggested that an additional member from the sponsoring national society also should be added to each OCIC, for example the Scientific Program Chairperson. The matter was not approved in 2001. It was carried forward for further discussion and rule-wording in the next Fiscal Period.

7.6. Chapter Bye-Laws

All three Chapters drafted their own Bye-Laws within broad guidelines for IFCN Bye-Laws and other IFCN policies and rules. Of general application across all Federation functions, the Federation Rules Committee is the arbiter of disagreements between Federation organization, and all Federation accounting is subject to annual accounting. The General Assembly is the organization with overall responsibility for Federation rules and functions. Within these broad guidelines, the intention is that the Chapters will function on their own and report their activities periodically to the other Chapters and the Executive Committee.

The three sets of Bye-Laws were reviewed by the Rules Committee and are in compliance with Federation Statutes and Bye-Laws. The Federation Council approved of all three sets of Bye-Laws.

8. Long-Range Planning Committee

The Long-Range Planning Committee (LRPC) was charged with defining long-term goals, means and finance. Several specific questions were posed including:

- Should we have a permanent central office and executive director?
- Should we become incorporated, should we obtain insurance?

- How should we distribute resources to economically disadvantaged regions?
- What should we do about societies who do not pay their dues?

Past President Carl Lücking (Germany) chaired the committee. Members included Dr. Giancarlo Comi (Italy), Dr. Daniel Cibils (Uruguay), Dr. Andrew A. Eisen (Canada), Dr. Nai-Shin Chu (Taiwan) and Dr. Erik Stålberg (Sweden) along with the elected members of the Executive Committee.

8.1. Accounting, financial planning, and reserve funds

Several questions were addressed: Should the Federation retain a professional financial advisor to review the investments and financial strategy? What should be the long-range financial plan? How should the large reserves be used? Should the dues structure change? Should current general account funds be set aside for fellowship funding or other specific purposes?

The Federation general funds accumulated a profit in most years. The general account balance had slowly expanded, doubling in 6 years to US $1.2 million. That is equivalent to 4 years of the Federation's budget. This was due in large part to profits from some Congresses, royalties from Elsevier, and careful monitoring of expenses by the Treasurer. The potential existed for adverse future years such as from a serious Congress fiscal loss or if Elsevier's royalty income were greatly reduced due to conversion to electronic publishing. There was also the ever present threat of lawsuits in the modern world. One or another of several governments could make tax payment demands. The LRPC recommended that the financial situation was tied up with the issues of the Federation's incorporation and clarification of the tax status and insurance, and that those issues must be resolved.

LRPC agreed to create an enrichment or special project account, and to set aside a portion of the general fund in this special account. The account would be used for support of education and training, such as donated books, journal subscriptions, fellowships, and similar activities.

The LRPC agreed with the de facto policy of investing a portion of our accounts in low-risk funds. A more formal policy written was desired. One was developed by Executive Committee member Mark Hallett and adopted by the Executive Committee to cover long-term financial planning in a general manner. Questions were raised about the Federation's investment in Elsevier, which created at least a perceived conflict of interest because the Federation depended on Elsevier for a contract and income. Questions also were raised about investing in vendors who exhibited at our meetings, such as equipment manufacturers. Future investments in those entities were discouraged.

8.2. Gifts, sponsorships and lecturers for meetings

This was covered above in the section on "Inclusiveness". The LRPC was involved in general direction for such activities, and in setting aside funds to cover these activities. The Executive Committee authorized US $7500 for sponsored subscription. From that allocation, 25 journal subscriptions were provided to 25 institutions of 8 countries. IFCN books also were distributed. Carl Lücking contacted many IFCN Delegates and other individuals to help to identify the best institutions for this program. Based on favorable results in the initial pilot project year, the program was authorized for an additional 5 years. Feedback from each institution was solicited annually so as to assure that a broad group of individuals could and did access these resources each year.

Requests to support local meetings were received frequently. In this Fiscal Period, several local courses received support, as reviewed in the section on IFCN Chapters. At first, the Chapter and LRPC discussed together to which local course to provide support. Later, this choice was turned over to the Chapter along with some funds to pay for the support.

8.3. Legal status, insurance and taxes

The LRPC recommended that the Federation retain an attorney to review the tax status and French nonprofit registration. At this time, the Federation was then a Registered Charity under a 1901 French law, but was not an incorporated organization. The Federation's Statutes declared the legal address of the Federation to be at the Centre Hospitalier Universitaire de la Timone, Marseilles, France. The administrative address of the Federation is that of the current President. No written document was found describing an incorporation of the Federation in Marseilles in 1949, only a Charitable Registration. It cannot be considered incorporated or as an equivalent.

The IFCN desired legal protection and appropriate status, clarification of the tax liability, and a desire for insurance to protect the Federation and its Executive Committee members from litigation and losses. To get insurance, an insurance agent informed the Executive Committee that we would need to incorporate and set up a permanent secretariat. An international business accounting firm would be needed to advise about tax status and international accounting practices.

Rules Committee member François Mauguière and IFCN Treasurer Paul Despland sought legal advice about this matter from an attorney in Lyon. French Law had changed, which would require a change in the formal status of the IFCN. The Lyon attorney investigated the implications and necessary actions. Incorporation seems necessary in order to obtain officers' and directors' insurance as well as potentially to take advantage of certain tax benefits.

In a French legal Instruction dated September 15, 1998, French fiscal administration stated that an Association would be subject to commercial taxes when it has privileged relations with companies drawing a commercial advantage from this collaboration. This would be the case if all members of IFCN member societies had an obligation to subscribe to the IFCN's journal, because this would constitute a protected market to the benefit of both the IFCN and Elsevier. Although this was obviously not the case, the attorney reviewed the 1983 contract between IFCN and Elsevier in this regard. He confirmed that there was no evident risk of the IFCN being in a taxable position with regard to French fiscal legislation.

The Executive Committee developed a policy about our financial objectives to protect our current tax-exempt status, one showing how we were using our funds for worthwhile social purposes. The Executive Committee asked the French attorney to help us incorporate as nonprofit charitable organization and to obtain directors' and officers' insurance. Unless there is a financial disadvantage, the incorporation would be in France. The issue of a permanent secretariat was brought back to the Executive Committee and LRPC.

The World Federation of Neurology (WFN) had dealt with some similar issues and had decided to incorporate. WFN Executive Board members received in this way some personal legal protection for their role in WFN matters. The WFN incorporation provided encouragement for IFCN to do the same. Insuring the IFCN directors and officers against liability was considered appropriate. The IFCN would need a permanent secretariat in order to incorporate. A properly incorporated nonprofit organization could receive the donations without incurring a tax liability and without needing separately to establish a Foundation.

Delegates were asked by mail and e-mail to contribute their thoughts on these matters. Active discussion with Delegates was held during the 1999 Prague ICEMGCN. Issues eventually carried over into the next Fiscal Period for incorporation and obtaining insurance.

8.4. Executive office

The matter of a central Executive office had been discussed for many years. The 1995 Kyoto ICEMGCN General Assembly raised the issue because the work required of Executive Committee officers was substantial. Each officer was using staff time at their home institution to do portions of the Federation's work, and each was personally doing an excessive amount of work that could have been delegated to properly trained central executive and office staff.

By the beginning of this Fiscal Period in early 1998, the Executive Committee evaluated the concept of a central officer executive director. There was no consensus about how this might work. The general idea seemed meritorious. The Executive Office could keep mailing lists, communicate with societies and delegates, conduct elections and other balloting, and organize the many meetings and minutes. This was referred to the LRPC.

LRPC noted that WFN and other international medical societies had established permanent secretariats in recent years. Mark Hallett, then Movement Disorder Society President, provided examples of how they used this central resource. Each Executive Committee member was asked to contribute to a list of duties they are currently performing that could be accomplished by a central executive office. A long consolidated list was collected. It seemed that this move was an inevitability, given the need for incorporation, insurance, legal protection, and relieving the officers from many organizational chores. The committee then sought more information about actual tasks accomplished by existing professional executive offices for other international medical organizations, which professional groups were used by others, and what options seemed to have the best advantages. By the end of this Fiscal Period, the Executive Committee recommended to hire or create an Executive Director and permanent office. The decision of whom to hire was left to the new Executive Committee at the beginning of the 2001–2006 term.

8.5. Dues

The Florence General Assembly discussed what to do about nondues paying societies. The Long-Range Planning Committee considered options. The committee recommended not to expel societies when economic problems precluded regular dues paying. For example some societies encountered national currency regulation problems. For others, dues were large compared to the daily income of typical member physicians. A few societies may have been dissolved but it is difficult to confirm that. One society was thought to have been dissolved, only to reappear and become active and paying dues again. There was a need to maintain good communications with Delegates and national societies so as to assure that correct contact information is used. The LRPC recommended that nondues paying societies lose their voting rights in the General Assembly and IFCN elections. Those societies would keep their eligibility for any office of IFCN and the capacity to get fellowships for their young members. Further work was needed to determine if a few societies have been dissolved.

An LRPC financial group task force included Andrew Eisen (Canada), Kjeld Andersen (Norway), François Mauguière (France) and Robert Miller (USA) to consider dues. The task force and LRPC group reported to the 1999 Prague General Assembly. The recommendation was not to change the dues amount.

9. Finances

Income and expenses varied considerably between the years because of the variable effects of International and Chapter congresses. Overall, a small to moderate profit was achieved every year. Paul Despland served as Treasurer since the 1993 Vancouver ICEEGCN. Over the succeeding 7 years, the Federation's assets more than doubled to US $1.3 million. The annual budget depended on congresses during that year; it averaged US $300,000 income and US $220,000 expenses. Gains in currency exchange values contributed to the positive asset change. Details of congress financing caused considerable gain/loss variability from year to year.

9.1. Income

During this Fiscal Period, the annual income averaged US $300,000. The major components were Elsevier royalties (US $193,400 to $231,200), National Society dues (US $42,140 to $67,807), Repayments from past congress profits (varied greatly), and Investment income (US $8200 to $35,800). In some years, the Elsevier royalties accounted for more than 75% of the income.

Elsevier royalties rose and fell with advertising revenues, expenses of publishing, number of new books released, and effects of electronic publishing. The contract called for the Federation to share in the profits rather than to get a preset annual amount.

9.2. Expenses

Annual expenses varied from US $204,000 to nearly $350,000, depending heavily on the kinds of congresses and projects accounted for in that year. The largest routine expense was the two Editors-in-Chief's offices, used for staff, mailing and other costs related to publishing the journal. This was budgeted at US $60,000 per year. Other variable expenses were for travel of the Executive Committee members to attend Executive Committee meetings, OCIC meetings, regional meetings, and Chapter Congresses. An expense was incurred for local costs of those meetings. Support for Fellowships to Congresses averaged US $44,000 per year but varied considerably. Support to the Congress budgets themselves varied from nothing in some years to US $100,000 in other years, much of which was a loan repayable from congress profits. Special projects were variable, for example US $42,000 to print the *Practice Recommendations* book. Executive Committee members were reimbursed for direct expenses of staff, mailing and other costs to their own institution to support Federation business. Executive Committee members personally never are paid a stipend, salary, or other payment for their time or effort. They are expected to pay Congress registration fees like any other registrant.

Chapter support started as a loan of US $3000 each year for each Chapter. The chapters were expected to report how the funds were spent, in part for the auditing process. Eventually this changed to an annual transfer, not a loan. In the next Fiscal Period the amount continued to change as the Federation assessed how best to support Chapter activities.

Office expenses were paid for the President, Secretary and Treasurer, while there were no expenses spent by the Past-President and Members-at-Large. The President's expense significantly decreased because of more frequent use of e-mail in lieu of airmail and faxes. The expense for one of the Editors-in-Chief was low because of expenses subsumed by the National Institutes of Health (NIH). As compared with the expenses in previous years, there was a significantly increased support for Congresses and Fellowships. The annual financial reports described substantial details and were accompanied by receipts. Expense details were made available for Delegates to examine and were presented to the external auditor for review.

9.3. Congresses

The International Congresses were operated by local organizations with oversight by the Federation. Those local organizations operated either as a part of the national society or by a PCO. The Federation contributed start-up funding as a loan to be repaid later from Congress profits. The Congress itself would raise most of its operating funds from local governments, charitable donations, exhibitor fees, and registration fees. Budgets were set to run a profit more than enough to repay the Federation start-up loan. The Organizing Committee of the International Congress (OCIC) is responsible for approving the budget and contracts as well as the scientific, social and other aspects of the Congress. The Federation held four of the seven votes on the OCIC, with the other three held by the national society.

The Federation gradually increased its Congress support as the Federation operating budgets allowed. This was meant to keep Congress registration fees from growing too high. On some occasions, the Federation gave funds without a requirement that it be repaid, instead taking an outcome stake, for example one-third of profits. In addition, budgets called for repayment of the fellowship grants out of Congress profits, if any. If no profit occurred, no fellowship repayment was expected. As a result of this variability in timing and repayments, the fiscal effect of each congress was spread over several years in the Federation budgets, and this was a cause of great variability in the Federation's annual financial profit or loss.

Obtaining good accounting of congresses was sometimes difficult. On one occasion, 3 years passed before the professional congress organizer business turned over accounting and repaid loans. That and many other lessons from previous congresses showed that great attention to detail was needed so as not to be taken advantage of by professional congress organizer businesses or convention centers.

Most congresses turned a profit, best when sufficient charitable donation were obtained. For example congresses regularly obtained unrestricted educational grants from vendors or local charities. On one occasion a very large donation was obtained from a national horseracing association, with whom an organizer had made some contact. These activities were an important part of organizing a financially successful congress. It also allowed for better quality social events, lunch breaks, or other ancillaries and, importantly, kept its registration fees lower.

Chapter congresses were handled differently. They were organized more directly by the Chapter or national society. In general, two members of the Federation Executive Committee were appointed to each Chapter congress organizing committee. Federation support started as loans and fellowship support similar to those for the International Congresses but often at smaller amounts. During future Fiscal Periods the organizational participation of two Executive Committee members remained, whereas financial support details gradually changed.

9.4. Audits

The 1997 Florence General Assembly approved a change in Federation external auditing and financial consulting arrangements. The recommendation was to retain an independent accounting firm with greater experience in international business. After a search, the Federation retained Mr. Alain Maillard of Geneva to provide independent auditing. Mr. Maillard was a member of the Swiss Institute of Certified Accountants and Tax Consultants. His auditing reports were shared with Executive Committee members. It was included with the finance materials brought to each General Assembly meeting, any Delegate who wished to review it, and the 1998 annual auditor's report was sent to all Delegates in June 1999. This communication was made much easier in the electronic communication era. Auditing for income, expenses, assets, liabilities, and balance sheet were generally satisfactory, with minor suggestions usually made for further improvements. Great details were kept of expenses along with receipts.

Areas of recommended improvement most often were for more detailed about Elsevier royalties. Those payments were often sparsely documented, even when the overall amounts were satisfactory. The Executive Committee and Treasurer pressed for more detail in publication royalties, income and expenses, as well as the list of journal subscribers. The journal title *Clinical Neurophysiology* is owned by the Federation, which gives greater leverage in negotiation. The contract with the publisher calls for payments to the Federation as a portion of profits, based on journal income and expenses. For that reason, those details would be relevant for auditing purposes.

The audits concluded each year that the balance sheet and profit–loss statement agreed with the books of account, the books of account have been properly kept, and the financial position, and the results of operations were presented in accordance with the principles and provisions of the Federation Statutes.

10. Nomination Committee

The Nomination Committee Chairman was Carl Lücking (Germany), as specified in the Statutes. Members were IFCN Delegates Americo Sakamoto (Brazil), Nobuo Yanagisawa (Japan), and Donald Sanders (USA).

In its usual procedure, the election was conducted in three stages. This complex process was specified in the Statutes and Bye-Laws so as to balance the Executive Committee geographically and by neurophysiology discipline.

Twelve societies were not allowed to vote because of failure to pay dues in the previous years. Forty-two societies were eligible to vote. In the several rounds of voting, 80–88% of those societies voted.

The results were

President	François Mauguière	France
Treasurer	Andrew Eisen	Canada
Secretary	Graham Harding	UK
Member-at-Large	Ryuji Kaji	Japan
Member-at-Large	Johannes Noth	Germany

Continuing members included

Past-President	Marc Nuwer	USA
Editor-in-Chief	Paolo Rossini	Italy
Editor-in-Chief	Mark Hallett	USA

Chapter 15

2001–2006

President: François Mauguière

This Fiscal Period marked several transitions in Federation operations. An Executive Office was established in London. Incorporation in Canada replaced the previous registration in France. The contract with Elsevier was updated resulting in a greater portion of revenue for the Federation. To supplement the Chapters' outreach to clinical neurophysiologists in unrepresented nations, a new Federation organization was established to serve their needs, the International Clinical Neurophysiology Society (ICNS). The Federation continued its transition to the new timing of International and Chapter congresses.

1. Executive Committee

The Executive Committee (ExCo) was comprised of President François Mauguière (France), Past-President Marc Nuwer (USA), Secretary Graham Harding (UK), Treasurer Andrew Eisen (Canada), Members-at-Large Johannes Noth (Germany) and Ryuji Kaji (Japan), and Editor-in-Chief Mark Hallett (USA). A second Editor-in-Chief, Paolo Rossini (Italy), also served during the first half of this term (see Appendix 11, Fig. 25). Concorde Ltd. Manager Wendy Holloway served as Executive Director for most of this term; Jane Hay succeeded her in the final year.

ExCo meetings sometimes included guests during portions of the meetings. Attorney Rod Kirkham from Hennan Blaikie joined by teleconference for some discussions of incorporation. Long-Range Planning Committee (LRPC) Chairman Carl Lücking joined for some discussions of that committee's work. Elsevier Publisher's Manager Peter Bakker participated in discussions of some publication issues.

This also marked the first time that the ExCo held some of its meetings by conference call instead of traveling for face-to-face meetings.

2. International Congresses

2.1. Numbering congresses

The combined congress series were renumbered. The 2001 Buenos Aires General Assembly authorized changing each congress's name to the International Congress of Clinical Neurophysiology (ICCN), dropping the designations as an EEG or EMG congress. The Executive Committee adopted a proposal to add together the numbers of two previous Congress series. The 1999 Prague meeting was called the XI International Congress of Electromyography and Clinical Neurophysiology. The 2001 Buenos Aires meeting was called the XV International Congress of Clinical Neurophysiology, already dropping the Electroencephalography designation.

According to this proposal, the 2003 Congress would be numbered the XXVII, and the 2006 Congress would be named the XXVIII International Congress of Clinical Neurophysiology. The numbering system continued to use Roman numerals.

2.2. XXVII International Congress of Clinical Neurophysiology, San Francisco 2003

The Prague ICEMGCN General Assembly appointed the American Association of Electrodiagnostic Medicine (AAEM) as host for the 2003 EMG congress. The year 2003 was AAEM's 50th Anniversary. The congress, planned for San Diego in September 2003, would be fully joint as equal partners, not just overlapping or consecutive. Such a fully joint meeting with a national society was similar to previous joint Federation meetings in Japan and Brazil. This 2003 congress would mark the last in the EMG series meetings, as spelled out in the plan to unify the Federation Congresses.

The Prague delegates considered this as an excellent opportunity to show the strength of clinical neurophysiology by holding a well-attended joint meeting, noting that AAEM is among the Federation's largest member societies. This would also mark the return of the Federation Congresses to an USA site after a long absence, 28 years since the previous 1975 Rochester, MN, International EMG Congress.

Under the able leadership of Convener Mark Hallett and Secretary Murray Brandstater, the Organizing Committee for the International Congress (OCIC) designed a joint meeting celebrating the AAEM anniversary. The meeting's treasurer was to be the AAEM treasurer at the time of the meeting, that is, Lois Nora. AAEM itself would serve as the professional congress organizer for the meeting. Others contributing substantially to the meeting organization included 2003 AAEM President Lawrence Phillips, 2003 American Clinical Neurophysiology Society (ACNS) President Donald Schomer, and Scientific Program Committee Chairperson Janice Massey.

The other US member society, the ACNS, initially declined the 1998 opportunity to co-sponsor this meeting. This meeting was a celebration of the AAEM's anniversary, and having a third joint partner might dilute their celebration. As an EMG series congress was not a topic in the core interest area for ACNS, formerly known as the American EEG Society. ACNS also preferred stand-alone meetings. Yet, with time, this position changed. The 1999 Federation General Assembly changed the scope of the meeting to cover all areas of clinical neurophysiology. The meeting was no longer to be designated as an EMG meeting, rather as an ICCN generically. The organizers invited ACNS to organize the EEG portions of the meeting. For these reasons the ACNS joined in toward the end of the congress planning as a third co-sponsor. This illustrates the complexity of the Federation's evolution toward unifying its goals, scope, congresses, and names.

That sponsorship change was not the only substantive alteration. The contracted hotel in San Diego was expanding to a larger size that would have sufficient meeting space for the congress. An economic recession in 2001 slowed construction progress, raising worries that it would not be ready on time. Site inspection by the Past-President revealed a large construction hole in the ground with no superstructure steelwork. After considering its options the OCIC approved moving the congress to San Francisco.

The OCIC sought to keep registration fees modest. AAEM usually subsidized its meeting registration fees through its annual membership fee. The Federation agreed with that concept and process to keep down registration fees. The OCIC and ExCo matched the AAEM plan by converting its repayable start-up funding into a non-repayable direct meeting subsidy. Furthermore the usual fellowship funding repayment would be taken out of the budget; no repayment would be expected unless the congress generated sufficient profits. Having decided that for the San Francisco congress, the ExCo agreed to extend that to other congresses starting with the 2001 Buenos Aires congress. This subsidy policy change benefited subsequent congresses and their registrants.

The Federation took a financial stake in this meeting, a change from its usual policy. In the past, the local organization was financially responsible and the Federation provided limited financial support. The Federation agreed to a contractual responsibility for this meeting for a portion of the profit or loss.

The usual 70 Young Investigator Fellowships were granted for this meeting for investigators below 35 years of age. These fellowship recipients were from 19 different countries. A new separate support was initiated at this meeting for national society Delegates from economically challenged nations who were otherwise unable to provide for their own travel support to the congress. This was initiated to encourage and make more practical that all official society Delegates would be able to attend the congress and its General Assembly.

Most Federation congresses have published their abstract books as supplemental issues of the journal. For this meeting, abstracts were published by *Muscle and Nerve* with the AAEM covering the cost of the publication. This change was helpful in keeping the budget modest; publication of abstracts in *Clinical Neurophysiology* would have cost the Congress approximately US $25,000. The *Clinical Neurophysiology Supplement Series* of books would publish the plenary talks and symposium lectures. These congress books have been labeled *Advances in Clinical Neurophysiology*, using as book editors some of the main congress organizers.

The Congress Scientific Program arranged for 130 faculty lecturers at invited symposia, workshops, and lectures. A plenary session on the early history of AAEM and EMG was presented in celebration of the AAEM anniversary. An unusually large number of named lectures were held because the three sponsoring organizations each traditionally had their own named lectureships. The named lectureships for plenary presentations included:

- IFCN Adrian Lecture on "Neurobiology of Pain" by Ronald Dubner.
- AAEM Reiner Lecture on "Microneurography" by Erik Torebjörk.
- AAEM Lambert Lecture on "Skin Biopsy" by William R. Kennedy.
- IFCN Kugelberg Lecture on "Reflex Dystrophy Syndrome" by Ralf Baron.
- ACNS Jasper Lecture on the "Role of the Thalamus" by Frederick Lenz.
- IFCN Berger Lecture on "Cortical Mechanisms" by Hiroshi Shibasaki.
- ACNS Gloor Lecture on the "Role of SII and the Insula" by François Mauguière.
- AAEM Anniversary Lecture on "Neuroimaging of Pain" by Karen Davis.
- AAEM Anniversary Lecture on "Rehabilitation" by Stanley A. Herring.

Continuing Medical Education (CME) was provided by AAEM. That process included the usual CME audience feedback forms. Attendees generally scored the meeting sessions very highly. Congress registration topped 2000. This meeting still holds the record as the largest Clinical Neurophysiology meeting.

2.3. XXVIII International Congress of Clinical Neurophysiology, Edinburgh, 2006

The British Clinical Neurophysiology Society hosted the 2006 XXVIII International Congress of Clinical Neurophysiology in Edinburgh, Scotland, in September 2006. National society organizers included Convener and Chairperson Jonathan Cole, Treasurer Ian Smith, Scientific Committee Chairperson Kerry Mills, Federation Secretary Graham Harding, as well as Roberto Guiloff, Robin Kennett, Nick Murray and Greg Moran. Concorde Ltd. was the Professional Congress Organizer.

Building on some policy changes implemented for the 2003 ICCN, the Federation contributed start-up funding and fellowships to the congress organization without considering that a loan. Instead the Federation took on responsibility for a portion of any profit or loss. Start-up funding was increased and the Federation accepted the risk that this would be recouped from congress profits. To financially support the congress, over £140,000 was raised from industry.

Over 704 abstracts were accepted from a wide number of countries. There were 76 invited speakers, 146 platform presentations, and 20 talking poster sessions. Brazier and Cobb Awards were given to two young investigators who published high quality research reports in the journal during the year before the congress. These awards included both a monetary award and the opportunity to present their work during a plenary platform session.

IFCN sponsored more than 80 Fellowship awards for young investigators. These Fellowship awards' value ranged US $500 for recipients from the UK, to $750 from the rest of Europe, and $1000 from elsewhere plus meeting registration. The usual age limit was 35 years for these Young Investigator Fellowship Awards. These awards went to candidates nominated by their national society, and for the first time the ICNS was able to nominate young investigators from otherwise unrepresented countries. The Federation needed to increase its budgeted support for these fellowships.

Delegates and some others from economically disadvantaged countries received support to help them attend the meeting. This support was called bursaries to distinguish it from fellowships that went to young investigators. For the bursaries the fellowship age limit did not apply. This was accomplished partially to assure Delegate representation at the General Assembly meeting. The best possible Delegate representation was desired for this meeting because of the discussion at that business meeting of the new constitution and Canadian incorporation.

The scientific program included both Federation named lectureship and lectures traditional for the British Society. The major plenary lectures were:

- Adrian Lecture: "How do we control movement?" by Prof. John Rothwell (UK).
- Kugelberg Lecture: "Human ion channels: in vivo investigation" by Prof. David Burke (Australia).
- Berger Lecture: "High frequency ("600 Hz") oscillations in EEG and MEG — what do they mean?" by Prof. Gabriel Curio (Germany).
- British Society Geoffrey Parr Lecture: "Magnetism and the nervous system" by Prof. Anthony Barker (UK).
- Keynote Lecture: "Genes and proteins: the impact of the new genetics on neuroscience" by Dr. Kenneth Fischbeck (USA).
- Keynote Lecture: "What can stem cells do now?" by Prof. Evan Snyder (USA).
- Keynote Lecture: "New developments in neonatal and pediatric epilepsy" by Prof. Perrine Plouin (France).
- Keynote Lecture: "Neural plasticity: what can we change and how?" by Prof. Ulf Ziemann (Germany).

Additional primary symposia were:

- The Neurophysiology of Movement and its Disorders, chaired by Prof. Berardelli.
- rTMS in Treatment: Review of the Mechanisms, chaired by Prof. Ulf Ziemann.
- Magnetoencephalography (MEG), chaired by Profs. Ian Holliday and Paul Furlong.

The social program was outlined including a welcome reception and a traditional Scottish gala dinner and Ceilidh (see Appendix 11, Fig. 32). An accompanying person's program and pre- and post-congress tours were available to explore Scotland and the surrounding areas around Edinburgh, and to visit Glenkinchie Distillery and the Edinburgh Crystal Company.

2.4. Competition for the 2010 congress

The bids for the 2010 Congress were received by the deadline of February 2005. The ExCo appointed members to investigate the feasibility of each bid. In addition, each bid was reviewed by the Concorde Ltd. staff who were experienced in congress organizing business. Bids were scored in a formal process to decide and prioritize each. Concorde also provided guidance on the bidding process for candidates. This was done proactively to organize details to give the General Assembly a thorough review of the strengths and weaknesses of each bid.

Initial inquiries were received from four societies. Each was invited to submit a complete bid using an organized application form. After extensive review, the ExCo voted to present the Singapore and Japanese Society bids to the ICCN Congress. Restrictions were placed on the length of General Assembly presentations, bidding society exhibit stands, and free gifts given to registrants that might influence votes at the Edinburgh General Assembly. Kobe, Japan, won the selection for the 2010 Congress.

3. Establishment of an executive office

At its first meeting in 2001, the ExCo discussed the previous Fiscal Period's LRPC's recommendations for a permanent secretariat. The previous ExCo left that recommendation for this new ExCo to review and implement. This plan was discussed with the General Assembly at several of its meetings.

The Secretary listed which functions a permanent secretariat could carry out (Table 15.1). A European would be most easily accessible for the current Secretary and President. The ExCo requested that the Secretary investigate potential services available in London, as this was felt to be the most convenient site. Mark Hallett provided documentation of an equivalent exercise undertaken recently by another organization. Federation Secretary Graham Harding was asked to bring information to the next ExCo for selection of a permanent secretariat.

After investigating possible businesses to provide this service, Prof. Harding recommended Concorde Services Ltd. This was the same organization that had recently been retained by the British Clinical Neurophysiology Society to serve as the professional congress organizer for the 2006 ICCN. A full contract was drafted and reviewed in detail by the ExCo. Detailed points were identified and the Secretary renegotiated these sections. The proposed cost of the service was £18,000 per year over a 4-year period. At its October 2001 meeting, the ExCo approved proceeding with a contract with Concorde pending negotiating the identified changes.

TABLE 15.1

ACTIVITIES FOR THE EXECUTIVE OFFICE

The following Executive Director tasks are taken from the list in use in 2002. Since then the list has gradually evolved.

Meetings of Executive Committee

The Executive Committee meets twice a year, and the Executive Director will:

- Attend meetings
- Organize meeting facilities, accommodations, and refreshments
- Obtain and circulate agenda information and attachment
- Circulate expense forms and forward receipts to Treasurer
- Take, circulate, revise and maintain minutes
- Undertake actions delegated at the meeting

Communications with Delegates

For the member societies and their Delegates, the Executive Director will:

- Invoice, receive, and track annual due payments in coordination with the Treasurer
- Send receipt acknowledgment letters
- Send dues reminders for later payments
- Maintain a dues database
- Maintain and update contact information database for all societies and their Delegates
- Solicit change information and track changes
- Prepare reports as required
- Send approved minutes and reports to delegates, with copies to the society and officer

(*to be continued on pp. 156 and 157*)

(*TABLE 15.1, cont.*)

Accounting
For Federation accounting, the Executive Director will:
- Invoice and track accounts receivable
- Pay accounts payable
- Maintain standard business practices for handling funds
- Pay annual insurance premiums, correspond with insurance carrier
- Keep Treasurer informed about accounts
- Work with Federation attorney regarding tax filing paperwork

Journal subscriptions
For the journal Clinical Neurophysiology, the Executive Director will:
- Receive journal subscriptions renewals and payments, organize and submit to the publisher
- Receive and reply to correspondence about subscriptions
- Track to which Society each subscriber belongs
- Process subscription payments, primarily by credit card
- Establish and maintain a bank account for payments
- Send combined payments to the Journal Publisher quarterly, as a bank transfer
- Handle change of address notifications
- Provide quarterly financial reports to the IFCN Treasurer

Journal Yellow Pages
For the journal's Yellow Pages, the Executive Director will:
- Receive news and information from Secretary and others
- Circulate to delegates requests for news
- Compile news items and send to Secretary for editing
- Send edited drafts camera-ready to Elsevier for printing
- Post confirmed Yellow Pages on the IFCN website

Mailing address
For the Federation, the Executive Director will:
- Act as a central mail address for IFCN information, and respond to inquiries
- Create and maintain central forms and stationery templates for Executive Committee members
- Mail or e-mail delegates, societies and officers as requested

Website
For the Federation's website, www.ifcn.info, the Executive Director will:
- Contact with webmaster regarding web page design
- Prepare page content updates
- Arrange for hyper-links as appropriate
- Update pages quarterly

Ballots and voting
For Federation elections for rules, officer and other issues, the Executive Director will:
- Prepare ballots and voting notices
- Circulate notices to all delegates via e-mail, fax or mail
- Receive and compile ballots
- Monitor responses, send reminders

Congresses
For Federation International and Chapter congresses and symposia, the Executive Director will:
- Attend Congress or Symposium when requested
- Organize facilities for Committee and Chapter meetings
- Staff IFCN secretariat room

(*TABLE 15.1, cont.*)

- Provide secretarial services
- Prepare exhibition stand and promotional material for IFCN
- Receive and reply to delegates' and member societies' requests

Young Investigator Fellowships
For Federation Fellowship Programs, the Executive Director will:

- Announce fellowships availability and request nominations from member societies
- Receive, compile, acknowledge, and screen societies' fellowship nominations
- Notify applicants of fellowship awards and rules
- Arrange for Treasurer's disbursements of fellowship funding at the congresses
- Prepare a formal certificate for each Fellow

General Assembly
For Federation General Assembly meetings, the Executive Director will:

- Formally notify societies and delegates
- Prepare and circulate agenda
- Receive committee and officer reports, reproduce and circulate
- Circulate previous General Assembly minutes
- Obtain a list of recent notable deaths
- Prepare hall and voting sheets for meeting
- Prepare attendance sheet and distribute
- Take, reproduce and circulate minutes following meeting
- Screen, evaluate proposals for future congresses

Statutes
For Federation Rules, the Executive Director will:

- Maintain records of Statutes and Bye-Laws, and any changes
- Notify delegates of any changes
- Post Statutes on the website
- Communicate with Federation attorney about rules changes

Archiving
For Federation record storage, the Executive Director will:

- Maintain archives according to the instructions of Executive Committee
- Store all past delegate records
- Retain samples of all print work
- Retain IFCN accounts

The IFCN Secretariat at Concorde Service Ltd. became operative on the 17th of January 2002, when the President, Secretary and Treasurer signed the contract. The fees for the provision of the above services would be £18,000 per annum, based upon the 4-year cycle, and to include out of pocket expenses, such as telephones, general postage, photocopying, fax and e-mails. The Contract was written to continue until the 31st of December 2005, near the end of this Federation Fiscal Period. The Secretariat took over production of the Yellow Pages. They began work as has been performed on a website and transfer of the previous web material from Kyoto to London. A pop-up exhibition stand was developed to provide the IFCN with a demountable stand for exhibit at meetings. In the previous Fiscal period, society executive Daniel Tjornehoj provided the Federation with individual membership subscription organizational services for the journal; with the signing of the Concorde contract, that function was transferred from Wisconsin to the new London office.

Soon thereafter, the new Executive Director Wendy Holloway began to attend Federation meetings. She attended the 2002 Barcelona European Chapter meeting. From that point the Executive Director attended Executive Committee meetings and Congress to help with the Federation business and organizational activities. In 2006, she was replaced by Jane Hay who staffed IFCN Edinburgh functions.

The Executive Committee asked for further services from Concorde Services Ltd. The Core Professional Organizer (PCO) staff was asked to review and score the 2010 ICCN bids. This was separately contracted for services from this firm. It included designing a form for congress candidates to complete and scoring reviewing the submitted bids. They also drafted a Memorandum Of Understanding (MOU) for each candidate to sign prior to the General Assembly in 2006. This was done to help attain better control over organizational actions that had previously pre-empted some OCIC control over Congress costs and organizational details. Concord agreed not to bid on the 2010 Congress so that they could serve as an independent reviewer in service to the Executive Committee and General Assembly.

4. Incorporation in Canada

4.1. Problems and possible solutions

Since its inception, the Federation was a non-profit foreign association registered in 1951 in the Préfecture des Bouches du Rhône in Marseilles, France. The registered name was Fédération Internationale de Neurophysiologie Clinique (formerly Fédération Internationale d'Electroencéphalographie et de Neurophysiologie). The registration number was 013/3/012674, accomplished under a 1901 French Law. The Federation's legal address was Hôpital Neurologique, Service de Neurologie Fonctionnelle et d'Epileptologie, 59 Boulevard Pinel, 69394 Lyon Cedex 03, France (formerly CHU La Timone, 13005 Marseilles, France). This needed to be updated with each new Executive Committee, and it was most recently updated in a communiqué provided to the Préfecture of Marseilles dated June 26, 2002.

In the years 1997–2001, problems became evident with that registration, problems that were discussed at the 2001 General Assembly. This 2001–2006 Executive Committee was charged with addressing these problems.

The LRPC and two successive Executive Committees had evaluated for a long time the issues of incorporation, legal status, insurance, and related uses.

The Federation carried no insurance. This was a drawback for publishing practice standards and guidelines, for journal and book publications, and for Congresses. Grieving parties might challenge the Federation in court. An attorney advised the Executive Committee to obtain insurance.

The President and Treasurer retained an attorney in Lyon with experience in non-profit organizations. They were told that in 1998 French Law had changed. The new law was more restrictive than the old statute under which the Federation had been established. The Federation would be unable to continue business as usual under the new French statute. The Federation might have tax liability for the journal income in the new French system. At least one Federation officer always must be French. Sufficiently broad insurance coverage would be difficult to obtain in France, and difficult to obtain elsewhere as a registered charitable organization based in France. Any rule and officer changes must be communicated promptly to the French authorities. Other constraints were discovered during consultation with the Lyon attorney.

French government authorities requested that the official registration be transferred from Marseilles to Lyon because the President is based in Lyon. The President wrote back pointing out that the presidency normally changed every 4 years, so there would therefore be no particular advantage to this transfer. Despite the objection, the authorities directed that the transfer go forward. The transfer of registration from Marseilles to Lyon was accomplished in 2002. The new official address was that of the current French Federation President, François Mauguière in

Lyon. The President confirmed that all official IFCN papers had been filed and received in Lyon.

It appeared that the Federation might escape from these new constraints if the organization were based elsewhere. Arrangements looked more advantageous for an international non-profit organization in the USA and the UK, where regulations were less restrictive and such a charity would not be liable for taxes. Executive Committee members investigated several possible options of new official homes in Europe and North America. The goal was to weigh the advantages and disadvantages of various home sites.

4.2. Opening a Canadian organization

The results of this comparison suggested that Canada would be the best new site. The non-profit organization laws were favorable there, and the Federation would have no tax liability. The organization did not need to have a Canadian officer at all times. Insurance was readily available for an organization such as the Federation. The Federation's founding president Herbert Jasper was from Montreal, so the move in a certain way would continue to honor the Federation's historical legacy. An important additional factor was the Canadian language policy, as an officially bilingual nation in French and English. The new Executive Office was already established in London, and a Canadian incorporation would balance this international organization's activity on a second continent. After reviewing the factors, the Executive Committee in 2002 unanimously recommended pursuing incorporation in Canada.

Treasurer Andrew Eisen, a Canadian, previously identified a law firm with the needed experience in non-profit corporations, the Vancouver law firm of Heenan Blaikie LLP. The original contact with them was to advise about insurance or legal protection for the Federation and its officers. This scope of work was later extended to include accomplishing Canadian incorporation. That firm transferred the Federation's legal representation from Lyon to Vancouver. Further contact with the French authorities was accomplished from Canada.

The General Assembly was briefed and a vote taken by mail regarding the movement to open an incorporation entity in Canada. The General Assembly ballot results were unanimous in favor of a move to Canada. The ballot included a quorum of responding societies. Consistent with the rules, the ballot was passed. All Delegates and societies were informed of the agreement to proceed.

Should the same Federation Statutes and Bye-Laws be adopted in Canada? The intention was to make as little change as possible. The attorney recommended new clauses about legal protections for the Federation and its officers. The existing Statutes and Bye-Laws would be reformatted with minor rewording. In other words, the French rules would continue in Canadian rules despite some reformatting and rewording.

There was a problem with the word *Statute*. In Canada only the Parliament makes statutes, a word meaning a law. The primary rules known in the French rules as *Statutes* now would be known officially in Canada as *Bye-Laws*. The lesser rules known in the French rules as *Bye-Laws* now would be known officially in Canada as *Rules and Regulations*. For historical reasons, the older traditional rules naming convention continued to be used colloquially in Federation internal business.

The Vancouver attorneys John Legge and Rod Kirkham of Heenan Blaikie LLP, the Rules Committee, and Executive Committee worked together on rules changes. Executive Committee members Graham Harding and Marc Nuwer worked on the Statutes. Marc Nuwer and Rules Committee member Hiroshi Shibasaki drafted the new Bye-Laws. The product was the new wording of Canadian rules. This is discussed more below in the Rules Committee section. The actions accomplished by the attorney also included closing the French registration and incorporation of the Federation in Canada. This process took an extended time because of the wish to be inclusive in seeking opinions and communicating about progress. To help with checking that the old rules were kept active in the new format, an extensive cross-walking table was created so that each portion the French rules could be compared with the new wording in the Canadian rules. This ensured that all substantive contents of the old document were included in the new. Sections were added for indemnification and liability protection for the Federation and officers. Amendment to the new rules could be accomplished by a majority vote of the General Assembly, less than the two-thirds needed in the French rules.

Since the new statutes would be in Canada, they would be written both in English and French. (The version printed in the appendix here is only the English version.) The Executive Committee also agreed that a version would be translated into Spanish. François Mauguière agreed to provide a translation from English to French.

The Canadian attorney, Executive Committee, and Rules Committee approved the revised documents. The General Assembly unanimously approved the new Canadian rules' documents by mail ballot. The documents were submitted to the Canadian government.

At the September 2005 Executive Committee meeting, the President announced that all legal formalities and preliminary conditions had been complied with and that Letters Patent had been issued by the Minister of Consumer and Corporate Affairs in conformity with the terms of the application for incorporation and bore the date of May 10, 2005. The Executive Committee, then still operating within the French Federation rules, took a break from its agenda to reconvene for an initial meeting of the new Canadian Executive Committee. A formal signing ceremony was held in which the official documents were signed. The two Executive Committee meetings were kept as separate minutes and agendas in conformity with legal formalities. This brief meeting marked the formal beginning of the new Canadian corporation entity. The meeting was organized at Aachen, Germany, the home city of IFCN Secretary Johannes Noth. It being a border city, the actual site of this Executive Committee meeting was adjacent to Aachen in the Hotel Kasteel Bloemendal, Vaals, The Netherlands on Monday September 19, 2005. Table 15.2 is the formal agenda item as presented and unanimously approved in Vaals.

TABLE 15.2

ACTION TAKEN AT THE SEPTEMBER 19, 2005 FIRST MEETING OF THE NEW ORGANIZATION'S EXECUTIVE COMMITTEE IN VAALS, THE NETHERLANDS

The Chairman announced that all the legal formalities and preliminary conditions relative to the incorporation of the Federation have been complied with and that Letters Patent had been issued by the Minister of Consumer and Corporate Affairs in conformity with the terms of the application for incorporation and bore the date of May 10, 2005.

Upon a motion duly made and seconded, it was unanimously RESOLVED:

THAT the Letters Patent dated the 10th day of May, 2005 and are hereby accepted as the Charter of the Federation

THAT the same be entered at length in the Minute Book of the Federation, the original thereof deposited with the corporate records of the Federation and duplicate copies thereof be lodged with the office of the Secretariat

The Chairman then presented to the Meeting the Bye-Laws of the Federation (to be defined and referred to as the "Statutes" of the Federation), in the form as submitted to the Department of Consumer and Corporate Affairs, and upon motion duly made and seconded, it was unanimously RESOLVED:

THAT the Statutes, as presented to this Meeting, and as submitted to the Department of Consumer and Corporate Affairs, be the same and are hereby enacted and adopted as the Statutes of the Federation, and that the Secretary be and is hereby ordered to enter the said Statutes in the Minute Book of the Federation and to lodge a duplicate copy thereof with the office of the Secretariat.

Upon motion made by the Treasurer, seconded (GH) and unanimously RESOLVED:
Messrs. Loewen Kruse, Chartered Accountants, were appointed the Auditors of the Federation to serve for such period as contemplated by the Statutes, under such terms and conditions as to their remuneration as shall be determined by the Directors of the Federation from time to time.

The Treasurer also submitted a form of Asset Transfer Agreement and Declaration of Trust and upon motion duly made and seconded, it was unanimously RESOLVED:

1. THAT the form of Asset Transfer Agreement and Declaration of Trust presented to this Meeting (the "Agreement") is hereby approved and confirmed by the Directors on behalf of the Federation
2. THAT the Agreement be executed and delivered by each of the Directors in their capacity as Director and member of the Executive Committee of the Federation on behalf of the Federation.
3. THAT the Treasurer is hereby authorized and directed, for and in the name of and on behalf of the Federation, to execute and deliver all such further agreements, instruments, certificates and other documents and to all such other things as such officer may determine to be necessary or advisable in connection with the transactions contemplated by the Agreement, the execution of any such document or the doing of any such other act or there being conclusive evidence of such determination.

There being no further business to transact, the Meeting was terminated upon motion duly made.
The Letters Patent establishing the Canadian IFCN was signed on May 10, 2005 by the Ministry of Industry.

4.3. Closing the old registered organization

Upon that action taken in Vaals, there were two societies in existence both in parallel to each other: the original International Federation of Clinical Neurophysiology, registered in France, and the new Canadian corporation of the same name. Steps taken under the attorneys' guidance included an "Asset Transfer Agreement and the Declaration of Trust", an "Application for Incorporation of a Corporation without Shared Capital under Part II of the Canada Incorporation Act", a "Statement on Registration of an Extraprovincial Society in British Colombia" and receiving "Letters Patent" from the Ministry of Industry. Bye-Laws ("Statutes" in Federation language) in their modified form were received (see Appendix 11, Figs. 27 and 28). The new legal address in Canada became in care of Heenan Blaikie LLP, 1055 West Hastings Street, Suite 2200, Vancouver, BC V6E 2E9, Canada.

This action was announced to interested parties. The President informed the Delegates and Societies of the actions, implications, and formalities. A further discussion would be held on the next occasion of the General Assembly's meeting in Edinburgh. If there were no problems raised at that discussion, the General Assembly would ratify the Canadian organization and give its permission to close the French organization. An announcement was made in the journal's yellow and white pages.

The Treasurer informed both Elsevier and Concorde of the change and the need to alter the contracts to show the new Federation as the contracting organization with them. This was important because the contracts were with the old French registered IFCN. A letter to the French authorities informed them that the IFCN was now incorporated in Canada. Due to some uncertainty of where the IFCN papers were held officially, letters were sent to authorities both in Marseilles and Lyon.

At the 2006 Edinburgh General Assembly, discussion was supportive and no serious problems were found (see Appendix 11, Figs. 29 and 30). The Assembly ratified the Canadian incorporation, authorized dissolving the French registration, and these actions were reflected in the minutes. These actions gave full legal clarity that the Canadian organization was the only organization in existence from that point forward. The attorneys submitted to the French authorities up a simple statement announcing the closure of the French registered company.

Treasurer Andrew Eisen investigated carriers who provided insurance to other medical organizations.

Directors and Officers, Liability, and Publications Insurance were obtained through the Lambert Group of Canada. The OCIC organizations will mandate that individual congresses purchase event liability insurance, including those meetings held under the auspices of the IFCN. Publications Insurance would cover anything the Federation publishes, journals and books, hard copy or electronic. Directors and Officers insurance would protect board and committee members when they acted on behalf of the Federation. General liability insurance provided coverage for other general business problems. The insurance would state that legal actions against the Federation must be considered in Canada under Canadian law.

Attorneys reported that the Canadian incorporation had proceeded smoothly. The audit report noted that all IFCN assets were tax exempt for Canadian purposes. The old organization's various assets had been transferred to the new organization.

Henceforth there was only one Federation organization instead of two parallel organizations as there had been for the previous 16 months. The actions included incorporation and liability protection, they clarified the tax and legal situation, and they avoided a need to alter the Federation's traditional rules.

5. Publications

This term marked a return to a single Editor-in-Chief. Conversion was completed to electronic manuscript submission. Impact factors remained high. Individual subscriptions increased. Two national societies contracted for subscriptions for all of their members. The Handbook and Supplement Series books continued to be published.

This term also saw Elly Tjoa retiring from Elsevier after working with the journal and the Federation for the past 36 years, more than half of the journal's life. She had become a centerpiece of our relations with Elsevier. Her career spanned eight Editors-in-Chief dating back to William Cobb and Mary A.B. Brazier, two giants of our Federation publishing history, both IFSECN presidents and founding organizers of the Federation. Elly Tjoa's retirement marked a generational change in Federation activity. She had been instrumental also in many of the additional Federation book publishing activities, and a knowledgeable resource for many members of the Federation as they dealt with publisher and publication issues.

5.1. Clinical Neurophysiology journal activity

Mark Hallett as the sole Editor-in-Chief beginning in 2003. European Office Editor-in-Chief Paolo Rossini finished his term with the journal at that time. New Associate Editors were appointed to help with the flow of manuscripts. These included Fabio Babiloni (Italy), Colin Binnie (UK), John Connolly (Canada), Gabriel Curio (Germany), Anders Fuglsang-Frederiksen (Denmark), and Hiroshi Shibasaki (Japan).

The flow of submissions continued to increase. Extra pages were added to the volumes to allow for additional manuscripts. The increased submissions also led to a more stringent threshold for acceptance. The acceptance rate dropped from 55% to 50%. In this way, the publication backlog still remained small and the speed of publication remained favorable.

Manuscripts were submitted by authors representing institutions worldwide. Asian countries' submissions notably increased. Areas of interest shifted. A progressive decline was seen in the number of evoked potential papers, accompanied by an increase in movement disorders and motor control, new EEG techniques, magnetoencephalographic technology, and psychophysiology.

The impact factor, a measure of citations of each journal articles by other subsequently published journal articles, remained good. This was a concern after the transition to a new journal name in 1999 and the consolidation of the three journals series into one. Those changes would have adversely impacted the citations rating at least temporarily. By 2003 *Clinical Neurophysiology's* impact factor was 2.485, making the journal the highest ranking of any in the discipline of clinical neurophysiology or its subspecialties.

Time was kept short for processing the received manuscripts, the mean time from the manuscript arrival to publication averaging 131 days. Usually the longest time was waiting for authors to revise their manuscripts. Time from acceptance to publication was less than 3 months. This was a positive factor for prospective authors.

5.2. Electronic publishing

Elsevier's new publishing software, Editorial Manager, aided submission and reviewing and cut the time for decisions about acceptance. That system replaced the previous electronic submission software, SmartWorks. Editorial Manager provided greater flexibility to submitters and editors. It also allowed authors to track their submissions through the editorial and publishing process. All manuscripts at this time must be submitted electronically. Authors and reviewers thought that this system worked well.

Clinical Neurophysiology is available on-line now through medical libraries that choose to subscribe. Individual subscribers also can access the journal on-line. Current issues can be accessed even before the printed copy arrives by mail. Back issues are posted on-line all the way back to Vol. 1 in 1949. Our journal has never been so accessible.

A change to electronic publishing was clearly taking place. *Clinical Neurophysiology* would be in Medicine Direct, an electronic subscription package of journals sold to institutions. It was noted that *Clinical Neurophysiology* was sold almost entirely to institutions at this time. Therefore this consolidated electronic subscription program would have a potentially large effect if libraries change to electronic versions. It may impede some users' access because print copies no longer would be on the shelves. It may aid others in journal access through their institutional libraries, since they could do so from off-site and easily access desired articles.

The US National Institutes of Health and the British Wellcome Trust demanded that their grant recipients post their accepted manuscripts in an open access forum. That would allow anyone to read or print those reports. The IFCN owns the copyright to the journal articles, which are released under subscriptions prices for viewing or printing. Although most *Clinical Neurophysiology* articles would remain unaffected, a decision should be made on how to move forward. After discussion the Executive Board agreed that authors may post in an open forum, but only at 12 months after publication as a matter of journal policy.

Abstracts from national society meetings had been published together in a single 13th issue each December. However, this was considered unfavorable for speed of publication, so the journal changed back to publishing society proceedings abstracts throughout each year. To save on print page space, society abstracts appeared in the on-line electronic version of the Journal. Book reviews and correspondence remain in the printed material. This seemed satisfactory to most users, since by this time most users had access to the electronic journal copies through their local medical libraries.

5.3. Editorial and liaison boards

Associated Editors were appointed in 2003 to supplement the Editor-in-Chief's work processing manuscripts. These Associated Editors were known as Field Editors because they brought to the Editor's office expertise in a variety of subspecialty areas. These were also chosen to represent a geographical balance, so as to keep the Editors informed of activities or problems in each of several regions. The proposed Fields Editors were: Fabio Babiloni (Italy), an expert in quantitative techniques, Colin Binnie (UK) an EEG expert, John Connolly (Canada), an expert in cognitive studies, Gabriel Curio (Germany), an expert on sensory physiology, Anders Fuglsang-Frederiksen (Denmark), an EMG expert, and Hiroshi Shibasaki (Japan), an expert on motor control. Appointment of Field Editors would be for 3-year terms with a possibility of renewal. All would have direct access to Editorial Manager to process manuscripts for review.

To engage national societies in journal activities, each society had been invited to nominate a member to serve as their representative on a Journal Liaison Board. That board aimed to promote the journal better within our member societies. The Board consists of a representative from each member society. It was separate from the Editorial Board that concerns itself with the science of review and the policies of the publication. Each society was invited to appoint one representative to the Journal Liaison Board. Terms were limited. Each representative was charged with reporting journal issues to their society, promoting increased individual subscriptions by society members, and reporting back to the Editor-in-Chief about journal-related issues from their society. The board also would meet from time to time at IFCN congresses. Each representative received a complimentary journal subscription.

This Journal Liaison Board concept was reviewed several years after its establishment. The Liaison Board was not working as well as it should have. The liaisons did not communicate with the journal. Each society's appointed person was not being rotating as required. The Editor-in-Chief was asked to review these issues with Liaison Board members when that panel met at the Edinburgh ICCN. One option would be termination of the program following that meeting.

5.4. Awards

Elsevier traditionally sponsored the Cobb and Brazier Awards for each quadrennial ICCN. The awards are given to investigators less than 40 years of age who had submitted winning manuscripts for publication in the journal *Clinical Neurophysiology*. The Awards are monetary plus a certificate presented at an ICCN ceremony. Often the award winners are given time to present an ICCN platform presentation on their work. The Awards should be based on merit alone, should be from different countries, and from different subspecialty areas of neurophysiology. After screening by the Editor-in-Chief, eight candidate applications for the Cobb and Brazier Awards were reviewed by the Executive Board.

5.5. Subscriptions

Continuing concern was about the relatively very small number of individual member subscriptions to the journal. It dropped from 2363 in the early 1990s, to 2262 in 1993, then 1896 in 1995, and further down to 1475 in 2000, and 1350 in 2001. The institutional subscriptions declined much less. The President wrote to delegates and officers of national societies pointing out the financial advantages of individual membership and asking them to promote the journal. The Federation continued to sponsor discounted individual journal subscriptions to members of Federation national societies. That program was organized through the Executive Office and previously was organized through an independent organizational executive office in Wisconsin. VAT was not applicable to these subscriptions in the UK. Elsevier was investigating whether the same tax arrangements held for the rest of Europe. Anyone interested in these subscriptions can make arrangements through the IFCN website.

Societies were offered the opportunity to enroll all their own members for journals subscriptions as part of their society membership dues. This would be at a deeply discounted price for all members of the society. The idea was based on a successful pilot program in the Italian society. The Japanese society also joined that program. Several other societies expressed interest. Each society would be able to state that the journal was the official journal of that society.

A different tactic was to provide an additional perquisite to encourage individual subscribers. An affinity group was formed for individual subscribers named the *Friends of the IFCN*

(FOIFCN). This club would hold receptions at congresses, ones to which only the individual subscribers were invited. Small tokens were developed including lapel pins for FOIFCN members. Other free gifts were sponsored at the Edinburgh FOIFCN reception, including water glasses and T-shirts with a logo. This also gave the editors and publisher a way to interact with individual subscribers to hear from them about their interests and concerns about the journal, and reasons for maintaining an individual subscription.

5.6. Journal contract with Elsevier

The journal's Executive Board renegotiated the contract with Elsevier. The new 6-year agreement was effective in January 2003.

The Federation's portion of profits increased with this new contract. The Federation owned the journal's trademark rights. The copyright notice in each issue of the Journal was: "Copyright 200x, International Federation of Clinical Neurophysiology." For administrative purposes, Elsevier managed copyright release and reprint requests. The trade name, seal and other identifying trademarks of the Federation also continued to be owned by the Federation.

5.7. Handbook of Clinical Neurophysiology

Under the leadership of Series Editors Jasper Daube and François Mauguière, the *Handbook of Clinical Neurophysiology*, with each volume about clinical neurophysiology in particular disease categories, was continued. This series replaced a previous book series entitled *Handbook of Electroencephalography and Clinical Neurophysiology*. Compared to the previous Handbook series, individual volumes would focus on a particular disease and then discuss neurophysiology techniques as they applied to the diagnosis or pathophysiology of that disorder. This disease-oriented approach contrasted with the technique-oriented Practice Guideline book. Affiliated physiological techniques can easily be included in the disease-oriented books, including techniques not covered in the Practice Guidelines book. The editors arranged to publish an average of two books per year for 5 years. A list of volumes produced is given in Appendix 3. Since the retirement of Elly Tjoa from Elsevier, the management of the Handbook Series was turned over to Michael Parkinson in Edinburgh.

5.8. Supplement series

The *Electroencephalography and Clinical Neurophysiology Supplement Series* continued to produce books, including the Congress Symposium book for the Prague 1999, Buenos Aires 2001, and San Francisco 2003 meetings. The IFCN Congress volumes are labeled as *Advances in Clinical Neurophysiology*. Other books published in this series were based on specific topics or other meetings of Federation member societies. Recent volumes included symposium books from the 2003 Transcranial Magnetic Stimulation and Transcranial Direct Current Stimulation symposium in Göttingen, Germany, the 2003 and 2006 Motor Unit Number Estimation (MUNE) symposia in Snowbird, UT, USA, and the 2004 8th Evoked Potentials and Related Techniques symposium in Fukuoka, Japan.

Topics were proposed ad hoc, some through the Federation and others coming from Elsevier, based on the interests of specific individuals. An advantage of this series for book editors and authors is that the series already has a wide existing distribution through subscription lists to individuals and medical libraries.

The series has no overall names editor. The Executive Committee approves new titles in the series. Individual volume editors then work directly with Elsevier to produce the book. A list of books published in this series is given in Appendix 4.

6. Rules Committee

The Rules Committee dealt in this term with amalgamation of the Council and General Assembly, incorporation in Canada, closing the

French organization, review of new member society applications, and establishment of the ICNS. The Rules Committee was composed of Marc Nuwer (USA) Chairperson, James Colebatch (Australia), Paul Despland (Switzerland), Roberto Reisin (Argentina), and Hiroshi Shibasaki (Japan).

6.1. Member societies

Three new societies joined the Federation as members: the Guatemalan Society of Clinical Neurophysiology, the Estonian Society of Clinical Neurophysiology, and the Singapore Society of Clinical Neurophysiology. The Yugoslav society changed its name to the Serbia and Montenegro Society of Clinical Neurophysiology.

In Colombia, the traditional member organization was the Valley Society of Clinical Neurophysiology. That organization went through reorganization and was replaced by a successor organization, the Colombian Clinical Neurophysiology Association (ACNC). The ACNC was recognized as the successor national society. A second society in Colombia applied for membership, one representing a different group of physicians, the Colombian Association of Electrodiagnostic Medicine (ACME). IFCN Statutes do allow for a second society as long as they represent mainly different members. One precedence was in the USA, where one society is primarily interested in EMG and peripheral neurophysiology, whereas the other society represents primarily EEG and central neurophysiology. A review of the two US societies showed only a 6% overlap of memberships. A similar disciplinary distinction occurred in Belgium, where two member societies were distinguished by discipline. China is recognized by the Federation as having two societies, one representing physicians on the mainland and the other physicians in Taiwan. (The Federation considers them the same country under a policy that defers to the United Nations General Assembly to decide when a region is a recognized nation. The Federation does not make those political decisions.)

The Federation rules call for negotiations with the two societies before accepting a second member society from the same nation. One goal would be to attempt to have the two societies work together or merge. The Rules Committee chairperson held electronic and face-to-face sessions with members of both societies to seek that end but without success. The two societies had different memberships, with one primarily composed of neurologists and the other composed of physical medicine physicians. In the end, the Rules Committee recommended accepting the second society into the Federation.

6.2. Journal changes

The General Assembly agreed with the change in journal title in 1999. The process to change Statutes and Bye-Laws is long, requiring several steps over time. During this term, the Federation's French Statutes and Bye-Laws were formally amended to change the journal's name throughout the documents.

The journal's Executive Board, that is, the Federation Executive Committee, had accepted the recommendations of Editors-in-Chief Gastone Celesia and Paolo Rossini to combine the two Editorial offices into one. The General Assembly deferred to the Executive Board about this matter. Rules changes were needed to accomplish this, one replacing the plural noun with the number neutral compound noun Editor(s)-in-Chief. This allowed the rules to be flexible, and gave the Executive Board clearer authority to make changes in number.

6.3. Organizing Committee for the International Congress (OCIC)

Adding the Editor-in-Chief to the OCIC would bring additional expertise to the OCIC about the scientific topics that currently are most active and the investigators who are most recently publishing new and exciting science. At the same time, there was a desire to maintain a relative balance of OCIC members representing IFCN and local organizers. To do so, adding to the OCIC one more local organizer was recommended, specifically the Scientific Program Committee Chairperson. The expanded OCIC would be comprised of the IFCN President, Past-President, Secretary, Treasurer, and one Editor-in-Chief, and four representatives from the member society hosting the Congress. The member society representatives were the Convener, Secretary, Treasurer, and the Scientific Program Committee Chairperson.

6.4. Consolidation of congresses

Another 1999 directive from the General Assembly was to discontinue having two separate International Congresses. In the sequential processes of rules changes, this wording of the new rules was drafted, reviewed, and approved during this term. The International Congress of EEG and Clinical Neurophysiology and the International Congress of EMG and Clinical Neurophysiology were consolidated into one quadrennial ICCN. The last EMG series meeting was held in 2003, renamed as an ICCN. To avoid one excessively long or short Executive Committee term, the quadrennial ICCN meetings were moved from odd-numbered years to even-numbered years beginning in 2006.

6.5. Chapter Bye-Laws

Chapter Bye-Laws are considered Bye-Laws of the Federation. They are subject to the same review as other Federation Bye-Laws, which needed Council approval.

The Latin American Chapter (LAC) made changes in their Bye-Laws to standardize at 2 months the timing of announcements prior to Chapter meetings. There had been three different times at 1, 2 and 6 months specified for announcing the date of the Chapter general Assembly, the nomination of officers, and other details. The uniform 2-month period makes congress organization easier. The Council agreed to this change.

That Chapter was saddened by the death of Chapter Executive Committee Member-at-Large A. Fernandez Guardiola (Mexico). This raised a rules question because there was no rule for replacing Executive Committee members through appointment or by-elections. To address that, the Chapter adopted new Bye-Laws rules that in the event of prolonged incapacity or death of the Secretary/Treasurer or a Member-at-large, the Nomination Committee would invite nominations to replace the incapacitated officer for the remaining of Fiscal the Period. Elections would take place soon after.

6.6. Disestablishment of the Council

Federation rules established two oversight bodies. The senior larger body, the General Assembly, was changed with meeting at the quadrennial EEG series congress, approving statute changes and budgets, recommending the next congress city, and other matters of greater importance. Council was charged with meeting not only during the quadrennial EEG congresses but also whenever called to meet in the interval in between. Council approved Bye-Law changes and advised the Executive Committee on lesser issues of routine business. The Executive Committee solicited advice from the Council between congresses by mail or e-mail. Traditionally this included meeting at the EMG series Congress. Council was composed of one Delegate from each member society. General Assembly was composed of 2–4 representatives from each member society, depending on the society's size. Occasionally when the two bodies gave differing opinions about items of business, the General Assembly's opinion was taken as more senior.

In 1999, the Council and General Assembly both agreed to hold just one organizational meeting during the ICCN meeting, not both. Members felt that the two bodies often discussed similar issues, and the matters were too redundant. A single organizational meeting would suffice. Council would continue to exist for advice and decisions by mail between congresses. General Assembly rules then did not permit mail or e-mail ballots. Bye-Laws were revised to hold just one business meeting at congresses, the General Assembly meeting. Council still existed for advice between congresses.

After further study of these rules, the Rules and Executive Committees recommended to disestablish Council altogether. This was not what had been discussed at the previous General Assembly. The role for Council could be filled by consulting with the Delegates directly and by the General Assembly for voting. This change was approved by Council by mail, then discussed and approved at the 2003 General Assembly meeting. At that point, Council ceased to exist as a Federation body. General Assembly became the sole broadly representative body.

General Assembly rules were changed to allow it to do business by mail, fax, or e-mail. This allowed Federation business to go forward without waiting for the quadrennial congress meetings. For example, this will allow the General Assembly to approve its minutes within weeks or months of each meeting, rather than waiting 4 years until its next meeting. The Delegates would still be consulted as much as before, and maybe even more now that e-mail made communications easier. Occasionally, the term *Council* still was mentioned when referring to the collection of Delegates, even though the official body had been dissolved.

The number of votes in the General Assembly seemed to be a never-ending question. Societies with fewer than 100 dues paying members were entitled to two votes and two representatives at each General Assembly meeting and mail ballot. Societies with 100–400 members were allowed three representatives and votes. Societies with 400 or more were allowed four representatives and votes. By the year 2001, several societies had more than 2000 dues paying members, and one had more than 5000. Should the cut-off numbers be changed? Discussions continued, but no changes were recommended.

How long should Delegates serve? Some had served for more than two decades. Concerns were raised about the lack of turnover. A mandated maximum length of Delegate service was considered but no action was taken.

6.7. Elections

The rules prohibited the Nomination Committee members from campaigning for or endorsing the candidacy for any one candidate in elections. The Nominations Committee was charged with overseeing the elections process. The national societies were to nominate and choose among the nominees. The nominees could contact Delegates soliciting their support, and the same could be done by national societies and others — except for the Nominations Committee members. This was different than in some other societies in which their nominations committees make up the slate of candidates, and sometimes only posted one candidate for each office.

Should the current Executive Committee members be allowed to endorse a candidate or contact Delegates seeking votes for one candidate? The belief was that the Federation should be more opened in its election processes so as not to discourage passing along offices among a smaller group of associates.

New rules' amendments prohibited electioneering by the current Executive Committee in the same way that it restricted the Nominations Committee.

6.8. International Clinical Neurophysiology Society (ICNS) and friends of the IFCN

The ICNS Bye-Laws were approved by the IFCN Council. The ICNS became an organization within the Federation. It provides an official IFCN home community for individuals from nations that did not have an IFCN member society. Individual were members of ICNS. The group is discussed in a separate section further below.

Some national societies excluded from their membership non-physicians. They did so for good reasons, sometimes for legal reasons in their own countries. Some engineers or others desire to participate in IFCN activities. The ICNS Bye-Laws were revised to allow those individuals to become ICNS members, but with a restriction. Any applicant for ICNS membership from countries with an existing IFCN member society cannot be a member of that existing society, cannot be eligible for membership in that society because of its membership restriction, and must obtain the member society's written support for the individual's request for ICNS membership. ICNS Bye-Laws were amended to that effect, and the IFCN Bye-Laws also were amended to include: "If a professional is excluded from membership in a national society, that society may officially support such excluded persons for ICNS membership."

The Friends of the IFCN was established as an affinity group to encourage individual subscriptions to the journal. This was discussed in an above section. Should that organization have a formal place in the Federation Bye-Laws? The Rules and Executive Committees decided that this could be handled more informally by Elsevier and the Editor-in-Chief and did not need to be incorporated into the formal rules.

6.9. Canadian Statutes and Bye-Laws

As discussed above, the move to Canada was accomplished in this term. The Rules Committee refined the new Canadian IFCN Statutes and Bye-Laws, formally known in Canada as the Bye-Laws and the Rules and Regulations. The Vancouver attorneys worked together with Executive Committee officers Graham Harding and Marc Nuwer to refine the new Statutes document, and with Marc Nuwer and Rules Committee member Hiroshi Shibasaki on the new Bye-Law documents. All went through the usual formal processes of rules' adoption.

Along the way, the rules were reformatted and streamlined without altering the content. A careful cross-walk of the old and new documents showed that old rules were carried forward and no new rules were inadvertently introduced. The Canadian rules were discussed again in Edinburgh even though they had been accepted by mail vote previously. At Edinburgh, the Canadian rules were endorsed.

Consistent with that concept, any new statements were identified for ratification. Statutes changes included:

- The journal name was changed from *Electroencephalography and Clinical Neurophysiology* to *Clinical Neurophysiology* in places not previously changed.
- A Corporate Seal of IFCN was newly added, as per Canadian custom.
- The IFCN head office was changed from France to Canada.
- Current Executive Committee members were named as founding Canadian corporate officers.
- New items related to the legal and liability issues were added to provide protection for the Federation and its officers, committee members, editors, and reviewers.
- Existence of IFCN Chapters was added.
- Council meetings were removed, and the word *Council* was replaced by *General Assembly* in some sections.
- Some sections previously in the Statutes were moved to Bye-Laws.
- Some sections previously in Bye-Laws were moved to the Statutes.
- Sections were re-ordered into groups, renumbered, with new headings and subheadings.
- Bye-Law references to Statute sections were renumbered.
- Associate Editors were added to the journal Editorial Staff.
- Rules were clarified about loss of a society's voting rights for non-payment of dues, and for removal of inactive or obsolete societies.

As the final part of moving from France to Canada, the Edinburgh 2006 General Assembly voted unanimously to disestablish the French registered IFCN organization. Federation attorneys were instructed to notify authorities French and Canadian authorities.

7. Practice Committee and Guidelines

7.1. "Practice Guidelines" book translations

The *Practice Guidelines* book, formally titled *Recommendations for the Practice of Clinical Neurophysiology: Guidelines of the International Federation of Clinical Neurophysiology*, was published two terms previously in 1999. That excellent book was edited and organized by Guenther Deuschl (Germany) and Andrew Eisen (Canada). National societies were given the opportunity to translate it into their own national language. The translation should be an official activity of the Society or Chapter. The Society producing the publication should involve as many societies as possible, which use the same language. The IFCN must be sent two copies for their archives. The IFCN owns the copyright to the original English-language guidelines. The translation must give credit to the Federation for the original version, and to the chapter authors for each chapter. The costs of the publication must be borne by the Society, and any profits may be kept by the Society. Neither IFCN nor Elsevier will charge any royalties. Permission to translate must be obtained from the IFCN President.

Several societies asked for authorization to proceed with translations. This included the societies from France, Mexico, Poland, Serbia and Montenegro, and Turkey. The Société de Neurophysiologie Clinique de Langue Française, working together with clinical neurophysiologists from other French speaking nations, published a guidelines translation. Jean-Marie Guérit, François Mauguière, and Perrine Plouin coordinated the translation and editing of *Guide Practique de Neurophysiologie Clinique*, printed through Elsevier, Oxford in 2002.

7.2. New and revised practice guidelines

Paolo Rossini (Italy) agreed to oversee development of new and revised IFCN guidelines. He was asked to propose to the Executive Committee specific topics and panel leaders. Each panel chairperson would suggest further panel members, subject to approval by the Executive Committee. Geographical diversity of panel members was desirable. Panels would be composed solely of clinicians. The target audience were physicians in training and in early stages of practicing clinical neurophysiology and the emphasis should be on commonly used clinical techniques. Reports would need to be reviewed by expert reviewers and approved by the Executive Committee. They would be published in the journal after the usual anonymous peer review and possible revisions. The collection of these reports eventually would be collected together into a next version of the Practice Recommendations book.

The previously approved guideline development on Clinical Use of TMS, under the leadership of Robert Chen, would be folded into this project. Paolo Rossini proposed to follow the evidence-based medicine guidelines, for example, as in the Cochrane rules. He made suggestions regarding guidelines and authors. Topics early in the development time line would include electroretinography (ERG), visual evoked potentials (VEPs), somatosensory evoked potentials (SEPs) and cognitive event-related potentials (ERPs). Considerations for additional near-term projects were magnetoencephalography, threshold tracking for peripheral nerve, EEG mapping and coherence, laser and pain evoked potentials, and nerve conduction studies (NCS).

8. Long-Range Planning Committee

Under the leadership of Carl Lücking (Germany), the LRPC commented on several projects previously recommended by the committee and which were now in the process of implementation. These projects included incorporation, insurance, and opening of an executive office. Along with Dr Lücking, the committee was composed of Daniel Cibils (Uruguay), Giancarlo Comi (Italy), Andrew Eisen (Canada), Nai-Shin Chu (Taiwan), Erik Stålberg (Sweden), the same committee membership as in the previous Fiscal Period.

The committee's charge and activities covered a broad range for the Federation. The committee provided additional advice and encouragement for the Federation to take several major steps. For Federation infrastructure changes, the LRPC recommendations pertained to incorporation, obtaining insurance, setting aside a special fund for education and training, and establishing a permanent secretariat. Action to implement those recommendations were taken during this and the next Fiscal Periods.

The committee continued to oversee donations of books and subscriptions to member societies and individuals in economically disadvantaged nations. The donated materials were to be made available for use by many individuals. ICNS members were considered eligible participants. From time to time, the committee gave a report to the Executive Committee and General Assembly on the scope and success of its projects.

A sum of US $7500 per annum had been allocated to provide journal subscriptions. Fifty-eight individuals at different institutions in 18 nations were receiving the journal. The committee proposed an additional 12 names bringing the total to 60. Most recipients provided the LRPC chairman with a detailed description of the location and availability of the journals, and the use that had been made at that facility. The Executive Committee agreed to continue support for this program for a further 5 years.

The Federation donated to the World Federation of Neurology (WFN) book program extra copies of Federation books that Elsevier was about to discard, mainly old issues from the Supplement Series books. They were sent instead to the WFN Secretariat for their program to provide books to economically disadvantaged neurology institutions. The WFN expressed appreciation for the books donated and asked the IFCN to keep in mind the WFN book program for any further excess book inventory.

The LRPC chairman has in his possession minutes, correspondence and photographs from 1970 onwards. The chairman suggested that important items be stored at the Secretariat after the LRPC chairman provided an index. The previous archives, the ones used by William Cobb (UK) for the earlier Federation History book, were given to a former Federation Secretary but they unfortunately are no longer available.

9. Chapters

9.1. Latin American Chapter

The Chapter in this term expanded to include two new members, conducted two Chapter Congresses, and sponsored several local Symposia on Clinical Neurophysiology topics. The LAC emphasized developing good communication among its member societies and their officers and delegates. The Chapter aimed to help other Latin American clinical neurophysiologists to form national societies and to be admitted to IFCN and become LAC members. In the absence of national societies in some locations, the LAC also complied contact lists of additional clinical neurophysiologists who could be invited individually to attend LAC events.

Finances for the LAC activities derived mainly from congress and symposium profits and from the Federation support to Chapters. Spanish and Portuguese language for clinical neurophysiology publications were considered, such as translation of the *Practice Guidelines* book, as another possible source of income to support the LAC.

Daniel Cibils (Uruguay) was chosen to serve as LAC president for the term from 2001 to 2005. His leadership was supported by Past-President Carlos Medina (Argentina) during the same term. LAC founder Nelly Chiofalo (Chile) continued to advise the LAC Executive Committee even after stepping down in 2001 from her formal role as

LAC Past-President. In 2005 at LAC elections Jose Xavier de Castro (Brazil) was chosen to serve as LAC President for the 2005–2009 term. Serving as Chapter Secretary–Treasurers during this term were Francisco Luccas (Brazil) 1999–2003 and Renato Verdugo (Chile) 2003–2007. The Federation's LAC Liaison Officer was Marc Nuwer (USA). Chapter Executive Committee members-at-large included Augusto Fernandez-Guardiola (Mexico) from 2001 until his unfortunate death in 2003, Olga Sanz (Argentina) 2001–2005, Juan Santoni (Dominican Rep.) 2003–2007, Henry Stokes (Guatemala) 2005–2009, and Jaime Ramos (Mexico) 2005–2009. The Chapter's Nominations Committee, Carlos Medina (Argentina), Mario Medici (Uruguay) and João Nobrega (Brazil) supervised elections during this term.

9.2. LAC congresses and symposia

The Chapter was actively involved in organizing congresses and local symposia. The principal LAC congresses each were titled Latin American Symposium of Clinical Neurophysiology. Two were held during this term, in Porto Seguro, Brazil in September 2002 and Santiago, Chile in October 2004. In keeping with the change in timing of major chapter congresses to a quadrennial schedule, the next congress was scheduled tentatively for 2008.

The III Congreso Latinoamericano de Neurofisiologia Clínica and IX Jornada Brasileña de Neurofisiologia Clínica, was held in Porto Seguro, Bahia, Brazil, in September 2002. The Brazilian Society of Clinical Neurophysiology hosted the meeting, which was held in an attractive seaside resort. José Fortunato Zanovello (Brazil) served as the local convener. Three hundred registrants attended, among which were young investigators who received meeting fellowship support.

The IV Latin American Symposium of Clinical Neurophysiology was held in Santiago, Chile in October 2004. This was a joint meeting with the host society, the Chilean Society of Clinical Neurophysiology. Local organizers were convener Renato Verdugo, Chapter President Daniel Cibils, Chilean Delegate Nelly Chiofalo, and Chilean society officer Perla David (see Appendix 11, Fig. 26). The congress registered 254 delegates from 10 of the 11 Latin American Chapter member societies and from several additional countries without an IFCN member society. Fifty submitted posters were presented, the IFCN granted funds for 34 fellowships for young investigators from six countries as well as three IFCN prizes.

In addition to the formal Chapter congresses, the LAC sponsored several local symposia. Two Executive Committee members attended a Brazilian Congress of Clinical Neurophysiology Recife, Brazil, October 2001. The Federation also lent its name and auspices to a 2003 a Latin American symposium in Rio de Janeiro on sleep monitoring. The Uruguayan Society organized a symposium on neuromonitoring held in 2006 in Montevideo. The societies of Brazil, Argentina and Chile collaborated in the organization of that meeting.

Toward the end of this Fiscal Period, the Federation Executive Committee turned over to the Chapters the responsibility to decide which Latin American local meetings should receive support. A pool of Federation funds was set aside for support of the chapter meetings during each 4-year Fiscal Period.

Overall, the LAC was active in sponsoring one or another Latin American symposium or other meetings almost annually. This provided an opportunity for interactions among clinical neurophysiologists that was seen as very positive and helpful for the senior leadership, the traditional practicing clinical neurophysiologist, and the trainees.

9.3. New member societies

During this term, two new member societies joined the Federation in the Latin American region and automatically became Chapter member societies. Guatemala joined under the leadership of society Delegate Henry Stokes. In Colombia, the existing national society changed. The Valley Society of

Clinical Neurophysiology was reorganized and replaced by a successor organization, the ACNC. The ACNC represented mainly neurologists practicing clinical neurophysiology. A second Colombian society applied for membership, the Colombian Association of Electrodiagnostic Medicine (ACME). The ACME represented mainly physical medicine physicians. After unsuccessful negotiations to encourage the ACNC and ACME to merge or band together, the Rules Committee agreed to recommend ACME for IFCN membership as the second Colombian society.

Other continuing member societies are from Argentina, Bolivia, Brazil, Chile, Cuba, Mexico, Peru, Dominican Rep., and Uruguay, bringing the total LAC membership to twelve. Contacts continue with clinical neurophysiologists in other unrepresented nations throughout the Latin American region.

9.4. Bye-Law changes

LAC Statutes Committee, Francisco Luccas (Brazil), Alicia Cueto (Argentina), Calixto Machado (Cuba), and Nelly Chiofalo (Chile) proposed several rules changes. Several different schedules were in use for informing Delegates about upcoming meetings and the topics for votes and discussion. The Bye-Laws were changed to standardize those notification times at 2 months.

After the untimely death of LAC Executive Committee Member-at-Large Augusto Fernandez-Guardiola (Mexico), the chapter decided to hold by-elections to fill the vacant position. This required a Bye-Laws change, as there was no process specified to replace a Member-at-Large. After formalizing this change, elections were held for that vacant position.

9.5. Translating the "Practice Guidelines"

Discussions were held at the Santiago LAC Congress about producing a translation of the IFCN *Practice Guidelines* into Spanish. The Mexican Society volunteered to look into this possibility, which would be in collaboration with other societies and the Chapter. Delegate Mario Shkurovich took the lead in this project, which was subsequently tabled when Shkurovich unfortunately fell ill during the next year and subsequently passed away.

10. European Chapter (EC-IFCN)

The European Chapter of the IFCN continued to be actively involved in sponsoring meetings, discussing the practice of clinical neurophysiology in Europe, and education of young physicians. The Chapter was organized during the previous Fiscal Period and held elections for a Chapter Executive Committee. The Chapter wrote Bye-Laws that were accepted by the Federation's Council. By 1998 the European Chapter was fully organized.

During the first two Chapter election cycles, the EC-IFCN Executive Committee included Chapter President Erik Stålberg (Sweden), Secretary-Treasurer Al de Weerd (The Netherlands), and Members-at-Large Giorgio Cruccu (Italy) and Teresa Sagalés (Spain). From 2001, Johannes Noth (Germany) served as the Liaison Officer for the Chapter and the IFCN Executive Committee. In 2005, Paolo Rossini (Italy) was elected Chapter President and Luis García-Larrea (France) was elected Secretary-Treasurer. Anders Fuglsang-Frederiksen (Denmark) and Jonathan Cole (UK) were chosen as Members-at-Large. The new terms began at the 2005 Stockholm European Congress of Clinical Neurophysiology (ECCN). Plans were made for future elections in which half of the Executive Committee positions would be elected every two years.

The Chapter continued to receive funding from the Federation general funds for the expenses of running the chapter. Additional support was made to Chapter congresses and certain other local symposia. In order to stay consistent with Federation requirements for Federation auditing, fiscal responsibility and oversight, the Chapter Treasurer sent annual reports and receipts to the

IFCN Treasurer. These were included in the annual Federation external auditing, the agreed upon method for properly accounting for all IFCN spending.

In other business, the journal *Clinical Neurophysiology* was adopted as the official journal of the European Chapter. The EC-IFCN maintained a website about its activities, congresses, symposia and officers. The IFCN authorized the French, Polish, Turkish and Slovenian societies to translate the Practice Guidelines into their respective languages. The French society worked with clinical neurophysiologists from other French speaking nations to publish the French translation.

A task force addressed the specialty status for clinical neurophysiology in Europe. The task force consists of Kjeld Andersen (Norway), Theresa Sagalés (Spain) and J.A. Jarrat (UK). The Chapter and its Task Force continued its discussions, as it had in the previous Fiscal Period, about the formal legal status of Clinical Neurophysiology in the European Community. A survey was initiated of the Clinical Neurophysiology training requirements and the board examinations given in various European nations.

10.1. Congresses and symposia

Chapter's 11th ECCN was held at the Congress Hall in Montjuich, Barcelona, August 24–28, 2002. The Convener was Teresa Sagalés. Joan Conill (Scientific Secretary), Isabel Moreno (Treasurer), Luis García-Larrea (Scientific Advisor), and François Mauguière (Past Convener) completed the Organizing Committee. The congress very successfully combined education, scientific and social events for the approximately 700 participants, from 48 countries. It included six symposia with a total of 29 speakers, six workshops, 12 courses, 31 platform sessions, 274 posters and 164 oral presentations. Total attendance to courses was 337 and to workshops 127. Altogether there were 111 invited speakers. All the courses, clinically oriented symposia and platforms were granted accreditation as Continuous Medical Education by the European Council (EACCME) of the European Union of Medical Societies. This was the first ECCN congress to have its own website, which was fully interactive for speakers and scientific committee reviewers. As a memorable social event, the gala dinner was held in a very interesting place, the "Hall of Mirrors" of the renowned Barcelona Opera House ("Liceu").

The Chapter's 12th ECCN was held in Stockholm in May 2005. The Congress met at the Stockholm City Congress Center Folkets Hus. Congress Convener Eva Svanborg and President Erik Stålberg arranged for Stockholm City to host a conference reception in the City Hall, where the annual Nobel Banquet takes place. The IFCN sponsored 34 fellowships for young investigators from throughout Europe. Six hundred registrants participated in the meeting that included educational courses, scientific symposia, and poster sessions.

Additional Chapter effort was applied to further educational activities. Courses on various aspects of EMG and neurography, pediatric EEG, epilepsy, and sleep were held under the auspices of the EC-IFCN in Spain, Romania, Czech Republic and Slovenia. The Chapter financially supported those local courses and Chapters Executive Committee members actively participated as faculty.

10.2. New societies

The European Chapter worked towards extending membership. The Baltic countries expressed interest in organizing their growing number of clinical neurophysiologists. The Estonian society was welcomed into the Federation in 2002 and formally joined the EC-IFCN activities at its 2005 ECCN. The Irish society began to participate in ECCN and Chapter activities and subsequently applied for formal membership in the Federation. Other countries advanced plans for membership and were in close contact with the EC.

11. Asian–Oceanian Chapter

At its 2000 Chapter meeting at the Manila II Asian–Oceanian Symposium of Clinical Neurophysiology, Prasert Boongird (Thailand) was chosen as the Chapter Chairman. Nobuo Yanagisawa (Japan) was re-elected as the Chapter Secretary. At the III Asian–Oceanian Symposium of Clinical Neurophysiology in 2005, toward the end of this 2001–2006 Fiscal Period, the Chapter Assembly elected Rawiphan Witoonpanich (Thailand) as Chapter President. Kwang-Woo Lee (Korea) was chosen as the Chapter Secretary. Ryuji Kaji (Japan) continued to serve as the Liaison Officer between the chapter and the IFCN ExCo.

Clinical neurophysiology activity across the Asian–Oceanian Chapter region continued most actively in Japan and Australia, where the national societies had strong annual meetings and agendas. The chapter continued its work on fostering mutual clinical neurophysiology activities and communications across the entire region and among the various national societies.

The Singapore Society of Clinical Neurophysiology was formed and joined the IFCN as a member society. This brought the Chapter membership up to 10 societies including Australia, India, Indonesia, Japan, Korea, Philippines, and Thailand. China was represented by societies in the Peoples Republic and in Taiwan. Contacts were made with individual clinical neurophysiologists in Iraq, Malaysia, Myanmar, and Sri Lanka.

11.1. Congresses and symposia

The III Asian–Oceanian Congress of Clinical Neurophysiology was held in Chiang Mai, Thailand on February 2–4, 2005. Regional organizing committee Chairperson Rawiphan Witoonpanich was supported by Secretary Siwaporn Chankrachang and Scientific Committee Chairman Yotin Chinvarun. All members of the IFCN Executive Committee were present and actively involved giving plenary lectures or organizing workshops. The program was composed of 10 Plenary Lectures, 13 Workshops, 10 Meet the Experts, three Lunch Symposia, two Platform Presentations, five Poster Sessions, two Video Case Discussions. The social program included a welcome reception and a gala dinner. The accompanying persons could participate in a City and Temple Tour and in visiting a home industrial village. The IFCN sponsored 24 fellowships for young investigators from 9 countries. The 340 registrants came from 21 countries. Nine prizes were awarded for the best poster and platform presentations. The abstracts of all presentations were published in a Supplement of the Neurology Journal of Thailand.

In addition to the Chiang Mai meeting, the 3rd Bangkok Symposium on Clinical Neurophysiology was held in March 2002. This was held just before The Neurological Society of Thailand annual meeting. This was third in a series of such local symposia held over the previous decade. Chapter support for this local meeting was because the interval between the 2000 and 2005 formal Chapter Congresses was long, and interim meetings would help foster the Chapter's organizational aims. In addition to the local Bangkok meeting, the Chapter supported a Symposium on Nerve Excitation and Threshold Tracking meeting in Japan in November 2004. After the Chapter's support, the Federation provided support for speakers and fellowships for young physicians to attend the 2nd Asian–Oceanian Workshop of Nerve Excitability Testing in Tokyo on November 2004. The Chapter and Federation planned an academic meeting, the International Consensus Meeting for Electrodiagnostic Criteria for Diagnosis of Amyotrophic Lateral Sclerosis (ALS). The meeting goal was a discussion of electrophysiologic criteria for the early diagnosis of ALS. Such a goal was important for planning and conducting drug studies as well as for patient care. The meeting took place in Awaji, Japan in December 2006. Ryuji Kaji and Andrew Eisen served as organizers.

A Myanmar medical organization requested Federation support for a local meeting on neurology and clinical neurophysiology. After consulting with the Chapter, the IFCN decided to send former President Carl Lücking to lecture at the meeting in Mandalay, Myanmar in January 2005. Inquiries were made as to the status on clinical neurophysiology in Myanmar, and encouragement was given to become active in Chapter activity.

The Chapter chose Seoul, Korea for its next formal Chapter Congress in May 2009. The Japanese and Singapore societies both intended to bid for the 2010 ICCN Congress.

Overall, the Chapter was on the road to fostering greater interaction, educational opportunities, and cooperation among the national clinical neurophysiology societies in the East Asian and Oceanian region. Ways to encourage greater participation from South Asian and Middle Eastern member societies was also given discussion within the Chapter.

12. North American region

The North American region had three societies but no formal Federation Chapter. To promote the Federation's presence and aims in this region, a special fellowships program was initiated, the IFCN International Exchange Fellowship Program. The concept was to foster an international program in this region. The program specifically sponsored fellowships for physicians and scientists from economically disadvantaged regions to attend North American meetings. The program was adopted and implemented by one regional society, AAEM. The society supplemented the program with support of its own, and providing the program for 4–9 fellows each year. The society and fellows both considered the program as very successful.

Discussion continued of forming a formal Chapter in this region.

13. International Clinical Neurophysiology Society

How could the Federation aid colleagues in countries that did not have a national society? It was suggested that a "Clinical Neurophysiology Society" could be formed, affiliated to the IFCN but without national boundaries. It would keep track of and encourage clinical neurophysiologists in those countries. When sufficient numbers practiced clinical neurophysiology in such a country, the Federation could encourage them to form their own national society and become a formal Federation member society.

At the 2003 Congress, the President reported on this new concept of the ICNS of members of non-affiliated countries (ICNS) to the General Assembly. The goal was to allow active neurophysiologists in non-affiliated countries to benefit from the activities of the IFCN and encourage communication among them and member societies. At the same meeting, the Secretary's report detailed Executive Committee's concern to promotion of the Federation's aims in parts of the world without member societies. To this point, active individuals in those countries were unable to benefit from the activities of the IFCN such as fellowships and communications about upcoming congresses.

The ICNS would be a professional association dedicated to fostering education in clinical neurophysiology and furthering the understanding of the nervous system designated for members from countries without an affiliated member society. The formally stated purposes were to:

- Promote personal contact between investigators and clinical neurophysiology and closely related fields, between the society and other similar societies throughout the world through the IFCN, thus facilitating exchange of scientific and professional information and opinions.
- Further the greater understanding and knowledge of clinical neurophysiology and disorders for which it is applied.
- Arrange for the exchange of journals or other written materials in these fields.
- Assist in the formation of committees for evaluation of standards, techniques, procedures, education, training or qualification of physicians or technologists.

- Achieve high standards for clinical practice of clinical neurophysiology.

ICNS members could apply for fellowships, reduced fees for journal subscriptions or international congresses. The Federation Secretary drafted a constitution for membership, which was approved by the Rules and Executive Committees and the General Assembly by mail ballot. The Executive Committee recommended Ryuji Kaji, a member-at-large, to shepherd this concept and eventually to serve as the organization's first president.

Members from Georgia, Pakistan, Vietnam, Sri Lanka, Syria, and Malaysia signed up for membership and paid the US $4 annual dues. Further members were sought by contacting national societies of neurology through the WFN. The clinical neurophysiologists contacted in Singapore found that they had sufficient local interest to form their own national society, which pursued as a route for IFCN participation.

By 2006, the ICNS was functioning. It met as an organization for the first time at the 2006 ICCN, ratified its Bye-Laws, elected its own IFCN Delegate, and discussed ways of broadening the inclusiveness of IFCN activities. As written in its Bye-Laws, the initial officers were drawn from the Federation Executive Committee. The ICNS Officers were President Ryuji Kaji (Japan), Secretary Graham Harding (UK), and Treasurer Andrew Eisen (Canada), the latter two in the same roles held in the Federation Executive Committee.

The plan was to limit the number of ICNS members that could be from any one nation. When a critical number is reached, they could be encouraged to form their own national society and move their memberships out of the ICNS.

14. Communications

The Secretary acquired a new internet worldwide web domain www.ifcn.info. The domain www.ifcn.org was already taken. Web site maintenance was delegated to the Executive Director and her office. A web designer redesigned the web pages to include links to national societies and chapters, rules, meeting announcements and the Yellow Pages from the journal, reports from the Executive Committee and other relevant information. Updates are posted every few months.

The Concorde Executive Office also developed a map of the world showing Federation chapters and national societies, as a useful and interesting graphic for the web page and the Federation exhibit booth display graphics. The banner and logo were also approved, but it was felt that it would be better if the color of the banners and the logo could reflect the colors of the journal.

Rules Committee Chairman Marc Nuwer provided an electronic copy of the Statutes. A link to the journal web page at Elsevier was useful for members who wished to contact the publisher.

The 1999 Practice Recommendations book did not exist in electronic format and the cost of putting this on the website was considered to be excessive. Instead, those Guidelines that had been published in the journal were available and included. As new guidelines are approved in the future, they would be added to the website. The President proposed that as Prof. Paolo Rossini would be retiring as Editor-in-Chief Europe he should be made responsible for updating the recommendations or guidelines, providing these for the website.

The Executive Committee decided not to post commercial advertisements on the website.

15. Finances

The Treasurer's office was moved from Switzerland to Vancouver at the start of this term. Over the 5 years, from 2001 to 2006, the Federation continued on average to operate in a surplus financial position, with annual performance depending on whether an ICCN was held in that year.

By 2006, the IFCN assets were approximately US $1.9 million, triple the value of 13 years earlier. Annual expenses averaged around US $250,000, or about 20% higher than 5–9 years earlier. The largest expenses were for the Editor's offices, the support of congresses and symposia, and the executive Secretariat. Income was primarily from Elsevier. Other lesser sources of income were from congress profits and repayments, society dues, and investment income. Because the aim of the Federation was to achieve scientific, professional, and educational goals — not to accumulate assets — the funding was gradually increased. Funding for Chapters increased substantially from US \$60,000 to \$100,000 in each 4-year term. Fellowship funding increased from US \$70,000 to \$100,000 for each 4-year term. Funding for additional workshops and symposia was increased to US \$60,000 for the next 4-year term. Bursaries were proposed at US \$40,000 in the next 4 years, which is support given to certain delegates from economically disadvantaged national societies. The plan was to reduce the Fiscal Period surpluses by investing in worthy projects. Budgeting for the next Fiscal period assumed continuing increases toward educational, scientific, and professional goals.

Chapters were more responsible for identifying funding needs in their own regions. Less reliance on the Federation Executive Committee was considered desirable. The Chapters themselves had been in operation for one term, and they had reached a stability of operations to turn over this responsibility to them. Requests for support from each region were to go through the respective Chapters.

Additional costs during this Fiscal period were for expenses of incorporating in Canada, establishing a permanent secretariat office, as well as purchasing insurance for publications, general liability and directors and officers. For the journal, the Federation was now paying Elsevier to manage the Editorial Manager electronic publishing software system. Tax statements were filed in Canada and France, but no significant taxes were due. Since the appointment of the Secretariat, the direct costs from the Officers decreased, resulting in the desired economies of scale and an overall reduction of costs.

Treasurer Andrew Eisen changed the Federation's investment advisors. The information received from the previous advisors was insufficient. The new advisors were more responsive and provided better information about account performances. The investment firm was instructed that the IFCN did not wish to invest in medical instrumentation or pharmaceutical products as it could give an appearance of conflict of interest. Likewise, the IFCN held stock in Elsevier. The Executive Committee directed that steps be taken to sell those stock holdings.

Each Executive Committee member was asked to provide to the Federation attorney a formal Declaration of Conflict of Interest. Mr. Kirkham reviewed what companies or directorships and what major stock investments were held. The attorney advised that no conflicts were reported concerning issues of the Executive Committee's business or actions.

Annual auditor's reports were circulated and approved by the Executive Committee, made available to Delegates, and posted on the IFCN website. No significant discrepancies or irregularities were described in the audits.

16. Nominations

IFCN Past-President Marc Nuwer (USA) chaired the Nominations Committee. Other committee members were Jeanette Farina (Brazil), Erik Stålberg (Sweden), and Kwang-Woo Lee (Korea). A timetable for elections was approved, one that began about 18 months before the next ICCN. This timetable allowed for sufficient time for three major rounds of nominations and balloting and allowed sufficient time for run-off ballots if needed.

Marc Nuwer expressed concern at the lack of effective contact details for some current IFCN Delegates and requested that the Secretariat continue to use all available resources and information to update this. This communication problem has been long standing within the Federation. During this election cycle all Delegates but one participated in the nominations and elections.

The Treasurer and Secretariat offices provided information on which societies were current on dues payments. Per Federation policy, those societies that had not been paying dues could nominate, but not cast ballots.

Societies were allotted the same number of votes that they were entitled to in the General Assembly, which is 2, 3, or 4, depending on their size. The Executive Committee member themselves have votes in the General Assembly, but not in officer elections.

The Executive Committee was reduced from eight members to seven because it no longer included two Editors-in-Chief. This would affect issues of geographic and disciplinary balance. The Nominations Committee was charged with assuring that each new Executive Committee would adhere to the prescribed geographic limitations and disciplinary balance. Those rules were designed when the Executive Committee had eight members: five for election in each quadrennial cycle, one Past-President carried over from the previous Fiscal Period, and two Editors-in-Chief. The Nominations and Executive Committees unanimously agreed to allow an EEG versus EMG disciplinary balance of 4:3 or 5:2 ratios, but not 6:1 or 7:0 ratios. These would be applied in either disciplinary direction. Discussion was held about how these disciplinary balance ratios were becoming anachronistic. But no move to change them was undertaken.

Geographic balance was separated into two regions. One region was Europe, Africa and Asia except for Japan. The other region was the Americas, Japan, and Australia.

The rules called for three major rounds of nomination and election. In the first round, the new President and Treasurer are selected. The new President was preferably from the geographic region different from the outgoing President. The outgoing President was from France, so the new President should be from the Americas, Japan, or Australia. No restrictions were placed on the Treasurer, other than a 2-term maximum that did not apply in this election cycle. Hiroshi Shibasaki (Japan) was elected President, and Andrew Eisen (Canada) was re-elected to a second term as Treasurer for 2006–2010.

The Secretary was to be from the opposite geographic region as the Treasurer. Since Dr. Eisen was from Canada, the new Secretary should be from Europe, Africa or Asia, except for Japan. Current Member-at-Large Johannes Noth (Germany) was elected as the new Secretary for the Fiscal Period 2006–2010.

Member-at-Large elections might need to be chosen carefully so as to attain the desired geographic and disciplinary balances. The two Member-at-Large positions were set as one from each geographic region. In that way the new Executive Committee would have four members from each of the two recognized regions. The three newly elected officers, the outgoing President and the Editor-in-Chief were already from an adequate mix of disciplines. As a very fortunate result, no disciplinary restrictions needed to apply to the Member-at-Large elections. Many nominations were received; 11 individuals agreed to serve if elected. The ballot listed seven candidates from Europe and four from the Americas. A run-off was necessary because no majority was reached for either position. In the run-offs between the top two vote recipients in each region, the societies chose Kerry Mills (UK) and Daniel Cibils (Uruguay) for the Member-at-Large positions for the 2006–2010 Fiscal Period.

The new Executive Committee at the beginning of the term 2006–2010 was:

President	Hiroshi Shibasaki	Japan
Past-President	François Mauguière	France
Secretary	Johannes Noth	Germany
Treasurer	Andrew Eisen	Canada
Member-at-Large	Kerry Mills	UK
Member-at-Large	Daniel Cibils	Uruguay
Editor-in-Chief	Mark Hallett	USA

Wave Length and Action Potentials: History of the IFCN
(Supplements to Clinical Neurophysiology, Vol. 61)
By: M.R. Nuwer and C.H. Lücking

Chapter 16

2006–2010

President: Hiroshi Shibasaki

In this term, the Federation continued to expand educational conferences and opportunities. The journal remained prominent and successful. Chapters developed and expanded their regional plans for activities. The Canadian incorporation was completed in the previous term, and now the Executive Office joined the legal address in Vancouver.

The Executive Committee was President Hiroshi Shibasaki (Japan), Past-President François Mauguière (France), Treasurer Andrew Eisen (Canada), and Members-at-Large Daniel Cibils (Uruguay) and Kerry Mills (UK). During the first year Secretary Johannes Noth (Germany) resigned to accept a position as Dean of Medical Faculty of Aachen Technical University. Reinhard Dengler (Germany) replaced him as Federation Secretary. Mark Hallett (USA) completed his 8 years as Editor-in-Chief during this term. David Burke (Australia) succeeded him (see Appendix 11, Figs. 31 and 33).

For the first time, the General Assembly approved its minutes by mail as allowed in the new rules. Official General Assembly minutes were available promptly instead of 4 years later. This allowed for timely publication in the journal.

In the previous Fiscal Period, the Executive Secretariat was contracted through Concorde Services Ltd (UK). The Executive Committee found it important to have the Secretariat nearer to one or another Executive Committee member's home city so as to allow for easier access and communication. A search was conducted for a replacement Secretariat. After having looked at several possibilities, Venue West of Vancouver was chosen because it best met the Federation's needs and budget. Venue West and the Federation signed a new 4-year Executive Secretariat contract in January 2007. The contract was set to run through 2011. Ms. Stephanie Hudson served as the IFCN Executive Director. All Federation materials relocated from Concorde to Vancouver shortly thereafter. Contact details for Venue West were:

International Federation of Clinical Neurophysiology, Venue West Conference Services Ltd., Suite 645 – The Landing, 375 Water Street, Vancouver, B.C., Canada V6B 5C6, congress@venuewest.com

This book was written in 2009 before the 2006–2010 term was completed. The reader should note that this chapter does not cover actions accomplished during the final 16 months of this Fiscal Period.

1. Congresses and meetings

This term included a growing number of meetings. Several additional sponsored meetings accompanied the standard International Congress of Clinical Neurophysiology (ICCN) and three Chapter Congresses. The Federation provided financial support for each Chapter for support of regional and local meetings in addition to the Chapter formal quadrennial congress. Individuals interested in organizing an educational course or workshop were encouraged to contact the respective Chapter.

1.1. XXIX International Congress of Clinical Neurophysiology

The ICCN is scheduled for October 28 to November 2, 2010 in Kobe, Japan. The Organizing Committee for the International Congress (OCIC) ExCo includes five members from the Federation Executive Committee and four from among the local organizers. The OCIC for the 2010 Kobe ICCN is Federation President Hiroshi Shibasaki (Japan), Past-President François Mauguière (France), and Treasurer Andrew Eisen (Canada) as well as the Editor-in-Chief Mark Hallett (USA), then David Burke (Australia) from ExCo, and the new Federation Secretary Reinhard Dengler (Germany). The Japanese organizing society includes Hiroshi Shibasaki as Convener, Ryuji Kaji as Congress Secretary General, Shin-ichi Niwa as Treasurer and Ryusuke Kakigi as Program Committee Chair.

The Executive Committee asked that each Chapter's President and Liaison Officers serve on the Congress's Scientific Program Committee. Thus, Paolo Rossini and Kerry Mills from the European Chapter, Jose Xavier de Castro and Daniel Cibils from the Latin American Chapter, and Rawiphan Witoonpanich from the Asian–Oceanian Chapter were invited and agreed to join that Committee. This will add a further international contribution to the Congress's scientific program planning and recognize the growing importance of Chapters in the Federation's activities.

Meeting preparation went smoothly except for some difficulty in the fund-raising because of the worldwide economic recession. Scientific Program Committee Chairperson Ryusuke Kakigi circulated the proposed program to international members of the Committee in February 2009, and suggestions made by the international members were taken into account as much as possible. General plans for the congress, venue, facilities, budget, program, and hotel rooms were satisfactory. The Second Announcement, circulated in July 2009, described a call for papers in October 2009 with an abstract submission deadline in January 2010. IFCN decided again to support fellowship grants for young investigators, age 40 or below, whose abstracts were accepted for presentation.

1.2. Chapter Congresses

The V Latin American Congress of Clinical Neurophysiology was held in Puebla, Mexico in October 2008. Jaime Ramos-Peek served as the Local Organizing Committee Chairman with organizing committee officers including Jorge Burgos-Centeno, Sergio de Jesus Aguilar-Castillo and Lilia de la Maza-Kreptowsky. The meeting had been originally scheduled for Varadero Beach, Cuba in March 2008, but was rescheduled for organizational reasons. Delegates from most South American national member societies attended despite the distance. This meeting marked the first occasion for a Chapter meeting in the northern portion of the Latin American region.

The XIII European Congress of Clinical Neurophysiology was held in May 2008 in Istanbul, Turkey. The Congress Convener Professor Onder Us welcomed 820 registrants. The meeting included more than 400 scientific contributions in lectures and posters. Eleven young investigators were recognized with a monetary prize given in the name of Prof. Korkut Yaltkaya, a highly respected Turkish neuroscientist. Besides the scientific activity, the Congress was also successful in offering a rich and lively social program, with the Faculty and Gala dinners taking place in enchanting and historical buildings of the old Istanbul, with terrific views of the Bosphorus and its coloured nocturnal life.

The IV Asian and Oceanian Congress of Clinical Neurophysiology (AOCCN) was held in April 2009 in Seoul, Korea. The Korean Society for Neurophysiology hosted the meeting with the theme "AOCCN in Cultural Variety: Momentum of Revival". Kwang-Woo Lee served as Convener, Juhan Kim as Secretary General and Jae-Moon Kim as Scientific Chairman. Over 700 clinical neurophysiologists participated from 37 countries around the world.

1.3. Other meetings

The International Consensus Meeting for Electrodiagnostic Criteria for Diagnosis of Amyotrophic Lateral Sclerosis (ALS) took place in Awaji, Japan in December 2006. Ryuji Kaji and Andrew Eisen organized the consensus conference. A draft of diagnostic criteria was prepared by the participants, circulated for comment and revisions, and was submitted to the journal *Clinical Neurophysiology*. The goal was to provide criteria useful not only to the practitioner but also for entry criteria in scientific therapeutic drug trials for proposed ALS treatments.

A Clinical Neurophysiology Symposium was held in conjunction with the 30th Annual Meeting of Taiwan Neurological Society in Taipei in April 2007. Yang-Chyuan Chang served as the convener. The IFCN Executive Committee members participated as speakers in the symposia and shared current topics of interest with local clinical neurophysiologists. This was the fourth time that the Federation participated in symposia in China, with the first three being in Beijing over the previous two decades.

IFCN President Hiroshi Shibasaki participated in the scientific meeting of Chinese Society of EMG & Clinical Neurophysiology. Li Ying Cui chaired the scientific meeting. Prof. Shibasaki also had the opportunity to meet with members of the Chinese society's executive committee.

A workshop on Clinical Neurophysiology was held in Bangalore, India in April 2007. Mustare Veerendrakumar served as the convener. The meeting was well attended and very successful. This was the first time that the Federation sponsored a meeting in India.

The Latin American Neurophysiological Monitoring Symposium was held in Montevideo, Uruguay in April 2007. This achieved a standing room only attendance from South American clinical neurophysiologists interested in surgical monitoring techniques and science.

The Second Latin American Symposium of Neurophysiological Monitoring was held 2 years later in Porto Alegre, Brazil. The Neurological and Neurosurgical Society of Rio Grande do Sul and the Brazilian Academy of Neurology also held sessions. The overall registration exceeded 500 (see Appendix 11, Fig. 34).

A Conference on Transcranial Magnetic Stimulation Safety was held in Siena, Italy in March 2008. Paolo Rossini served as the convener for this conference, which was held under Federation sponsorship. The results of this meeting formed the basis for an IFCN Practice Guidelines on this topic.

More detail on some of these meetings is given below in the section on the Chapters.

2. Publications

The journal *Clinical Neurophysiology's* impact factor has steadily increased. It reached 2.972 in 2009, a record high for this journal and exceeding the previous record high of 2.86 that this journal reached in the late 1990s. In the impact factor rankings, the journal continues to place it higher than any other in this specialty or subspecialty.

The Italian and Japanese Societies each have adopted *Clinical Neurophysiology* as its official journal. Society members were required to subscribe to the journal. In this arrangement, the societies received a deep discount on the subscription price. Some other societies also planned to adopt *Clinical Neurophysiology* as the society's official journal with discounted member subscriptions.

The IFCN Secretariat handled the regular individual journal subscriptions that were available at a specially discounted rate for members of IFCN national societies. The arrangement changed so that Elsevier directly processed renewals and collections of subscription fees. The Federation Secretariat became responsible for ascertaining that the individuals were members in good standing of their respective national societies. The electronic access to *Clinical Neurophysiology* changed to access through Science Direct rather than through the IFCN web site. These changes facilitated easy administration.

The Yellow Pages society information section printed in *Clinical Neurophysiology* was used less in these days of readily available on-line information. Because of the more popular use of the IFCN website for society, Federation and meeting information, the Yellow Pages were canceled starting from the 2007 April issue of the journal.

2.1. Editor-in-Chief

The Editor-in-Chief position of *Clinical Neurophysiology* was opened for a worldwide search. Outgoing Editor-in-Chief Mark Hallett completed his 8-year term at the end of 2007, and was ineligible to serve another term. The Federation terms for the Editor-in-Chief are 4 years, renewable once. The Federation Executive Committee, in its role as the journal's Executive Board, appoints the Editor-in-Chief as well as the subsidiary editors. The Executive Board published a call for candidates in as many sources as possible and made an announcement of this opening in many forums. Applications were received from nine excellent candidates by January 2007 deadline. David Burke (Australia) was selected as the next Editor-in-Chief for the term beginning January 2008. Prof Burke previously had served the Federation as an Executive Committee Member-at-Large during the 1997–2001 term.

Several Associate Editor positions were revised. In part this was to limit service to 6 years. The Associate Editors serve several functions. They have special expertise in particular areas of clinical neurophysiology and can bring that expertise to decision making about acceptance of submissions. They also represent different geographic locations, so as to keep the journal aware of developments in those locations. The Associate Editors were Fabio Babiloni (Italy), Anders Fuglsang-Frederiksen (Denmark), Matthew Kiernan (Australia), Christian Krarup (Denmark), Cees J. Stam (Netherlands), Craig Tenke (USA), Y. Ugawa (Japan), Josep Valls-Solé (Spain), and Ulf Ziemann (Germany). The position of Book Review Editor was abolished at this point because of the smaller number of reviewed books being received.

2.2. Other publication issues

The program of Friends of IFCN was established in the previous Fiscal Period for individual subscribers to *Clinical Neurophysiology*. It provided a forum for direct feedback to the editors from individual subscribers as well as prerequisites for those subscribers. It was designed to encourage the growth of individual subscribers to the journal. This program's impact and financial advantages were modest at best, both for IFCN and individual subscribers. As a result, the Executive Board decided to discontinue the program.

The Reed Elsevier Group was actively engaged in the International Arms Fairs Exhibitions for a number of years. Elsevier Science Publishers is a business branch of Reed Elsevier. The journal's Executive Board found this situation inadvisable for the Elsevier Publisher, which publishes materials related to life science and medicine. The Executive Board wrote to the Chairman of the Reed Elsevier Group signed by the IFCN President and the Editor-in-Chief. The Federation's letter asked them to discontinue their military activity. Other medical and scientific societies wrote similar letters. In 2009 Reed Elsevier announced their decision to exit the defense exhibition sector.

The Federation sponsors two book series, the *Handbook of Clinical Neurophysiology* and the *Clinical Neurophysiology Supplement Series*. In 2008, the Executive Committee commissioned a history book with the preliminary title "History of the IFCN". The goal was to extend the previous Federation history work written nearly three decades earlier by former Federation President and journal Editor-in-Chief William Cobb (UK). That book, entitled *Wavelength: A History of the IFSECN*, was given to each registrant at the London 1985 International Congress of EEG and Clinical Neurophysiology. The new work will be provided to all participants in the Kobe 2010 XXIX International Congress of Clinical Neurophysiology. It will also be made available online to all journal subscribers and published as a *Clinical Neurophysiology Supplement Series* book.

3. Societies and Chapters

3.1. Member societies

By this point the Federation had expanded to 60 member national societies from 56 countries. Four countries, Belgium, China, Colombia and the United States, each have two member societies. The Executive Committee explored other countries with sufficient clinical neurophysiologists, and which might be encouraged to join the Federation. New member societies accepted in 2008 were Irish Society of Clinical Neurophysiology and the Clinical Neurophysiology Section of Malaysian Society of Neurosciences. An Icelandic society was attending European Chapter activities but was not yet a member society of IFCN. New Zealand joined the Australian Society, which changed its name to Australia–New Zealand Association of Clinical Neurophysiologists.

At the beginning of this Fiscal Period, communication was difficult with member societies in Greece, Iran, Slovak Republic, Jordan, and China PRC. At the 2006 Edinburgh ICCN, contact was re-established with Professor Cui Li Ying, the Delegate of the Chinese Society, and Shahriar Nafissi represented the Iranian Clinical Neurophysiology Branch of the Iranian Neurological Association. IFCN President Hiroshi Shibasaki visited Beijing subsequently and met with the members of the Chinese Society Executive Committee. Maintaining good, open communication with each member society has always been a priority for the Federation. Yet it is also a big challenge because of unreported changes of delegates or their contact information.

3.2. International Clinical Neurophysiology Society

The International Clinical Neurophysiology Society (ICNS) is a member organization approved by General Assembly that plays a role as if it were a national society. This brought a total to 60 member societies. That includes 59 member national societies plus the ICNS.

The main role for ICNS is to serve as a home base for clinical neurophysiologists from countries that do not have their own national member society. Individuals can apply for membership in the ICNS. Once a country has 10 clinical neurophysiologists in ICNS, the intention is that they would form their own national society and apply for Federation membership. During this term the ICNS President was Daniel Cibils (Uruguay). An application form was available on the IFCN website. Members of ICNS may sign up for journal subscriptions at the discounted rate, may nominate institutions for Federation sponsored journal subscriptions. The ICNS also may nominate individuals for young physician and investigator scholarships for training or research experiences abroad, and nominate young investigators for travel fellowships to attend ICCN or Chapter meetings.

The ICNS actively encouraged individual membership from clinical neurophysiologists in countries such as Latvia, Lithuania, Georgia, Iraq, Pakistan, Sudan, Senegal, Ethiopia, South Africa, Saudi Arabia, Sri Lanka, Vietnam, Ecuador, Honduras, and Venezuela. ICNS served as a means to communicate with these individuals.

3.3. European Chapter

The Chapter expanded its scope to include member societies in the Middle East and Africa. With the expanded region covered by the Europe, Middle East and Africa Chapters, the existing societies from Egypt, Jordan and Iran joined the Chapter. As a new society, Ireland joined the Federation and the Chapter. During this term, the Executive Committee from 2005 to 2009 included President Paolo Rossini (Italy), Secretary/Treasurer Luis García-Larrea (France), Liaison Officer Professor Kerry Mills (UK), and Member-at-Large Anders Fuglsang-Frederiksen (Denmark). For the other Member-at-Large position, Teresa

Sagalés' (Spain) term ended in 2008. She was replaced by Jonathan Cole (UK).

The XIII European Congress of Clinical Neurophysiology attracted 820 registrants to Istanbul, Turkey in 2008. The Congress Convener Professor Onder Us organized the meeting along with Dr Tullin Taridag. The scientific and educational sessions included 412 original scientific contributions and 100 invited speakers. A total of 60 fellowships were awarded to assist young physicians and investigators to attend the meeting. The Congress awarded 11 prizes to the best scientific presentations. The General Assembly of the European Chapter has also voted the site of the next congress after having highly appreciated the nice presentations of Prof. Topka of the Austrian Society supporting Innsbruck and of Prof. Comi of the Italian Society supporting Rome. The Delegates expressed their votes (22–15) in favor of having the next congress in Rome in 2011.

The Chapter developed Bye-Law changes for elections that took into account the new quadrennial cycle for Chapter congresses and the 1-year delay in the cycle for International Congresses. These would clarify the overlap of terms of office of Chapter Executive Committee members so that only some were replaced or re-elected in each election cycle.

The European Union of Medical Specialists (UEMS) oversees specialty organizations in Europe. Eva Svanborg (Sweden) represented Clinical Neurophysiology in European discussions about medical specialties. One goal was to develop uniform training standards, and a core curriculum for Clinical Neurophysiology was published in 2008. The recommended duration of training was 5 years for an independent medical specialty, and fewer years in national systems in which clinical neurophysiology is a subspecialty. Whether to have a European board examination was discussed, as opposed to relying solely on each nation to develop and maintain its own examinations in Clinical Neurophysiology. That remained a topic of discussion. Uniform standards for Continuing Medical Education were also discussed.

Chapter Secretary Luis García-Larrea conducted a survey of Educational Programs of Clinical Neurophysiology in European Countries. This was based on previous work by G. Cruccu, T. Sagalés, A. de Weerd and E. Stålberg. The survey assessed the types and length of training, a national board, content of training, and status of the specialty.

The 4-year interval between ECCN meetings led to further consideration of holding a smaller, single topic meeting during each 4-year term. The EC-IFCN has supported many regional conferences on particular topics. Most included 1–2 days of teaching or training. Both audio-conferences and regional courses have been sponsored. EC-IFCN financial contributions went toward defraying costs of faculty travel and preparations of handout materials. From 2005 through 2008, these meetings included: Evoked Potentials (Haifa, Israel), Motor Control (Madrid, Spain), Sleep Medicine (Copenhagen, Denmark and Vilnius, Lithuania), rTMS Safety (Siena, Italy), Cortical Stimulation (Paris, France), Laser EPs (Lyon, France), EMG (Prague, Czech Rep.), EMG–ENG (Granada, Spain and Belgrade, Serbia), and Clinical Neurophysiology (Lisbon, Portugal).

The election cycles were discussed. With the change in ECCN timing from every 2 years to every 4 years, it threw off the timing of the elections for Chapter Officers. Bye-Law changes were planned to rectify that situation. Depending on the outcome of those discussions and voting, three of the current Executive Committee members' terms will end either in 2009 or in 2011. The year 2009 is 4 years since they were elected. The year 2011 is the time set for the next ECCN in Rome.

The Chapter website moved to the Neuroscience Federative Institute in Lyon. The revised web pages included direct links to national societies, posting of meetings that may be of interest to clinical neurophysiologists, a job search site, minutes of meetings, contact information on societies and delegates, and Chapter Statutes.

3.4. Latin American Chapter

The Chapter was active especially for meetings during this term. The V Latin American Congress of Clinical Neurophysiology was held in Puebla, Mexico in October 2008. Jaime Ramos-Peek served as the Local Organizing Committee Chairman. Armando Tello served as the International Scientific Committee Chairman. All the IFCN Executive Committee members participated in the scientific sessions in this attractive city located at driving distance south of Mexico City and its archeological attractions for visitors. The meeting had been originally scheduled for Varadero Beach, Cuba in March 2008, but was rescheduled for organizational reasons. Delegates from most South American national member societies attended despite the distance. This meeting marked the first occasion for a Chapter meeting in the northern portion of the Latin American region.

The Latin American Neurophysiological Monitoring Symposium was held in Montevideo, Uruguay in April 2007. Daniel Cibils served as the convener. The meeting covered topics about the science and clinical techniques for intraoperative monitoring and testing. This achieved a standing room only attendance from South American clinical neurophysiologists interested in surgical monitoring techniques and science. The attendees recommended that further such meetings be held every few years.

The Second Latin American Symposium of Neurophysiological Monitoring was held 2 years later in Porto Alegre, Brazil. It was held together with three other neurological and neurosurgical symposia in May 2009. The joint meeting was entitled the 5° Congresso Gaúcho de Neurologia e Neurocirurgia, Sul Neuro 2009. Ricardo Ferreira organized the Latin American Symposium of Neurophysiological Monitoring portion of this meeting. Latin American Chapter President José Xavier de Castro and Executive Committee member Daniel Cibils represented the Chapter in this organization. The Neurological and Neurosurgical Society of Rio Grande do Sul and the Brazilian Academy of Neurology also held sessions. The overall registration exceeded 500: & white; (see Appendix 11, Fig. 34).

In the 2009 Chapter elections, Renato Verdugo (Chile) succeeded Jose H. Xavier de Castro (Brazil) as Chapter President. Jorge Gutierrez (Colombia) was elected as the Chapter Treasurer. Member-at-Large election results still were uncertain when this book went to press. Those two new officers will join the continuing Chapter Executive Committee members Secretary Alberto Yorio (Argentina) and Member-at-Large Jaime Ramos Peek (Mexico). The Liaison officer between the Chapter and the Federation Executive Committee continued to be Professor Daniel Cibils (Uruguay).

3.5. Asian–Oceanian Chapter

This Chapter's activity concentrated on congresses and other local meetings. The major meeting was the IV AOCCN held in April 2009 in Seoul, Korea. The meeting, whose theme was "AOCCN in Cultural Variety: Momentum of Revival", was hosted by the Korean Society for Neurophysiology. Kwang-Woo Lee served as the Convener, along with Juhan Kim as Secretary General and Jae-Moon Kim as the Scientific Chairman. Over 700 clinical neurophysiologists participated from 37 countries around the world. Over 3 days the congress held four plenary lectures, eight workshops, eight meet the expert sessions, 11 clinical and scientific symposia, three luncheon symposia, and 236 individual presentations.

The Chapter in 2009 elections chose outgoing Chapter Secretary Kwang-Woo (Korea) to serve to succeed Rawiphan Witoonpanich (Thailand) as the Chapter President for the 2009–2013 term. Bob Santoso Wibowo (Indonesia) was elected as the next AO Chapter Secretary/Treasurer. Hiroshi Shibasaki (Japan) will continue to serve as the Liaison Officer. The Chapter Assembly chose Bali, Indonesia as the site of the AOCCN during the next Fiscal Period.

During this term, Dr. M. Veerendrakumar organized a regional meeting held in Bangalore,

India in April 2007. The Chapter agreed to provide some Federation funding and sponsorship for the meeting.

3.6. North American Chapter

The three Federation member societies in North America were American Association of Neuromuscular and Electrodiagnostic Medicine (AANEM), American Clinical Neurophysiology Society (ACNS) and Canadian Society of Clinical Neurophysiologists. This region had not had a formal Federation Chapter. The Executive Committee had agreed to make funding available for the region. In the previous term that funding was support for international fellows to attend meetings. The Executive Committee proposed that the three societies form a North American Chapter. The three societies agreed in principle. AANEM Chapter Bye-Laws that were subsequently approved by the three societies, the IFCN Rules and Executive Committees and the General Assembly. Delegates from the here mentioned societies formed a Chapter Executive Committee. Andrew Eisen (Canada) served as the Liaison Officer. The Chapter Executive Committee was charged with defining the Chapter's activities and processes of achieving the Federation's goals.

4. Rules Committee

Amendments approved by the Edinburgh General Assembly were filed with the Canadian Minister of Industry. Further amendments of IFCN Statutes and Bye-Laws were under discussion during this term. François Mauguière (France) served as the Rules Committee Chairman. Marc Nuwer (USA), James Colebatch (Australia), Ricardo Reisin (Argentina) and Rawiphan Witoonpanich (Thailand) served on the committee.

In accordance with the incorporation of IFCN under Part II of the Canada Corporations Act, the Statutes were largely re-structured. These new Statutes were approved by the General Assembly during the previous Fiscal Period. At the Edinburgh General Assembly, the Editor-in-Chief and host society's Scientific Program Committee Chairman were added to the OCIC. ICNS membership criteria were expanded. New rules allow for mail or e-mail approval of the General Assembly minutes.

4.1. Geographic balance

In December 2007, the General Assembly approved the North American Chapter Bye-Laws. That change resulted in four IFCN Chapters: Latin America, Asia–Oceania, North America, and Europe, including Middle East and Africa. In contrast, the IFCN Statutes recognize two geographical areas: (1) North and South America, Australasia and Japan, and (2) Europe, Asia (except Japan) and Africa. This was felt to be inequitable. The situation prompted the Executive Committee to explore adopting a new system, expanding the number of geographical areas from 2 to 4. They would correspond to the Chapters. The new four geographic areas would be used for nomination of Federation officers. A Task Force was formed to explore this important issue of geographical balance in Executive Committee election. The Task Force comprised representatives from four Chapters, the Rules Committee, the Executive Committee, and the IFCN attorney Roderick Kirkham. Luis García-Larrea (France) represented the European Chapter, Donald Sanders (USA) represented the North American Chapter, Jose Xavier de Castro (Brazil) represented the Latin American Chapter, and Kwang-Woo Lee (Korea) represented the Asian–Oceanian Chapter.

In the system in 2009, Federation Executive Committee elections were carried out in three steps. A first round elects the President and Treasurer. A second round elects the Secretary. A third round elects two Members-at-Large. The President and Past-President should be from different geographical regions, and cannot be from the same geographical region in more than two consecutive elections. The Secretary and Treasurer should be from different geographical regions. The two Members-at-Large should be from different geographical regions, and from countries different from the President, Past-President, Treasurer, and Secretary.

The system in 2009 also required the Nominations Committee to determine whether a candidate is from the EEG or the EMG discipline. The Executive Committee cannot have more than five members from one discipline. The delicate balancing of geography and discipline has been the problem requiring a three-stage election process. The Member-at-Large election stage was an opportunity to limit the candidates' disciplines so as to meet the disciplinary rule.

After careful discussion, the Task Force recommended increasing the geographical regions from 2 to 4. The regions would correspond to the four Chapters: Asia–Oceania, Europe, including Middle East and Africa, Latin America, and North America. The particular rule recommended stated: "No region should have more than two Executive Committee officers, excluding the Editor-in-Chief", and "Each region should have at least one officer".

In such a new system each Chapter would have an equal opportunity in the election process. The Task Force recognized that the Chapters do differ in number of member societies, total number of individual members, and votes in elections. The Member-at-Large election step would serve as an opportunity for one or two unrepresented regions to gain an Executive Committee seat.

The Task Force's plan would be in consideration by the 2010 General Assembly.

4.2. Votes per society

The General Assembly is composed of the Executive Committee, the Delegates, and additional representatives from each member society. Each member society has one Delegate, who is the principal person serving as a liaison between the Federation and his or her member society. The number of each member society's additional General Assembly Representatives corresponded to the number of that society's dues-paying members. Societies with 1–99 members had one additional representative. A society with 100–399 was entitled to two additional representatives. A society with 400 or more was entitled to three additional representatives.

The Executive Committee recommended a change in the number of each society's General Assembly votes and voting Delegates and Representatives. In 2009 each society's total number of votes was 2, 3 or 4 depending on the number of members in the society. The plan was to change this to 1, 2 or 3. The Task Force agreed with that recommendation, and that it should apply both to elections and General Assembly meetings. This issue was scheduled for presentation at the 2010 Kobe General Assembly.

4.3. Eligibility to vote and nominate

Member societies are eligible to vote in Federation elections and at the General Assembly unless they have failed to pay their dues. That policy has been followed for decades in the Federation. In recent times about a half dozen societies were ineligible to vote because of failures to pay their society dues. Two rules questions remained under discussion. The first question was whether a member of an ineligible society was allowed to run in an election. The second was whether an ineligible society was allowed to nominate a candidate.

The Statute in 2009 stated: "Even if a society is not eligible to vote, its individual members may still nominate persons for any position, and its members remain eligible for nomination". The Rules Committee recommended changing that rule to: "Even if a society is not eligible to vote, its members remain eligible for nomination; such nominees should take membership in the ICNS before becoming eligible".

The ICNS rules also would need a change to allow for that. The ICNS membership rule in 2009 was: "The society shall consist of honorary fellows, fellows, members and junior members from non-affiliated countries. Additional members may be from countries with an affiliated society if the individual cannot be a member of that affiliated society, and that society provides written support for the individual's request for ICNS membership". The Rules Committee recommended to change the first part of that rule to: "The society shall consist of fellows, members and junior members from non-affiliated countries or countries where their society is ineligible to vote at the General Assembly".

That would allow an individual to run for an Executive Committee office even if his or her national society did not pay its dues. It also clarified that an ineligible society could not make a nomination in Federation elections.

The broader issue also was discussed about societies that regularly do not pay their dues. The reasons vary. One or two societies may have disappeared entirely. Others have difficulty with the amount of the dues, which is US $4 per member per year. Some cited currency restrictions. The Executive Committee recommended a rule: "A member society failing to pay its annual dues for four years shall be deemed delinquent and that society will be recommended to the General Assembly for removal as a member society of the IFCN, according to Statutes 2.3". The Rules Committee would need to discuss this suggestion.

4.4. Nomination Committee

Composition of Nomination Committee was discussed. In 2009 the Nominations Committee was composed of the Past-President as chairperson, and three Federation Delegates as committee members. The Executive Committee appointed the three Delegates.

The Executive Committee recommended that others be allowed to serve on the Nominations Committee, not just formal Delegates. Where the rule about the Nomination Committee composition mentions "three delegates", the language could be changed to "three persons from member societies".

5. Practice Committee

Several IFCN Practice Guidelines were developed during this term. Giorgio Cruccu (Italy) chaired a committee to develop "Guidelines on Somatosensory Evoked Potentials". His committee also included M.J. Aminoff, G. Curio, J.M. Guérit, R. Kakigi, F. Mauguière, P.M. Rossini, R.D. Treede, and L. García-Larrea. Connie Duncan (USA) chaired a committee to develop "Guidelines on Event-Related Potentials". The latter committee included C.C. Duncan, R.J. Barry, J.F. Connolly, C. Fischer, P.T. Michie, R. Näätänen, J. Polich, I. Reinvang, and C. van Petten. Their specific topic was "Event-related potentials in clinical research: guidelines for eliciting, recording, and quantifying mismatch negativity, P300, and N400". Both were presented and accepted by the Federation and appeared in the journal *Clinical Neurophysiology*.

Graham Holder (UK) chaired a committee to develop "Guidelines on Visual Evoked Potentials and Electroretinography". The Executive Committee accepted a proposal by Donald Schomer of the ACNS. He proposed that the IFCN and ACNS jointly prepare a guideline on "Monitoring EEG for Pre-surgical Epilepsy Evaluation". Hartwig Siebner (Germany) chaired another committee to develop "Guidelines on Transcranial Magnetic Stimulation", one that would emphasize ways to conduct those techniques.

Professor Simone Rossi served as chairperson for a conference on TMS safety and ethics, which was held in Sienna, Italy in March 2008 under the sponsorship of IFCN. S. Rossi, M. Hallett, P.M. Rossini and A. Pascual-Leone summarized the results of that conference as a guidelines document under the title "Safety, Ethical Considerations, and Application Guidelines for the Use of Transcranial Magnetic Stimulation in Clinical Practice and Research. A Consensus Statement from the International Workshop on Present and Future of TMS: Safety and Ethical Guidelines."

6. History project

The history of the Federation should be preserved and made available for review by IFCN society members and future Clinical Neurophysiologists. In the mid-nineties, then IFCN President Carl Lücking first took the initiative to establish IFCN archives. He wrote to the first President Herbert Jasper and had contact with and received documents from William Cobb and Robert Naquet, both former Federation Presidents in the seventies. In the eighties William Cobb had proposed archives located at the National Hospital in London, but no action followed. Therefore Carl Lücking suggested to establish IFCN archives once a permanent Secretariat would be installed. As Chairman of the Long-Range Planning Committee in the previous term, he recommended a process to identify and maintain archives and otherwise make the story of the Federation available. The Executive Committee considered ways to archive and create a historical document. Previously William Cobb (UK) wrote a book titled "Wave Length: a History of the IFSECN". The Federation distributed it to all participants to the London 1985 ICEEGCN. That book detailed Federation history from its beginning to 1982. It had been more than a quarter century since that work was completed. To follow the subsequent history of the Federation, the Executive Committee invited Marc Nuwer (USA) and Carl Lücking (Germany) to write a monograph for this purpose in 2008–2009. Those two authors invited pictures and information from the Chapter officers and Executive Committee members among others. They themselves had witnessed much of the interval since 1985, and brought a depth of experience to this project. Marc Nuwer served as a Practice Guidelines chairman starting in 1986, subsequently served three terms on the Rules Committee and 13 years on the Executive Committee, including one term each as Federation President (1997–2001) and Past-President (2001–2006). Carl Lücking served two terms on the Rules Committee, 8 years on the Executive Committee as Federation President (1993–1997) and Past-President (1997–2001), followed by five more years as Chairman of the Long-Range Planning Committee until 2006. Together they have had considerable personal knowledge to carry on the Federation story after the years covered by William Cobb work. The plans are for a soft covered book as the second edition to the Cobb book, one that can be distributed to registrants at the ICCN 2010 in Kobe. A hard covered edition will be published as a *Clinical Neurophysiology Supplement Series* book.

7. Sponsorships and donations

For the previous several Fiscal Periods, the Federation has had a committee charged with identifying societies and individuals who merit a donation of sponsorship by the Federation. For several terms, this was the Gift Committee under the chairmanship of Fernando Lopes da Silva (The Netherlands) and others. In subsequent terms, this was folded into the responsibilities of the Long-Range Planning Committee under the leadership of Carl Lücking (Germany). Those committees assessed not only to whom donations might be given but also the broader issues of identifying needs and recommending relevant Federation policy and process changes. In this term, the Executive Committee felt that there is no need for a Long-Range Planning Committee at that moment, and that the committee could be appointed as necessary in the future. The donations and sponsorship activity were assumed by the Executive Committee members working together with the Executive Secretariat in Vancouver.

7.1. Sponsored subscriptions and books

Under a system launched during the Fiscal Period 1997–2001, the sponsored subscription program provided financially disadvantaged societies and medical centers with free *Clinical Neurophysiology* journal subscriptions. In 18 countries sponsored subscriptions were given to 58 key persons who made the Journal accessible for a multitude of neurophysiologists. Additionally the program provided Federation books such as the *Practice Guidelines* book and *Clinical Neurophysiology Supplement Series* books.

The secretariat office in this term contacted all recent sponsored subscribers to check how the journal and books were used. The program's goal was to have these resources available to many physicians and scientists at each institution, not just for the private use of one individual. The contact person during this term was IFCN Secretary, Professor Reinhard Dengler.

The program was authorized through 2009 for subscribers who acknowledged that the program was meeting the defined use goal. After that, an expanded formal application and review process were implemented. In that process, sponsored assistance applications were submitted through IFCN member societies. Individuals from countries without a member society were encouraged to join the ICNS to become eligible for this program. In this way, the national societies were given a greater voice about which sites would receive the sponsored books and journal subscriptions, and the Federation routinely would receive information on the program's effectiveness at each site.

7.2. Equipment donations

A new assistance program, launched in 2007 sought to meet equipment needs in economically disadvantaged member nations. The program aimed at matching institutions and individuals with surplus equipment with others who need equipment, even older generation pieces. That equipment then could be shipped to the needed site. Various technical difficulties slowed the progress of this program. This project continued under the leadership of Member-at-Large Daniel Cibils (Uruguay). Information about the program was posted on the IFCN website or could be obtained by contacting the IFCN secretariat in Vancouver.

The IFCN would facilitate the exchange of information among parties, but not the actual transfer or cost of shipping neurophysiologic equipment. The IFCN would not be responsible for insurance, customs, maintenance, repair, supplies or any other expenses associated with the equipment exchange. Members of national societies and of the ICNS were invited to send messages about needs and available equipment to the IFCN secretariat. Appropriate messages would be posted on a web page dedicated to these equipment needs messages.

7.3. International scholarships for young investigators

A new program supported two scholarships annually to support young researchers of developing geographic areas. This was to support training or research in clinical neurophysiology in distinguished institutions abroad. Each scholarship was valued at approximately US $25,000. Detailed information is available on the IFCN website (http://www.ifcn.info).

In 2009, the program's first year, 10 applications were received. A physician from Azerbaijan was chosen for EEG and epilepsy training in Great Ormond Street Hospital for Children in London, UK. A physician from Armenia was chosen for training in EMG and nerve conduction techniques at the Hospital for Sick Children in Toronto.

8. Inclusiveness

To foster clinical neurophysiology worldwide, the IFCN works both with its member societies and with other international organizations. The Federation has for decades had an excellent working relationship with the World Federation of Neurology (WFN). Jun Kimura (Japan), Federation President in the term 1990–1993, went on to serve subsequently for a 4-year term as WFN President. The two organizations have held their quadrennial congresses jointly on several occasions, most recently in Vancouver in 1993. The IFCN has held a seat on the WFN Research Committee that meets annually. That committee has several goals, such as contributing ideas for topics and faculty to the WFN Congress organizers and facilitating interactions among the various international organizations. President Hiroshi Shibasaki and Member-at-Large Daniel Cibils represented the IFCN at meetings of the WFN Research Committee during this term.

The Federation has enjoyed good working relationships with many subspecialty- and technique-oriented societies over many decades. Joint meetings and collaborations have included not only the WFN but also the Movement Disorder Society, the International Pharmaco-EEG Working Group (IPEG), the International Evoked Potential Symposia series, the International Spinal Cord Monitoring Symposia work group, and the International Society for Transcranial Stimulation (ISTS). With the rapid growth in size and number of societies dealing with functional neuroimaging, the Executive Committee recognized the importance of having a close association with neuroimaging groups. The German Society of Clinical Neurophysiology successfully formed relationships with other societies involved in functional neuroimaging and took over the leadership of training in this domain. Consequently, the society changed her name into Deutsche Gesellschaft für Klinische Neurophysiologie und funktionelle Bildgebung (German Society for Clinical Neurophysiology and Functional Imaging). Secretary Reinhard Dengler reported to the Executive Committee on this process to facilitate further discussion of how the IFCN could follow a similar mutually beneficial or collaborative path.

It remained important for each member society to keep in close contact with the IFCN Executive Office and Executive Committee. Keeping current on contact information remained a problem for the IFCN. Too often Delegates changed without proper notification of addresses or e-mail addresses changed without notifying the Federation. Good contact information was needed not just for voting and fellowship nominations, but also for information exchange. Thoughts or suggestions to promote clinical neurophysiology always have been welcomed. Regular informational e-mailed reports to the societies and their delegates were sent out to the known contact addresses, reports that reviewed the ongoing issues, meeting information, and activities for the Federation committees.

9. Finances

IFCN finances remained healthy despite of the world economic recession during this term. A decline in investment earnings and a loss on foreign exchange caused economic constraints. Overall assets declined to US $2.2 million by the end of 2008. This was still higher than at the beginning of this Fiscal Period in 2006. Canadian law requires posting the annual audit statement on the IFCN website at the beginning of each new fiscal year. These were available back through fiscal year 2001. This positive fiscal picture has been due to careful planning and spending by the several Executive Committees and diligent work of Treasurers Manuel Meyer, Paul Despland, and Andrew Eisen over the past two dozen years. This is enormously better than the situation in the early 1980s when the Federation had serious financial difficulties.

The journal and book publications' royalties from Elsevier remained the largest source of Federation income, comprising more than half of the average annual revenue. Society dues, congress profits and investment income were the remainder of the income.

The main expenditures remained for congress meetings, both the ICCN and the Chapter Congresses. The funding given each Chapter was increased at the end of the last term from US $60,000 to US $100,000 per 4-year Fiscal Period. This funded not only the quadrennial Chapter Congresses but also other regional symposia and Chapter organizational expenses. In addition, the Federation undertook a policy to subsidize publication of the Chapter Congress abstracts, which previously was an expense borne by each meeting budget.

Organizational support for the Editor's Office and for the Secretariat in Vancouver continued. Payments to an external financial advisor, the attorney's office and for insurance also continued. Executive Committee expenses were mainly for travel to their meetings. Those Executive Committee meetings were scheduled at the time of Federation sponsored Chapter Congresses or symposia so as to allow the officers to lecture at those meetings at no cost to the meetings' budgets.

A new initiative funded two scholarships annually, each of approximately US $25,000 for young researchers. This was described above. The Treasurer budgeted for this annually, beginning in 2009. The Federation continued funding journal subscriptions and books for economically disadvantaged regions.

10. Nominations

The work of the Nomination Committee was initiated very early in this term because of the resignation of Secretary Johannes Noth (Germany) during the first year. He resigned in 2007 to accept the position of Dean of the Medical Faculty of Aachen Technical University. A by-election was held to fill the open position. Six nominations were submitted and four of those candidates agreed to stand for election. Reinhard Dengler (Germany) was elected to serve as Secretary for the remainder of the term.

The complex quadrennial election cycle began in early 2009 for nomination and election of the next Executive Committee officers for the Fiscal Period 2010–2014. As set forth in the rules, the process sought to balance geography and discipline. The rules define EEG and EMG as the two recognized disciplines, even though clinical neurophysiology had grown into a much more complex field. The geographic regions remained (a) Europe, Africa, and Asia except Japan, and (b) the Americas, Japan, and Australia. There was discussion about changing the election process to one that recognized four geographic regions in place of the two regions — one for each Chapter's region. That was still a matter of discussion during this term. The 2009 elections cycle was conducted using the traditional two-region rule.

To accomplish the delicate balance of the geography and discipline, the election was carried out in three steps. In the first round, two candidates for the President and three candidates for the Treasurer were nominated. Paolo Rossini (Italy) was elected President and Reinhard Dengler (Germany) was elected as the new Treasurer. Paolo Rossini previously served as Editor-in-Chief and President of the European Chapter. Reinhard Dengler was currently serving as Federation Secretary when he was elected to serve as Treasurer. The second round of the election was set to choose a Secretary, followed by a third round to choose two Members-at-Large. In the second round, the societies chose Daniel Cibils (Uruguay) as Secretary. In the final round, the societies chose Lawrence Phillips (USA) and Mamede de Carvalho (Portugal) as the two Members-at-Large for the 2010–2014 term.

The Nomination Committee is charged with overseeing the elections process. The committee itself does not make nominations or chose candidates. Past-President François Mauguière (France) chaired the committee. Other members were Donald Sanders (USA), Dr. Jeanette Farina (Brazil) and Mustare Veerendrakumar (India).

Section II

Appendices

Wave Length and Action Potentials: History of the IFCN
(Supplements to Clinical Neurophysiology, Vol. 61)
By: M.R. Nuwer and C.H. Lücking

Appendix 1

International and Chapter congress series and sites

The Federation has had several series of official Congresses. These are in addition to numerous additional symposia held regionally on specific topics. The Congresses have been held in six series. For many years, two separate series of major International Congresses were held, one with EEG and one with EMG as its major area of interest.

In the early years, the EEG series was known generally as the International Congress. By 1969, the EEG Congresses were known as the International Congress of Electroencephalography and Clinical Neurophysiology. The EMG Congress series initially was known as the International Congress of EMG. By 1992, the EMG Congresses were known as the International Congress of Electromyography and Clinical Neurophysiology. The latter names are used below for simplicity of presentation.

Since 1999, the two International Congress series have been combined into a unified International Congress of Clinical Neurophysiology (ICCN). The latter now are held every 4 years. To recognize its roots in the two separate series International Congresses, the ICCN continued its count from the sum of the two previous series.

Between the quadrennial worldwide congresses, three Chapters hold their own regional Chapter congresses. The North American Chapter does not hold such congresses. The European Congress series predates formation of the European Chapter itself. Some congresses formally were named Symposia.

International Congress of Clinical Neurophysiology

2010	Kobe, Japan (29th)
2006	Edinburgh, Scotland, UK
2003	San Francisco, CA, USA
2001	Buenos Aires, Argentina

International Congress of EEG and Clinical Neurophysiology (ICEEGCN)

1997	Florence, Italy (14th)
1993	Vancouver, BC, Canada
1990	Rio de Janeiro, Brazil
1985	London, UK
1981	Kyoto, Japan
1977	Amsterdam, The Netherlands
1973	Marseilles, France
1969	San Diego, CA, USA
1965	Vienna, Austria
1961	Rome, Italy
1957	Brussels, Belgium
1953	Boston, MA, USA
1949	Paris, France
1947	London, UK

International Congress of EMG and Clinical Neurophysiology (ICEMGCN)

1999	Prague, Czech Rep. (11th)
1995	Kyoto, Japan
1992	Jerusalem, Israel
1987	Sorrento, Italy
1983	Munich, Germany
1979	Stockholm, Sweden
1975	Rochester, MN, USA
1971	Brussels, Belgium
1967	Glasgow, Scotland, UK
1963	Copenhagen, Denmark
1961	Pavia, Italy

European Congress of Clinical Neurophysiology (ECCN)

2008	Istanbul, Turkey (13th)
2005	Stockholm, Sweden
2002	Barcelona, Spain
1998	Ljubljana, Slovenia
2000	Lyon, France
1996	Munich, Fed. Rep. Germany
1994	Budapest, Hungary
1992	Lisbon, Portugal
1990	Paris, France
1987	Amsterdam, The Netherlands
1983	Basel, Switzerland
1979	Salzburg, Austria
1976	Venice, Italy

Asian and Oceanian Congress of Clinical Neurophysiology (AOCCN)

2009	Seoul, Korea (4th)
2005	Chiang Mai, Thailand
2000	Manila, Philippines
1996	Beijing, People's Rep. of China

Latin American Congress of Clinical Neurophysiology (LACCN)

2008	Puebla, Mexico (5th)
2004	Santiago, Chile
2002	Porto Seguro, Brazil
1997	Buenos Aires, Argentina
1995	Guatemala City, Guatemala

Appendix 2

Federation published standards, guidelines, recommendations, and reports

The Federation has produced a considerable number of reports, assessments, guidelines, standards, recommendations and similar printed products. These have covered technology, education, science, and clinical practice topics. These were generally the product of Federation committees commissioned by the Executive Committee and the General Assembly. All were reviewed by the Executive Committee and other experts in those fields, many were peer-reviewed by the journal, and many were endorsed by the Council or General Assembly.

In addition to the written reports mentioned below, the Federation has produced other reports. Some were not included here because of their generality and brevity. Others were soon superseded by newer or more complete reports that are included here. Some of the earliest reports are not included for that reason. Our apologies to those who have published reports that were not included in this list. The process of identifying and compiling a list is complex, as there has been no previous such list on which to rely. "In press" citation refers to the time that this book went to press.

The published reports are presented here in three parts:

- Those published in the journal;
- Those published in the 1983 *Practice Guidelines* book;
- Those published in the 1999 *Practice Guidelines* book.

Journal publications

Safety, ethical considerations, and application guidelines for the use of Transcranial Magnetic Stimulation in clinical practice and research. A consensus statement from the international workshop on present and future of TMS: safety and ethical guidelines. S. Rossi, M. Hallett, P.M. Rossini, A. Pascual-Leone. *Clinical Neurophysiology* 2009;120:2008–2039.

Event-related potentials in clinical research: Guidelines for eliciting, recording, and quantifying mismatch negativity, P300, and N400. C.C. Duncan, R.J. Barry, J.F. Connolly, C. Fischer, P.T. Michie, R. Näätänen, J. Polich, I. Reinvang, C. van Petten. *Clinical Neurophysiology* 2009;120:1883–1908.

The clinical diagnostic utility of transcranial magnetic stimulation: report of an IFCN committee. R. Chen, D. Cros, A. Curra, V. Di Lazzaro, J.P. Lefaucheur, M.R. Magistris, K. Mills, K.M Rösler, W.J. Triggs, Y. Ugawa, U. Ziemann. *Clinical Neurophysiology* 2008;119:504–532.

Recommendations for the clinical use of somatosensory-evoked potentials. G. Cruccu, M.J. Aminoff, G. Curio, J.M. Guérit, R. Kakigi, F. Mauguière, P.M. Rossini, R.D. Treede, L. García-Larrea. *Clinical Neurophysiology* 2008;119:1705–1719.

IFCN Standards for digital recording of clinical EEG. M.R. Nuwer, G. Comi, R. Emerson, A. Fuglsang-Fredericksen, J.M. Guérit, H. Hinrichs, A. Ikeda, F.J. Luccas, P. Rappelsberger, *Electroencephalography and Clinical Neurophysiology* 1998;106:259–261.

IFCN recommended standards for electrophysiologic monitoring in comatose and other unresponsive states. G.E. Chatrian, B. Bergamasco, A. Bricolo, J. Frost, P. Prior, *Electroencephalography and Clinical Neurophysiology* 1996;99:103–126.

Central EMG and tests of motor control. M. Hallett, A. Berardelli, P. Delwaide, H. Freund, J. Kimura, C. Lücking, J. Rothwell, B. Shahani, N. Yanagisawa. *Electroencephalography and Clinical Neurophysiology* 1994;90:404–432.

Human reflexes and late responses. J. Kimura, J. Daube, D. Burke, M. Hallett, G. Cruccu, B. Ongerboer de Visser, N. Yanagisawa, M. Shimamura, J. Rothwell, *Electroencephalography and Clinical Neurophysiology* 1994;90:393–403.

Non-invasive electrical and magnetic stimulation of the brain spinal cord and roots. Basic principles and procedures for routine clinical application. P. Rossini, A.T. Barker, A. Berardelli, M. Caramia, G. Caruso, R. Cracco, M. Dimitrijevic, M. Hallett, C. Lücking, A. Maertens de Noordhout, C. Marsden, N. Murray, J. Rothwell, M. Swash, C. Tomberg. *Electroencephalography and Clinical Neurophysiology* 1994;91:79–92.

IFCN recommended standards for long-latency auditory event related potentials. D. Goodin, J. Desmedt, K. Maurer, M.R. Nuwer. *Electroencephalography and Clinical Neurophysiology* 1994;91:18–20.

IFCN recommended standards for brainstem auditory evoked potentials. M.R. Nuwer, M. Aminoff, D. Goodin, S. Matsuoka, F. Mauguière, A. Starr, J.F. Vibert. *Electroencephalography and Clinical Neurophysiology* 1994;91:12–17.

IFCN recommended standards for short latency somatosensory evoked potentials. M.R. Nuwer, M. Aminoff, J. Desmedt, A. Eisen, D. Goodin, S. Matsuoka, F. Mauguière, H. Shibasaki, W. Sutherling, J.F. Vilbert. *Electroencephalography and Clinical Neurophysiology* 1994;91:6–11.

IFCN guidelines for topographic and frequency analysis of EEGs and EPs. M.R. Nuwer, D. Lehmann, F.H. Lopes da Silva, S. Matsuoka, W. Sutherling, J.F. Vibert. *Electroencephalography and Clinical Neurophysiology* 1994;91:1–5.

Long-term monitoring for epilepsy. J. Engel, J. Burchfield, J. Ebersole, J. Gates, J. Gotman, R. Homan, J. Ives, D. King, J. Lieb, S. Sato, R. Wilkus. *Electroencephalography and Clinical Neurophysiology* 1993;87:437–458.

Recommended standards for electroretinograms and visual evoked potentials. G. Celesia, I. Bodis-Wollner, G. Chatrian, G. Harding, S. Sokol, H. Spekreijse. *Electroencephalography and Clinical Neurophysiology* 1993;87:421–436.

Neuromonitoring during surgery. M.R. Nuwer, J. Daube, C. Fischer, J. Schramm, C. Yingling. *Electroencephalography and Clinical Neurophysiology* 1993;87:263–276.

Basic mechanisms of cerebral rhythmic activities. M. Steriade, P. Gloor, R.R. Llinás, F.H. Lopes da Silva, M. Mesulam. *Electroencephalography and Clinical Neurophysiology* 1990;76:481–408.

Kindling: basic mechanisms and clinical validity. M. Sato, R. Racine, D. McIntyre. *Electroencephalography and Clinical Neurophysiology* 1990;76:459–472.

Committee on standards of clinical practice of EEG and EMG. O. Magnus, J. Daube, S. Gomes Lins, I. Hausmanowa-Petrusewicz, F. Isch, D. Klass, S. Kubicki, J. Kugler, K. Mechelse, J. Payan, G. Scollo-Lavizzari, E. Stålberg. *Electroencephalography and Clinical Neurophysiology* 1982;54:9–10.

Committee on quantification in electromyography. R.G. Willison, I. Petersén, M. Meyer, P. Pinelli, J.E. Desmedt, K. Kunze, R.G. Lee, I. Hausmanowa-Petrusewicz, F. Isch, A. Arrigo. *Electroencephalography and Clinical Neurophysiology* 1982;54:12–14.

Report of committee on cessation of cerebral function, in the Xth international congress of electroencephalography and clinical neurophysiology: proceedings of the General Assembly. E. Walker, D.R. Bennett, A. Bricolo, L. Cigánek, A.M. Gurvich, N. Chiofalo. *Electroencephalography and Clinical Neurophysiology* 1982;54:9.

Appendix A: EEG instrumentation standards (revised 1977): Report of the committee on EEG instrumentation standards of the international federation of societies for electroencephalography and clinical neurophysiology. J.S. Barlow, A. Kamp, H.B. Morton, A. Ripoche, H. Shipton, D.B. Tchavdarov. *Electroencephalography and Clinical Neurophysiology* 1978;44: 144–150.

Appendix C: EEG instrumentation standards: report of the committee on EEG instrumentation standards of the international federation of societies for electroencephalography and clinical neurophysiology. J.S. Barlow, A. Kamp, H.B. Morton, A. Ripoche, H. Shipton. *Electroencephalography and Clinical Neurophysiology* 1974;37:549–553.

Appendix B: A glossary of terms most commonly used by clinical electroencephalographers. G.E. Chatrian, L. Bergamini, M. Dondey, D.W. Klass, M. Lennox-Buchthal, I. Petersén. *Electroencephalography and Clinical Neurophysiology* 1974;37:538–548.

Report of the committee on EMG instrumentation, in the VIIIth international congress of electroencephalography and clinical neurophysiology, proceedings of the General Assembly. R.G. Willison. *Electroencephalography and Clinical Neurophysiology* 1974;37:532–534.

Report of the committee on EMG instrumentation: technical factors in recording electrical activity of muscle and nerve in man, submitted to the General Assembly, VIIth international congress of IFSECN. C. Guld, A. Rosenfalck, R.G. Willison. *Electroencephalography and Clinical Neurophysiology* 1970;28:399–433.

Terminology of electromyography. J.A. Simpson. *Electroencephalography and Clinical Neurophysiology* 1969;26:224–226.

Appendix A: Proposal for an EEG terminology by the terminology committee of the International Federation of Societies for Electroencephalography and Clinical Neurophysiology. W. Storm van Leeuwen, R. Bickford, M. Brazier, W.A. Cobb, M. Dondey, H. Gastaut, P. Gloor, C.E. Henry, R. Hess, J.R. Knott, J. Kugler, G.C. Lairy, C. Loeb, O. Magnus, L. Oller Daurella, H. Petsche, R. Schwab, W.G. Walter, L. Widén. *Electroencephalography and Clinical Neurophysiology* 1966;20: 306–310.

Report of the committee on apparatus: recommendations to manufacturers, in the proceedings of the IVth international EEG congress. J.R. Knott, H.W. Shipton, F. Buchthal, C. Henry, C. Marshall, W. Storm van Leeuwen, A. Rémond. *Electroencephalography and Clinical Neurophysiology* 1958;10:378–380.

Appendix: The ten–twenty electrode system of the International Federation. H. Jasper. *Electroencephalography and Clinical Neurophysiology* 1958;10:371–375.

Report of the committee on methods of clinical examination in electroencephalography, 1957. W. Cobb, C. Ajmone-Marsan, H. Gastaut, R. Hess Jr., R. Jung, J.R. Knott, O. Magnus, H. Petsche, R. Schwab, H. Terzian, L. Widén. *Electroencephalography and Clinical Neurophysiology* 1958;10: 370–371.

Published in the 1983 practice guidelines book

Recommendations for the Practice of Clinical Neurophysiology. International Federation of Societies for Electroencephalography and Clinical Neurophysiology. Elsevier, 1983.

Electroencephalography

The ten–twenty electrode system of the International Federation
H.H. Jasper

A glossary of terms most commonly used by clinical electroencephalographers
G.E. Chatrian, L. Bergamini, M. Dondey, D.W. Klass, M. Lennox-Buchthal and I. Petersén

EEG instrumentation standards (revised 1977): report of the Committee on EEG Instrumentation Standards of the International Federation of Societies for Electroencephalography and Clinical Neurophysiology
J.S. Barlow (Chairman), A. Kamp, H.B. Morton, A. Ripoche, H. Shipton and D.B. Tchavdarov

Report of committee on cessation of cerebral function
A.E. Walker (Chairman), D.R. Bennett, A. Bricolo, L. Cigánek, A.M. Gurvich and N. Chiofalo. Committee on standards of clinical practice of EEG and EMG

Appendix I. Standards of clinical practice of EEG

IA: Standards of clinical practice in the EEG department

IB: Standards of clinical practice of EEG of newborns

Standards of clinical practice of EEG of newborns—Annex. The 12.5–25 system of electrode positions

IC: Standards of clinical practice of EEG in intensive care units

ID: EEG monitoring during open-heart and carotid artery surgery. A.J.R. Simon

IE: Standards of clinical practice of EEG in cases of suspected “cerebral death”. G.E. Chatrian

IF: Standards of clinical practice for the recording of evoked potentials (EPs). M. Halliday

Electromyography

Report of the committee on EMG instrumentation. Technical factors in recording electrical activity of muscle and nerve in man
C. Guld, A. Rosenfalck and R.G. Willison

Report of the committee on EMG instrumentation
C. Guld, A. Rosenfalck and R.G. Willison

Committee on quantification in electromyography
R.G. Willison (Chairman), I. Petersén, M. Meyer, P. Pinelli, J.E. Desmedt, K. Kunze, R.G. Lee, I. Hausmanowa-Petrusewicz, F. Isch and A. Arrigo

Appendix II. Committee on standards of clinical practice of EMG

IIA: Principles of clinical practice of EMG
IIB: Standards of instrumentation and application of EMG
IIC: EMG terminology

The Constitution

Constitution de la Fédération Internationale des Sociétés d'Electroencéphalographie et de Neurophysiologie Clinique

Published in the 1999 practice guidelines book

Recommendations for the Practice of Clinical Neurophysiology: Guidelines of the International Federation of Clinical Neurophysiology (2nd Revised and Enlarged Edition). Edited by Günther Deuschl and Andrew Eisen. *Electroencephalography and Clinical Neurophysiology Supplement,* Vol. 52, Elsevier, 1999

Section 1. EEG (technical standards and glossary)

The ten-twenty electrode system of the International Federation
G.H. Klem, H.O. Lüders, H.H. Jasper and C. Elger

EEG instrumentation
A. Ebner, G. Sciarretta, C.M. Epstein and M.R. Nuwer

IFCN standards for digital recording of clinical EEG
M.R. Nuwer, G. Comi, R. Emerson, A. Fuglsang-Frederiksen, J.-M. Guérit, H. Hinrichs, A. Ikeda, F.J.C. Luccas and P. Rappelsberger

IFCN guidelines for topographic and frequency analysis of EEGs and EPs
M.R. Nuwer, D. Lehmann, F. Lopes da Silva, S. Matsuoka, W. Sutherling and J.F. Vibert

A glossary of terms most commonly used by clinical electroencephalographers and proposals for the report for the EEG findings
S. Noachtar, C. Binnie, J. Ebersole, F. Mauguière, A. Sakamoto and B. Westmoreland

Appendix 3

Handbook series books

The Federation has commissioned two major Handbook series of books plus one 6-volume update that appeared between those two.

The first Handbook series dealt with techniques for recording physiological data in the various forms of EEG, EMG, and other common and special technologies. In addition, it covers clinical applications of those techniques. It was commissioned at the 1969 International Congress. Volumes appeared individually from 1972 to 1979. Former Federation President Antoine Rémond served as series Editor-in-Chief. The collection of volumes was arranged from the beginning to cover the technologies in use at the time, 1969, when the work was commissioned.

The Revised series followed the original Handbook series, mainly by describing techniques that were new since the time of the original series. Initially Antoine Rémond served in an encore reprisal of his previous role as Editor-in-Chief. Eventually the individual volume editors themselves took on an independent role in producing their volume. These volumes appeared between 1986 and 1999.

The new Handbook series was commissioned in 1997. Under the capable leadership of Jasper Daube and François Mauguière, this series took a different approach. Instead of technology-based topics, it organized the books into disease-based topics. Each covered the various clinical disorders and situations, and described the current, new and advanced clinical neurophysiology techniques that applied in those clinical disorders and circumstances. Some volumes in this series still were in press or in preparation at the time that this book went to press. Eventually the list of volumes will be longer than described here. These volumes began appearing in 2003 and continue to be in press at the time of this writing.

The names of the series and their volumes are presented below in chronological order:

- Handbook of Electroencephalography and Clinical Neurophysiology
- Handbook of Electroencephalography and Clinical Neurophysiology, Revised Series
- Handbook of Clinical Neurophysiology

Handbook of Electroencephalography and Clinical Neurophysiology

Editor-in-Chief: Antoine Rémond

Volume 1. Appraisal and Perspective of the Functional Exploration of the Nervous System
Editor: W.A. Cobb
(A) Evolution of Clinical Neurophysiology since Hans Berger
Editor: W.A. Cobb
(B) Frontiers of Neurophysiology
Editor: W.A. Cobb
(C) Values of Clinical Neurophysiology
Editor: W.A. Cobb

Volume 2. Electrical Activity from the Neuron to the EEG and EMG
Editor: O. Creutzfeldt
(A) Morphological Basis of EEG Mechanisms
Editor: O. Creutzfeldt
(B) Basic Neurophysiology of Neuronal and Glial Potentials
Editor: C.F. Stevens
(C) The Neuronal Generation of the EEG
Editor: O. Creutzfeldt
(D) Basic Mechanisms of the EMG
Editor: A. Struppler

Volume 3. Techniques and Methods of Data Acquisition of EEG and EMG
Editor: M.R. De Lucchi
(A) Acquisition of Bioelectrical Data: Collection and Amplification
Editor: R.J. Broughton
(B) Graphic and Magnetic-Tape Recording of Bioelectrical Phenomena
Editors: J.D. Frost Jr. and J.S. Barlow
(C) Traditional Methods of Examination in Clinical EEG
Editor: B.B. MacGillivray
(D) Activation and Provocation Methods in Clinical Neurophysiology.
Editor: R. Naquet

Volume 4. Evaluation of Bioelectrical Data from Brain, Nerve and Muscle, I
Editor: M.A.B. Brazier
(A) Sampling, Conversion and Measurement of Bioelectrical Phenomena
Editor: F.H. Lopes da Silva
(B) Digital Processing of Bioelectrical Phenomena
Editor: D.O. Walter

Volume 5. Evaluation of Bioelectrical Data from Brain, Nerve and Muscle, II
Editors: M.A.B. Brazier and D.O. Walter
(A) Frequency and Correlation Analysis
Editor: M. Matoušek
(B) EEG Topography
Editor: H. Petsche

Volume 6. The Normal EEG Throughout Life
Editor: G.C. Lairy
(A) The EEG of the Waking Adult
Editors: G.E. Chatrian and G.C. Lairy
(B) The Evolution of EEG from Birth to Adulthood
Editor: G.C. Lairy

Volume 7. Physiological Correlates of EEG
Editors: E.K. Killam and K. Killam
(A) EEG and Sleep
Editor: P. Passouant

(B) Influence on the EEG of Certain Physiological States and Other Parameters
Editor: R. Cooper
(C) Effect of Drugs on the EEG
Editor: V.G. Longo

Volume 8. Electrical Reactions of the Brain and Complementary Methods of Evaluation
Editor: P. Buser
(A) Visual, Auditory and Somesthetic Evoked Potentials and CNV
Editors: W. Storm van Leeuwen, F.H. Lopes da Silva and A. Kamp
(B) Complementary Electrophysiological Techniques and Methods for Evaluation of the CNS
Editor: J.S. Barlow

Volume 9. Somatic Sensation
Editor: W.A. Cobb

Volume 10. Direct, Cortical and Depth Evaluation of the Brain
Editor: C. Ajmone Marsan
(A) Slow Potential Shifts Recorded Directly from the Cortex
Editor: H. Caspers
(B) Stereoencephalography
Editor: J. Bancaud
(C) Electrocortigraphy
Editor: C. Ajmone Marsan

Volume 11. Clinical EEG, I
Editor: W.A. Cobb
(A) Semiology in Clinical EEG
Editors: M. Dondey and J. Gaches
(B) EEG Interpretation in Clinical Medicine
Editor: W.A. Cobb

Volume 12. Clinical EEG, II
Editors: R. Harner and R. Naquet
(A) Altered States of Consciousness, Coma, Cerebral Death
Editors: R. Harner and R. Naquet

Volume 13. Clinical EEG, III
Editor: H. Gastaut
(A) Epilepsies
Editors: H. Gastaut and C.A. Tassinari
(B) Mental Diseases
Editor: M. Dongier

Volume 14. Clinical EEG, IV
Editor: O. Magnus
(A) Cardiac and Vascular Diseases
Editor: J.H.A. Van der Drift

(B) Traumatic Disorders
Editor: J. Courjon
(C) Brain Tumours and Space Occupying Processes
Editor: R. Hess

Volume 15. Clinical EEG, V
Editor: D.D. Daly
(A) Infections, Inflammatory and Allergic Reactions and Degenerative Diseases
Editor: F.J. Radermecker
(B) Hereditary, Congenital and Perinatal Diseases
Editors: C. Dreyfus-Brisac and R.J. Ellingson
(C) Metabolic, Endocrine and Toxic Diseases
Editor: G.H. Glaser

Volume 16. EMG
Editor: F. Buchthal
(A) Nervous and Muscular Evoked Potentials
Editor: H.E. Kaeser
(B) Neuromuscular Diseases
Editor: J.A. Simpson

Handbook of Electroencephalography and Clinical Neurophysiology: Revised Series

Editor-in-Chief: Antoine Rémond

Volume 1. Methods of Analysis of Brain Electrical and Magnetic Signals
Editors: A.S. Gevins and A. Rémond

Volume 2. Clinical Applications of Computer Analysis of EEG and Other Neurophysiological Signals
Editors: F.H. Lopes da Silva, W. Storm van Leeuwen and A. Rémond

Volume 3. Human Event-Related Potentials
Editor: T.W. Picton

Volume 4. Clinical Neurophysiology of Epilepsy
Editors: J.A. Wada and R.J. Ellingson

Volume 5. Electromyography
Editor: H.P. Ludin

Volume 6. Event-Related Desynchronization
Editors: G. Pfurtscheller and F.H. Lopes da Silva

Handbook of Clinical Neurophysiology

Editors-in-Chief: Jasper R. Daube and François Mauguière

Volume 1. Movement Disorders
Editor: M. Hallett

Volume 2. Clinical Neurophysiology of Disorders of Muscle and Neuromuscular Junction Including Fatigue
Editor: E. Stålberg

Volume 3. Presurgical Assessment of the Epilepsies with Clinical Neurophysiology and Functional Imaging
Editors: F.H. Rosenow and H.O. Lüders

Volume 4. Clinical Neurophysiology of Motor Neuron Diseases
Editor: A. Eisen

Volume 5. Disorders of Visual Processing
Editor: G. Celesia

Volume 6. Clinical Neurophysiology of Sleep Disorders
Editor: Ch. Guilleminault

Volume 7. Peripheral Nerve Diseases
Editor: J. Kimura

Volume 8. Intraoperative Monitoring of Neural Function
Editor: M.R. Nuwer

Volume 9. Vertigo and Imbalance: Clinical Neurophysiology of the Vestibular System
Editors: S.D.Z. Eggers and D.S. Zee

Appendix 4

Supplement Series books: Supplements to Electroencephalography and Clinical Neurophysiology and Supplements to Clinical Neurophysiology

This book series was initiated to provide an available and durable resource for materials that did not fit into the regular journal publication. A variety of content has been accepted into this book series. That first was a compendium of references on EEG. Many have been congress proceedings, most for the Federation International Congresses but also some for other congresses or symposia. The series is also a convenient home for books on particular topics relevant to clinical neurophysiologists. On average one new book appeared each year. An advantage for publishing in this series is that many libraries already subscribe to the book series.

Notice that this is different from supplemental journal issues. Those issues appear from time to time, often on a particular short topic or as abstracts for a scientific meeting. As an example, the abstract books for some Chapter meetings are published as supplemental issues of the journal. The supplemental journal issues usually mark their pages with the letter S followed by the page number. The Supplement series books do not do so.

The Supplement Series of books changed its name in 1999. Before that it was known as *Supplements to Electroencephalography and Clinical Neurophysiology* series. Since that time, the series has been known as *Supplements to Clinical Neurophysiology* series.

Organizations interested in publishing in this series should contact either Elsevier or the IFCN Executive Committee.

The titles in this series are:

Volume 1. Bibliography of Electroencephalography. Edited by Mary A.B. Brazier, 1950, 178 pp.

Volume 2. 2e Congrès International d'EEG: Rapports – Conférences – Symposium. Edited by H. Fischgold, 1950, 137 pp.

Volume 3. Third Congress, Cambridge, MA, Abstracts. 1953, 94 pp.

Volume 4. Third Congress, Cambridge, MA, Symposia. 1953, 260 pp.

Volume 5. Encéphalites et Encéphalopathies. Edited by J. Radermecker, 1956, 243 pp.

Volume 6. Conditionnement et Réactivité en Electroencéphalographie. Edited by H. Fischgold and H. Gastaut, 1957, 475 pp.

Volume 7. Fourth EEG Congress and First Congress of Neurological Sciences. Symposia and Proceedings. Edited by L. Van Bogaert and J. Radermecker, 1959, 750 pp.

Volume 8. EEG Researches in the Soviet Union. Edited by V.S. Rusinov and N.Y. Rabinovich, 1958, 36 pp.

Volume 9. Proceedings of the 6th Annual Meeting of the Japan EEG Society. Edited by Takashi Minoshima, 1958, 141 pp.

Volume 10. A Symposium on Dendrites: American Society of Electroencephalographers (abstracts). 1958, 76 pp.

Volume 11. Obnubilations, Comas et Stupeurs. Edited by H. Fischgold and P. Mathis, 1959, 126 pp.

Volume 12. 7th Annual Meeting of the Japan EEG Society and 11th Annual Meeting of the Japan EMG Society. Edited by Kentaro Shimizu, 1959, 155 pp.

Volume 13. Moscow Colloquium on Higher Nervous Activity. Edited by G.D. Smirnov and H. Jasper, 1960.

Volume 14. The Barbiturate Withdrawal Syndrome. Edited by M. Hurtel Wulff, 1959, 173 pp.

Volume 15. A Seizure Atlas. Edited by C. Ajmone Marsan and K. Abraham, 1960, 215 pp.

Volume 16. Exploration du Cerveau Humain par Electrodes Profondes. Edited by M. Ribstein, 1960, 130 pp.

Volume 17. Rayon X, Radio-isotopes et EEG dans l'Epilepsie. Edited by H. Fischgold and H. Gastaut, 1960, 226 pp.

Volume 18. 8th Annual Meeting of the Japan EEG Society and 12th Annual Meeting of the Japan EMG Society. Edited by Kentaro Shimizu, 1959, 124 pp.

Volume 19. EEG and Cerebral Tumours. Edited by O. Magnus, W. Storm van Leeuwen and W. A. Cobb, 1961, 248 pp.

Volume 20. Computer Techniques in EEG Analysis. Edited by M.A.B. Brazier, 1961, 98 pp.

Volume 21. Progress in Electromyography. 1st International EMG Congress, Pavia, 1961. Edited by P. Pinelli, F. Buchthal and F. Thiébaut, 1962, 184 pp.

Volume 22. Stagnant Anoxia and Carbon Monoxide Poisoning. Edited by N. Bokonjic, 1963, 102 pp.

Volume 23. The Physiology Basis of Mental Activity. Edited by H. Hernandez Peón, 1963, 283 pp.

Volume 24. A Selected Bibliography of EEG in Human Psychopharmacology. Edited by M. Fink, 1964, 68 pp.

Volume 25. Recent Advances in Clinical Neurophysiology. Symposia of the 6th Congress, Vienna, 1965. Edited by L. Widén, 1967, 308 pp.

Volume 26. The Evoked Potentials. Edited by W. Cobb and C. Morocutti, 1967, 218 pp.

Volume 27. Advances in EEG Analysis. Edited by D.O. Walter and M.A.B. Brazier, 1969, 78 pp.

Volume 28. Hans Berger on the EEG of Man. Edited by P. Gloor, 1969, 350 pp.

Volume 29. A KWIK Index 1966–1969. Edited by P.L. Walter, 1970, 548 pp.

Volume 30. A KWIK Index 1964–1966. Edited by M. Wineburg and P.L. Walter, 1971, 392 pp.

Volume 31. Recent Contributions to Neurophysiology. Edited by J.-P. Cordeau and P. Gloor, 1972, 208 pp.

Volume 32. Febrile Convulsions. Edited by M.A. Lennox-Buchthal, 1973, 138 pp.

Volume 33. Event-Related Slow Potentials of the Brain. Edited by W.C. McCallum and J.R. Knott, 1973, 390 pp.

Volume 34. Contemporary Clinical Neurophysiology. Edited by W.A. Cobb and H. Van Duijn, 1978, 578 pp.

Volume 35. Henry Gastaut and the Marseilles School's Contribution to the Neurosciences. Edited by R.J. Broughton, 1982, 448 pp.

Volume 36. Kyoto Symposia. Edited by P.A. Buser, W.A. Cobb and T. Okuma, 1982, 758 pp.

Volume 37. Long-Term Monitoring in Epilepsy. Edited by J. Gotman, J.R. Ives and P. Gloor, 1985, 444 pp.

Volume 38. Cerebral Psychophysiology: Studies in Event-Related Potentials. Edited by W.C. McCallum, R. Zappoli and R. Denoth, 1986, 566 pp.

Volume 39. The London Symposia. Edited by R.J. Ellingson, N.M.F. Murray and A.M. Halliday, 1987, 425 pp.

Volume 40. Current Trends in Event-Related Potential Research. Edited by R. Johnson, Jr., J.W. Rohrbaugh and R. Parasuraman, 1987, 770 pp.

Volume 41. New Trends and Advanced Techniques in Clinical Neurophysiology. Edited by P.M. Rossini and F. Mauguière, 1990, 382 pp.

Volume 42. Event-Related Brain Research. Edited by C.H.M. Brunia, G. Mulder and M.N. Verbaten, 1991, 393 pp.

Volume 43. Magnetic Motor Stimulation: Basic Principles and Clinical Experience. Edited by W.J. Levy, R.Q. Cracco, A.T. Barker and J.C. Rothwell, 1991, 393 pp.

Volume 44. Perspectives of Event-Related Potentials Research. Edited by G. Karmos, M. Molnari, V. Csepe, I. Czigler and J.E. Desmedt, 1995, 464 pp.

Volume 45. Continuous Wave-Form Analysis. Edited by R.M. Dasheiff and D.J. Vincent, 1996, 162 pp.

Volume 46. Functional Neuroscience: Sensory, Motor and Cognitive Systems. Edited by C. Barber, G.G. Celesia, G.C. Comi and F. Mauguière, 1996, 364 pp.

Volume 47. Visualization of Information Processing in the Human Brain. Edited by I. Hashimoto, Y.C. Okada and S. Ogawa, 1996, 461 pp.

Volume 48. Electrocorticography: Current Trends and Future Perspectives. Edited by L.F. Quesney, C.D. Binnie and G.-E. Chatrian, 1998, 158 pp.

Volume 49. Functional Neuroscience: Evoked Potentials and Magnetic Fields. Edited by C. Barber, G.G. Celesia, I. Hashimoto and R. Kakigi, 1999, 330 pp.

Volume 50. Clinical Neurophysiology: From Receptors to Perception. Edited by G. Comi, C.H. Lücking, J. Kimura and P.M. Rossini, 1999, 608 pp.

Volume 51. Transcranial Magnetic Stimulation. Edited by W. Paulus, M. Hallett, P.M. Rossini and J.C. Rothwell, 1999, 375 pp.

Volume 52. Recommendations for the Practice of Clinical Neurophysiology: Guidelines of the International Federation of Clinical Neurophysiology. Edited by G. Deuschl and A. Eisen, 2000, 304 pp.

Volume 53. Clinical Neurophysiology at the Beginning of the 21st Century. Edited by Z. Ambler, S. Nevšímalová, Z. Kadaňka and P.M. Rossini, 2000, 469 pp.

Volume 54. Advances in Clinical Neurophysiology. Edited by R.C. Reisin, M.R. Nuwer, M. Hallett and C. Medina, 2002, 527 pp.

Volume 55. Motor Unit Number Estimation (MUNE). Edited by Mark B. Bromberg, 2003, 342 pp.

Volume 56. Transcranial Magnetic Stimulation and Transcranial Direct Current Stimulation. Edited by W. Paulus, F. Tergau, M.A. Nitsche, J.C. Rothwell, U. Ziemann and M. Hallett, 2003, 452 pp.

Volume 57. Advances in Clinical Neurophysiology. Edited by M. Hallett, L.H. Philips, II, D.L. Schomer and J.M. Massey, 2004, 760 pp.

Volume 58. Brainstem Function and Dysfunction. Edited by Giorgio Cruccu and Mark Hallettt, 2006, 287pp.

Volume 59. Functional Neuroscience: Evoked Potentials and Related Techniques. Edited by C. Barber, S. Tsuji, S. Tobimatsu, T. Uozumi, N. Akamatsu and A. Eisen, 2006, 339 pp.

Volume 60. Motor Unit Number Estimation (MUNE) and Quantitative EMG. Edited by Mark B. Bromberg, 2009, 298 pp.

Volume 61. Wave Length and Action Potentials: History of the International Federation of Clinical Neurophysiology. By Marc R. Nuwer and Carl H. Lücking, 2010, 294 pp.

Wave Length and Action Potentials: History of the IFCN
(Supplements to Clinical Neurophysiology, Vol. 61)
By: M.R. Nuwer and C.H. Lücking

Appendix 5

List of IFCN Chapters and member societies

The following is a listing of the IFCN member societies. This is up to date through 2009. The list is separated by Chapter region. There are four chapters. In addition to the regular member societies representing national clinical neurophysiology organizations, the International Clinical Neurophysiology Society (ICNS) is treated as if it were a national member society.

The societies are given below within each chapter in alphabetic order by their nation's name as listed on the Federation website. The member societies are:

Europe, Middle East and Africa Chapter

The Austrian Society for Clinical Neurophysiology

Belgian Society of Clinical Neurophysiology

Belgian Society EMG & Clinical Neurophysiology

Bulgarian Society for EEG, EMG & Clinical Neurophysiology

Croatian Federation for EEG and Neurophysiology

Czech Society for Clinical Neurophysiology

Danish Society of Clinical Neurophysiology

Dutch Society for Clinical Neurophysiology

Egyptian Society of Electrodiagnosis Medicine & Clinical Neurophysiology

Estonian Society of Clinical Neurophysiology

Finnish Society of Clinical Neurophysiology

Societé de Neurophysiologie Clinique de Langue Française

Deutsche Gesellschaft für Klinische Neurophysiologie und funktionelle Bildgebung

Hellenic Society of EEG & Clinical Neurophysiology

Hungarian Society of Clinical Neurophysiology

Iranian Neurological Association

Irish Society of Clinical Neurophysiology

Israeli Society for Clinical Neurophysiology

Italian Society of Clinical Neurophysiology

Jordanian Society of Clinical Neurophysiology

Société Luxembourgeoise de Neurologie

Norwegian Society of Clinical Neurophysiology

Polish Society of Clinical Neurophysiology

Portuguese Association of EEG & Clinical Neurophysiology

Romanian Society of Electrodiagnostic Neurophysiology

I.P. Pavlov Russian Physiological Society

Serbia and Montenegro Society of Clinical Neurophysiology

Slovak Society of Clinical Neurophysiology

Slovenian Society of Clinical Neurophysiology

Spanish Society of Clinical Neurophysiology

Swedish Society for Clinical Neurophysiology

Swiss Society of Clinical Neurophysiology

Turkish Society of Clinical Neurophysiology

British Society for Clinical Neurophysiology

Asia–Oceania Chapter

Australian and New Zealand Association of Neurologists (ANZAN)

Chinese Society of EMG & Clinical Neurophysiology

Indian Academy of Neurology, Clinical Neurophysiology Subsection

Pokdi Neurofisiologi (Indonesian Society for Neurophysiology)

Japanese Society of Clinical Neurophysiology

Korean Society for Clinical Neurophysiology

Malaysian Society of Neuroscience, Clinical Neurophysiology Section

Philippine Society of Clinical Neurophysiology

Clinical Neurophysiology Society of Singapore

Taiwan Society of Clinical Neurophysiology

Thai Society of Clinical Neurophysiology

Latin America Chapter

Argentinian Society of EEG and Clinical Neurophysiology

Bolivian Society of Clinical Neurophysiology

Brazilian Society of Clinical Neurophysiology

Chilean Society of Clinical Neurophysiology

Colombian Association of Electrodiagnostic Medicine (ACME)

Colombian Association (ACNC)

Cuban Clinical Neurophysiology Society

Dominican Society of EEG & Clinical Neurophysiology

The Guatemalan Society of Clinical Neurophysiology

Mexican Society of Clinical Neurophysiology

Peruvian Society of Clinical Neurophysiology

Uruguayan Society of Clinical Neurophysiology

North America Chapter

American Association of Neuromuscular and Electrodiagnostic Medicine (AANEM)

American Clinical Neurophysiology Society (ACNS)

Canadian Society of Clinical Neurophysiologists (CSCN)

Appendix 6

IFCN Chapter officers and meetings

Chapter Executive Committee members are elected by the Chapter General Assembly, except for the Liaison Officer. The Federation Executive Committee appoints the Liaison Officer who acts as a liaison to the Chapter.

European Chapter of the International Federation of Clinical Neurophysiology (EC-IFCN)

EC-IFCN Executive Committee 1997–2005: Elected Members

- Erik Stålberg (Sweden) Chairman
- Al De Weerd (The Netherlands) Secretary-Treasurer
- Theresa Sagalés (Spain) Member-at-Large
- Giorgio Cruccu (Italy) Member-at-Large

EC-IFCN Executive Committee 2005–2009: Elected Members*

- Paolo Rossini (Italy) Chapter Chairman 2005–2009
- Luis García Larrea (France) Secretary-Treasurer 2005–2009
- Anders Fuglsang-Frederiksen (Denmark) Member-at-Large, 2005–2009
- Theresa Sagalés (Spain) Member-at-Large until 2008
- Jonathan Cole (UK) Member-at-Large, 2008–2012

EC-IFCN Liaison Officer

- François Mauguière (France) 1995
- Paolo Rossini (Italy) 1996–2001
- Johannes Noth (Germany) 2001–2006
- Kerry Mills (UK) 2006–2010

European Congresses of Clinical Neurophysiology (ECCN)

2011	Rome (14th)
2008	Istanbul
2005	Stockholm
2002	Barcelona
2000	Lyon
1998	Ljubljana
1996	Munich
1994	Budapest
1992	Lisbon
1990	Paris
1987	Amsterdam
1983	Basel
1979	Salzburg
1976	Venice

Latin American Chapter of the International Federation of Clinical Neurophysiology (CLA-IFCN)

CLA-IFCN Executive Committee

President

1995–1997	Nelly Chiofalo (Chile)
1998–2000	Carlos Medina (Argentina)
2000–2004	Daniel Cibils (Uruguay)
2004–2008	Jose Xavier de Castro (Brazil)
2009–2013	Renato Verdugo (Chile)

Secretary

1995–1998	Daniel Cibils (Uruguay)
1999–2002	Francisco Luccas (Brazil)
2003–2006	Renato Verdugo (Chile)
2007–2011	Alberto Yorio (Argentina)

*These terms might be extended until the next ECCN in 2011.

Treasurer

2009–2013	Jorge Gutierrez (Colombia)

Members-at-Large

1996–1999	Pedro Valdez (Cuba)
1996–1999	Jose Xavier de Castro (Brazil)
2001–2004	Olga Sanz (Argentina)
2001–2003	Augusto Fernandez Guardiola (Mexico) (died 2003)
2003–2007	Juan R. Santoni (Rep. Dominicana)
2005–2008	Henry Stokes (Guatemala)
2007–2011	Jaime Ramos (Mexico)
2009–2013	Lilia Morales (Cuba)

Liaison Officers

1995–2002	Gastone Celesia
2002–2006	Marc Nuwer
2006–2014	Daniel Cibils

Latin American Congresses of Clinical Neurophysiology

2011	Montevideo, Uruguay
2008	Puebla, Mexico
2005	Santiago, Chile
2002	Porto Seguro, Brazil
1997	Buenos Aires, Argentina
1995	Guatemala City, Guatemala

Asian and Oceanian Chapter of the International Federation of Clinical Neurophysiology (AOC-IFCN)

AOC-IFCN Executive Committee 1996–2000

Xiao-Fu Tang (People's Rep. of China) Chairperson
Nubuo Yanagisawa (Japan) Secretary
Xiao-Fu Tang also served as Liaison Officer 1996–1997
Hiroshi Shibasaki (Japan) Liaison Officer 1997–2001

AOC-IFCN Executive Committee 2000–2005

Prasert Boongird (Thailand) Chairman
Nobuo Yanagisawa (Japan) Secretary
Ryuji Kaji (Japan) Liaison Officer 2001–2006

AOC-IFCN Executive Committee 2005–2009

Rawiphan Witoonpanich (Thailand) Chairman
Kwang-Woo Lee (Korea) Chapter Secretary
Hiroshi Shibasaki (Japan) Liaison Officer 2006–2014

AOC-IFCN Executive Committee 2009–2013

Kwang-Woo Lee (Korea) Chairman
Bob Santoso Wibowo (Indonesia) Secretary
Hiroshi Shibasaki (Japan) Liaison Officer 2006–2014

Asian and Oceanian Congress of Clinical Neurophysiology (AOCCN)

2009 Seoul, Korea
2005 Chiang Mai, Thailand
2000 Manila, Philippines
1996 Beijing, People's Rep. of China

North American Chapter of the International Federation of Clinical Neurophysiology

Chapter Officers 2008–

Donald B. Sanders (AANEM)
M. George Elleker (CSCN)
John S. Ebersole (ACNS)

Wave Length and Action Potentials: History of the IFCN
(Supplements to Clinical Neurophysiology, Vol. 61)
By: M.R. Nuwer and C.H. Lücking

Appendix 7

Executive Committees of the International Federation

The Executive Committee composition has changed over the years. Initially, when the number of societies was few, each society was represented directly on the Executive Committee. Those representatives were Federation Vice-Presidents during the first three terms. Eventually a separate Council of Delegates was created. The positions of Vice-President then were discontinued.

An EMG Commission existed from 1961 to 1990 to represent the interests of the EMG community in the Federation. The EMG Commission Chairman was a member of the Executive Committee during those terms. Eventually EMG became an integral part of the Federation as a whole, and the need disappeared for a separate EMG Commission.

A Member-at-Large position was created in 1965 to increase the diversity of representation of the Executive Committee. A second Member-at-Large position was added in 1985 for the same reason.

1949–1953

President	Herbert Jasper	Canada
Vice-Presidents	Robert Schwab	USA
	William Grey Walter	UK
	Fritz Buchthal	Denmark
Secretary	Henri Gastaut	France
Treasurer	Antoine Rémond	France

1953–1957

President	William Grey Walter	UK
Past-President	Herbert H. Jasper	Canada
Vice-Presidents	F. Buchthal, A. Fessard, F. Gibbs, R. Granit, D. Hill, R. Jung, G. Moruzzi, K. Motokawa, S. Obrador-Alcalde, R. Schwab	
Secretary	Henri Gastaut	France
Treasurer	Mary A.B. Brazier	USA

1957–1961

President	Henri Gastaut	France
Past-President	William Grey Walter	UK
Vice-Presidents	H. Fischgold, M. Gozzano, M.R. Hess, J.R. Knott, E. Kugelberg, O. Magnus, A. Mosovich, G. Pampiglione, H. Petsche, J. Radermecker, V.S. Rusinov, S.A. Sarkisov, R. Schwab, N. Yoshii	
Secretary	Mary A.B. Brazier	USA
Treasurer	William Cobb	UK

1961–1965

President	Mary A.B. Brazier	USA
Past-President	Henri Gastaut	France
Secretary	Robert Naquet	France
Treasurer	William Cobb until 1962	UK
	W. Storm van Leeuwen from 1962	The Netherlands
Editor-in-Chief	Herbert H. Jasper	Canada
Chairman EMG Commission	Fritz Buchthal	Denmark

1965–1969

President	Antoine Rémond	France
Past-President	Mary A.B. Brazier	USA
Secretary	Robert Naquet	France
Treasurer	W. Storm van Leeuwen	The Netherlands
Editor-in-Chief	William Cobb	UK
Member-at-Large	Michael G. Saunders from 1966	Canada
Chairman EMG Commission	Edwin Lambert	USA

1969–1973

President	Cosimo Ajmone Marsan	USA
Past-President	Antoine Rémond	France
Secretary	Robert Ellingson	USA
Treasurer	M.R. Hess	Switzerland
Editor-in-Chief	William Cobb	UK
Member-at-Large	David Ingvar	Sweden
Chairman EMG Commission	Fritz Buchthal	Denmark

1973–1977

President	William Cobb	UK
Past-President	Cosimo Ajmone Marsan	USA
Secretary	Robert Ellingson	USA
Treasurer	Max Dondey	France
Editor-in-Chief	Mary A.B. Brazier	USA
Member-at-Large	Helmuth Petsche	Austria
Chairman EMG Commission	Albrecht Struppler	Germany

1977–1981

President	Robert Naquet	France
Past-President	William Cobb	UK
Secretary	Robert Ellingson	USA
Treasurer	Max Dondey	France
Editor-in-Chief	Mary A.B. Brazier	USA
Member-at-Large	Johann Kugler	Germany
Chairman EMG Commission	John Desmedt	Belgium

1981–1985

President	Robert Ellingson	USA
Past-President	Robert Naquet	France
Secretary	Morton Low	Canada
Treasurer	Max Dondey until 1983	France
	Pierre Buser from 1983	France
Editor-in-Chief	Mary A.B. Brazier until 1984	USA
	Hans van Duijn from 1984	The Netherlands
Member-at-Large	Carlo A. Tassinari	Italy
Chairman EMG Commission	John Desmedt	Belgium

1985–1990

President	John Desmedt	Belgium
Past-President	Robert Ellingson	USA
Secretary	Bram Ongerboer de Visser	The Netherlands
Treasurer	Manuel Meyer	Switzerland
Editor-in-Chief	Hans van Duijn until 1987	The Netherlands
	François Mauguière from 1987	France
Editor-in-Chief	Timothy Pedley 1987	USA
	Gastone Celesia from 1988	USA
Member-at-Large	Jhun Wada	Canada
Member-at-Large	Roberto Low	Brazil
Chairman EMG Commission	Stéphane Métral	France

1990–1993

President	Jun Kimura	Japan
Past-President	John Desmedt	Belgium
Secretary	Barry Tharp	USA
Treasurer	Manuel Meyer	Switzerland
Editor-in-Chief	François Mauguière	France
Editor-in-Chief	Gastone Celesia	USA
Member-at-Large	Jagjit Chopra	India
Member-at-Large	Jerzy Majkowsky	Poland

1993–1997

President	Carl Lücking	Germany
Past-President	Jun Kimura	Japan
Secretary	Giuseppe Caruso	Italy
Treasurer	Paul Despland	Switzerland
Editor-in-Chief	François Mauguière until 1995	France
	Paolo Rossini from 1995	Italy
Editor-in-Chief	Gastone Celesia	USA
Member-at-Large	Xiao-Fu Tang	People's Rep. of China
Member-at-Large	Marc Nuwer	USA

1997–2001

President	Marc Nuwer	USA
Past-President	Carl Lücking	Germany
Secretary	Hiroshi Shibasaki	Japan
Treasurer	Paul Despland	Switzerland
Editor-in-Chief	Gastone Celesia through 1999	USA
	Mark Hallett from 2000	USA
Editor-in-Chief	Paolo Rossini	Italy
Member-at-Large	David Burke	Australia
Member-at-Large	Günther Deuschl	Germany

2001–2006

President	François Mauguière	France
Past-President	Marc Nuwer	USA
Secretary	Graham Harding	UK
Treasurer	Andrew Eisen	Canada
Editor-in-Chief	Paolo Rossini until 2003	Italy
Editor-in-Chief	Mark Hallett	USA
Member-at-Large	Johannes Noth	Germany
Member-at-Large	Ryuji Kaji	Japan

2006–2010

President	Hiroshi Shibasaki	Japan
Past-President	François Mauguière	France
Secretary	Johannes Noth until 2007	Germany
	Reinhard Dengler from 2007	Germany
Treasurer	Andrew Eisen	Canada
Editor-in-Chief	Mark Hallett until 2008	USA
	David Burke from 2008	Australia
Member-at-Large	Daniel Cibils	Uruguay
Member-at-Large	Kerry Mills	UK

2010–2014

President	Paolo Rossini	Italy
Past-President	Hiroshi Shibasaki	Japan
Secretary	Daniel Cibils	Uruguay
Treasurer	Reinhard Dengler	Germany
Editor-in-Chief	David Burke	Australia
Member-at-Large	Lawrence Phillips	USA
Member-at-Large	Mamede de Carvalho	Portugal

Wave Length and Action Potentials: History of the IFCN
(Supplements to Clinical Neurophysiology, Vol. 61)
By: M.R. Nuwer and C.H. Lücking

Appendix 8

Honorary Fellows and Past-Presidents

Any person who has rendered important services to the Federation may be appointed an Honorary Fellow of the Federation by a supermajority of the General Assembly. All Federation former Presidents become Honorary Past-Presidents of the Federation after they finish their term on the Executive Committee as immediate Past-President. All Honorary Fellows and Honorary Past-Presidents hold such title for life, are entitled to attend all Congresses, and serve the Federation as non-voting members of the General Assembly.

Honorary Fellows

Lord Adrian of Cambridge
Frédéric Bremer (Brussels)
Mario Gozzano (Rome)
Herbert Jasper (Montreal)
Horace Magoun (Los Angeles)
Wilder Penfield (Montreal)
Giuseppe Moruzzi (Pisa)
Henri Gastaut (Marseilles)
Naosaburo Yoshii (Hyogo)
William Cobb (Beaulieu)
Hallowell Davis (St. Louis)
Willem Storm van Leeuwen (Bilthoven)
Antoine Rémond (Paris)
Fritz Buchthal (Copenhagen)
Edward Lambert (Minneapolis)
Yasuo Shimazono (Tokyo)
Pierre Gloor (Montreal)
John Desmedt (Brussels)
Jun Kimura (Kyoto)
Robert Ellingson (Omaha)
Robert Naquet (Paris)
Gastone Celesia (Chicago)

Honorary Past-Presidents

Herbert Jasper (Montreal)
W. Grey Walter (Bristol)
Henri Gastaut (Marseilles)
Mary A.B. Brazier (Los Angeles)
Antoine Rémond (Paris)
Cosimo Ajmone Marsan (Miami)
William Cobb (Beaulieu)
Robert Naquet (Paris)
Robert J. Ellingson (Omaha)
John E. Desmedt (Brussels)
Jun Kimura (Kyoto)
Carl Lücking (Freiburg)
Marc Nuwer (Los Angeles)
François Mauguière (Lyon)

Appendix 9

Registration and incorporation documents

The Federation was officially registered as a Registered Charity in France in 1951. Figure 25.1 is the official registration document from that governmental action. The official name was the Fédération Internationale d'Electroencéphalographie et de Neurophysiologie Clinique.

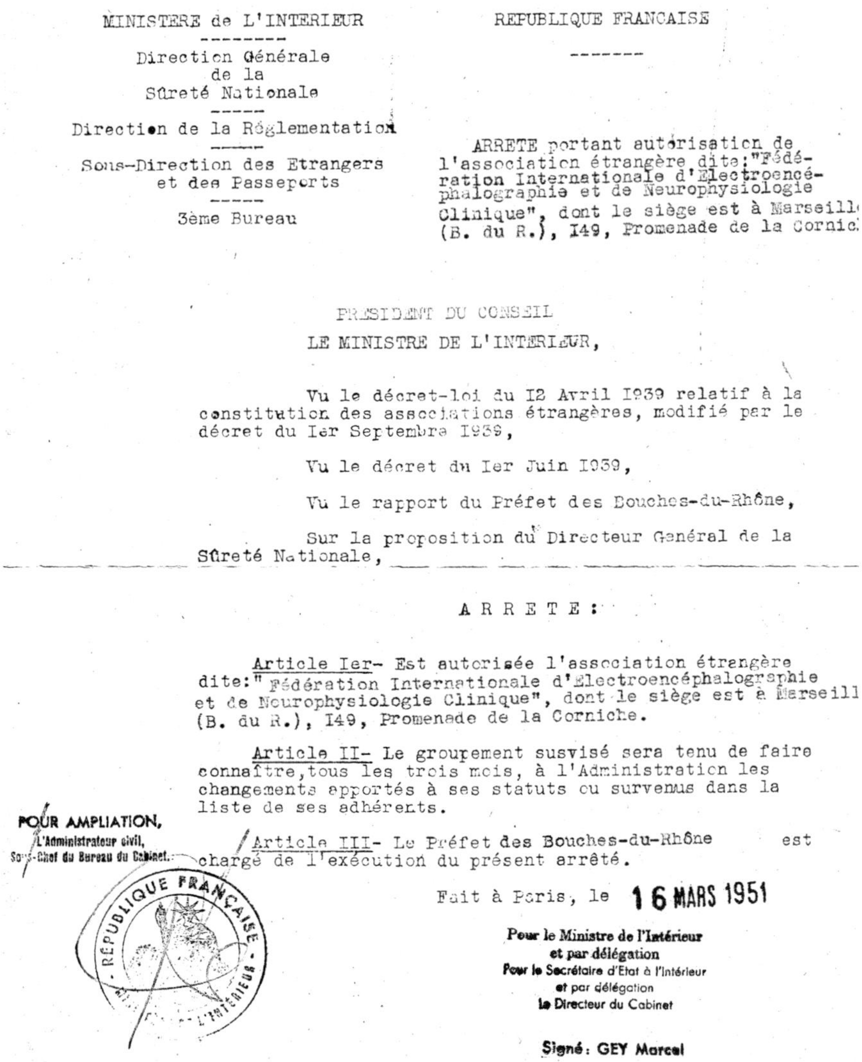

MINISTERE de L'INTERIEUR

Direction Générale
de la
Sûreté Nationale

Direction de la Réglementation

Sous-Direction des Etrangers
et des Passeports

3ème Bureau

REPUBLIQUE FRANCAISE

ARRETE portant autorisation de l'association étrangère dite:"Fédération Internationale d'Electroencéphalographie et de Neurophysiologie Clinique", dont le siège est à Marseill (B. du R.), I49, Promenade de la Cornic

PRESIDENT DU CONSEIL
LE MINISTRE DE L'INTERIEUR,

Vu le décret-loi du I2 Avril I939 relatif à la constitution des associations étrangères, modifié par le décret du Ier Septembre I939,

Vu le décret du Ier Juin I939,

Vu le rapport du Préfet des Bouches-du-Rhône,

Sur la proposition du Directeur Général de la Sûreté Nationale,

A R R E T E :

Article Ier- Est autorisée l'association étrangère dite:" Fédération Internationale d'Electroencéphalographie et de Neurophysiologie Clinique", dont le siège est à Marseill (B. du R.), I49, Promenade de la Corniche.

Article II- Le groupement susvisé sera tenu de faire connaître, tous les trois mois, à l'Administration les changements apportés à ses statuts ou survenus dans la liste de ses adhérents.

Article III- Le Préfet des Bouches-du-Rhône est chargé de l'exécution du présent arrêté.

Fait à Paris, le 16 MARS 1951

POUR AMPLIATION,
L'Administrateur civil,
Sous-Chef du Bureau du Cabinet.

RÉPUBLIQUE FRANÇAISE
... L'INTÉRIEUR

Pour le Ministre de l'Intérieur
et par délégation
Pour le Secrétaire d'Etat à l'Intérieur
et par délégation
Le Directeur du Cabinet

Signé: GEY Marcel

Fig. 25.1. French registration documentation for the Fédération Internationale d'Electroencéphalographie et de Neurophysiologie Clinique.

Industry Canada   Industrie Canada

Canada
Corporations Act

Loi sur les
corporations canadiennes

C A N A D A

LETTERS PATENT

WHEREAS an application has been filed to incorporate a corporation under the name

International Federation of Clinical Neurophysiology
Fédération Internationale de Neurophysiologie Clinique

THEREFORE the Minister of Industry by virtue of the powers vested in him by the *Canada Corporations Act*, constitutes the applicants and such persons as may hereafter become members in the corporation hereby created, a body corporate and politic in accordance with the provisions of the said Act. A copy of the said application is attached hereto and forms part hereof.

Date of Letters Patent - May 10, 2005

GIVEN under the seal of office of the Minister of Industry.

for the Minister of Industry

File Number: 430120-0

Canadä

Fig. 25.2. Canadian incorporation document for the International Federation of Clinical Neurophysiology, Fédération Internationale de Neurophysiologie Clinique.

On May 10, 2005, the Federation was incorporated in Canada. Figure 25.2 is the official incorporation document from that governmental action by the Ministry of Industry. The two official names are International Federation of Clinical Neurophysiology and Fédération Internationale de Neurophysiologie Clinique. In 2006 the General Assembly authorized closing the French Registered Charity.

Wave Length and Action Potentials: History of the IFCN
(Supplements to Clinical Neurophysiology, Vol. 61)
By: M.R. Nuwer and C.H. Lücking

Appendix 10

Federation Statutes and Bye-Laws

The International Federation of Clinical Neurophysiology (IFCN) is governed by several enabling documents. These now are commonly referred to as the Statutes and Bye-Laws.

The Statutes are the primary organizational rules that govern the Federation. They are the principal document filed with the Canadian Ministry of Industry. They contain the major rules for overall conduct of Federation business as well as statements of its mission.

The Bye-Laws are subsidiary organizational rules that govern portions of the Federation. There are six sets of Bye-Laws:

- Bye-Laws of the IFCN
- Bye-Laws of the European Chapter
- Bye-Laws of the Latin American Chapter
- Bye-Laws of the Asian and Oceanian Chapter
- Bye-Laws of the North American Chapter
- Bye-Laws of the International Clinical Neurophysiology Society (ICNS)

These are considered Bye-Laws of the Federation even though some are labeled as Statutes of the individual chapter organization.

Under Canadian Law, the actual official names of these documents are different. The legal name of the Federation's Statutes is the "Bye-Laws", since in Canada a Statute refers to an Act of Parliament. The Federation's six sets of Bye-Laws are the "Rules and Regulations", in keeping with the standard terminology in use legally in Canada. Nevertheless, it remains allowable for the Federation to continue to refer to its own documents internally by their traditional and familiar names as the Statutes and Bye-Laws. That is how they are presented here. Together the collection of Statutes and Bye-Laws sometimes is referred to as the Constitution.

The original 1949 Constitution is printed in *Electroencephalography and Clinical Neurophysiology*, 1951, 3: 517–522. A series of changes and additions were made in new Bye-Laws over the next three decades. The revised full Constitution was printed in *Electroencephalography and Clinical Neurophysiology,* 1978, 45: 151–171. With a few further small changes, it also is printed in Recommendation for the 1983 book, *Practice of Clinical Neurophysiology*, pages 151–191.

Following that, a series of changes were made in the subsequent two decades, culminating in a complete reformatting at the time of Canadian incorporation. The primary goal then was not to change the rules but rather to reformat them. At that time, some items were moved from the Bye-Laws into the Statutes, and vice versa. The logo was added, as was an item about indemnification and legal protection.

The rules are voted upon by the General Assembly on recommendations brought to them by the Rules Committee. For the most part the rules below are as approved through the 2006 General Assembly meeting.

The official rules are bilingual or multilingual. The official Statutes and Bye-Laws are in both English and French. The Latin American Chapter Bye-Laws also are in Portuguese. Only the English version is printed below because of printed page space considerations.

A full copy of the current Statutes and Bye-Laws is printed below. The reader should recall that these are a living set of rules that do change over time. Before the ink is dry on these pages, some changes may have been made.

Statutes of the International Federation of Clinical Neurophysiology

The following shall constitute the Bye-Laws of the INTERNATIONAL FEDERATION OF CLINICAL NEUROPHYSIOLOGY (the "Federation") which have been drafted, to the extent possible, in a manner consistent with the Statutes of the predecessor Federation formed under French law and shall be referred to herein and in the conduct of the business of the Federation as the "Statutes".

In order to provide for terminology consistent with that employed by the predecessor Federation, thereby providing for greater continuity in the operations of the Federation, the rules and regulations contemplated under Article 13.1 of these Statutes shall be referred to herein and in the conduct of the business of the Federation as the "Operational Bye-Laws".

The official languages of the Federation shall be English, French and Spanish and the translation of these Statutes from one language to the other shall be organized as much as possible to give, if not the whole text, at least a summary. The English text of these Statutes is authoritative. All official communications of the Federation shall be conducted in English.

1. Mission and objects

1.1. Main object

The mission of the Federation is to strive, in all countries, to promote education and the attainment of the highest level of knowledge and understanding in the field of clinical neurophysiology in so far as such activities shall be of a wholly non-profit making nature. (The term "clinical neurophysiology" shall not be interpreted in a restrictive sense.)

1.2. Intended goals

To that end but without restricting the foregoing main object of the Federation, and in so far as the same shall be wholly charitable, the Federation intends:

(a) To foster and encourage scientific research, investigation and demonstration in the field of clinical neurophysiology;
(b) To improve the quality of instruction in the professions dealing with these sciences;
(c) To supply information to, to cooperate with and to advise, through its committees, any society, institution or individual interested in these problems;
(d) To propose guidelines for the practice of clinical neurophysiology and to give advice concerning criteria for methods, techniques and for the interpretation of results; and
(e) To establish and maintain an efficient collaboration with international and national learned societies, governmental organizations, professional associations and other groups, societies, institutions and individuals who contribute to progress in the field of clinical neurophysiology.

1.3. Stated means

The means of attaining these ends shall consist more particularly in:

(a) Organizing international congresses and chapter and regional meetings of clinical neurophysiology to be held in one of the countries represented in the membership of the Federation;
(b) Appointing special committees, commissions, groups or individuals for the purpose of studying all problems related to the aims of the Federation;
(c) Fostering and facilitating, in all countries, the proper methods of study and promote meeting and exchange of ideas concerning progress attained in clinical neurophysiology;

(d) Printing and publishing, and controlling the printing and publishing, of a journal, book, or reprint, and using all other ways of disseminating information. In particular, publishing, in conjunction with such publishing house with which the contract is for the time being in force, the international journal "Clinical Neurophysiology" (the "Journal"). Appointing the officers of the same and determining through them the policies of the Journal;
(e) Making known its activities as well as those of congresses and chapter or regional meetings, and those of its committees, by all appropriate means and, in particular, through the medium of the Journal and the Federation website; and
(f) Collaborating with the United Nations Educational, Scientific and Cultural Organization, and with other institutions insofar as they endeavor to improve human health in the field of normal and pathological physiology of the nervous system, including the World Health Organization.

2. Membership

2.1. Member societies

The Federation is a corporation without share capital incorporated under Part II of the *Canada Corporations Act* composed of member societies of clinical neurophysiology and related neurological sciences, whose names appear on Appendix "A" to these Statutes or whose application for membership shall have been accepted by a majority vote of the General Assembly as specified in Article 6.5 below. Only members of such societies may hold office or serve on committees or commissions of the Federation.

Application for membership must be made in writing to the President and be accompanied by a list of current officers and members of the applying society with a copy of its constitution.

2.2. Right of withdrawal

Any member society may withdraw from the Federation by delivery to the Federation of a written resignation to the Secretariat of the Federation.

2.3. Removal

Any member society may be required, on a reasoned proposal of the Executive Committee (ExCo), to resign by a vote of three-quarters of the General Assembly, provided that a member of such society shall be granted an opportunity to be heard at a meeting of the General Assembly.

2.4. Annual dues

Each member society shall pay annual dues. The amount shall be determined by the General Assembly and the dues of each member society shall be in proportion to the number of its members. Payment shall be made in advance on the first day of January of each year. Failure of a member society to pay its annual dues within 1 year following the date on which they are due, shall result in the suspension of the right of that society to vote in the General Assembly or in the election of IFCN Directors, until such payment has been made.

2.5. Honorary fellows and other non-voting members

Any person who has rendered important services to the Federation may be appointed an Honorary Fellow of the Federation by a two-thirds (2/3) majority of the General Assembly. All Past-Presidents of the Federation other than the immediate Past-President, who continues to serve as a member of the Executive Committee, are Honorary Past-Presidents of the Federation. All Honorary Fellows and Honorary Past-Presidents hold such title for life and are entitled to attend all congresses without paying registration fees and attend meetings of the General Assembly; however, they are not entitled to vote thereat.

3. Corporate seal

3.1. Form of seal

The seal, an impression of which is stamped in the box below, shall be the seal of the Federation:

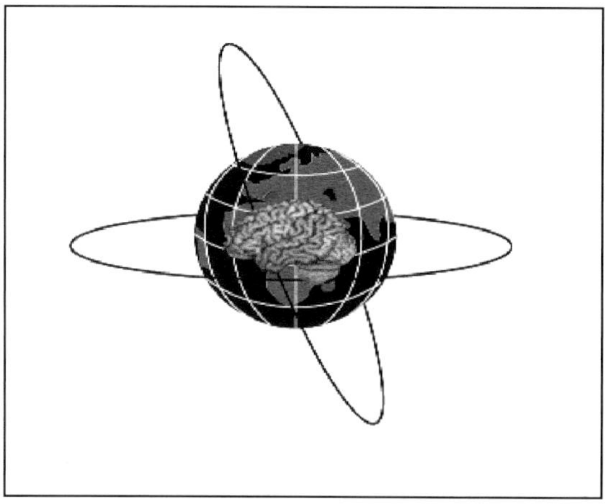

4. Head office

4.1. Head office

The head office of the Federation shall be in the City of Vancouver in the Province of British Columbia which shall serve as the office of record for acceptance of all correspondence contemplated under Part II of the Canada Corporations Act and other applicable legislation. The head administrative office of the Federation shall be the office of the Secretariat of the Federation as determined by the Executive Committee (as defined below) from time to time.

5. Executive Committee

5.1. Powers and composition

The property and business of the Federation shall be managed and administered by an executive committee (the "Executive Committee") composed of the President, the immediate Past-President, the Secretary and the Treasurer of the Federation, the Editor(s)-in-Chief of the Journal, and two additional Members-at-Large. Included in the powers of the Executive Committee is the responsibility to act as the executive board of the Journal with full power to appoint and remove all members of the Journal's editorial staff.

5.2. Directors

Each member of the Executive Committee is also a director of the Federation.

5.3. First directors and Executive Committee

The applicants for incorporation named below shall become the first directors of the Federation, holding the following offices until their successors are duly elected or appointment in accordance with these Statutes:

Name	*Office*
François Mauguière	President
Marc R. Nuwer	Past-President
Andrew Eisen	Treasurer
Graham F.A. Harding	Secretary
Mark Hallett	Editor-in-Chief
Johannes Noth	Member-at-Large
Ryuji Kaji	Member-at-Large

5.4. Term

The term of office of all subsequent Executive Committees shall be one Fiscal Period (as defined below).

5.5. Limitation on term of office

The President, Secretary, and Members-at-Large may serve only one term in office. The Treasurer is eligible for re-election once only. The term of office of the Editor(s)-in-Chief of the Journal shall not extend more than 2 years into the next Fiscal Period following the Fiscal Period in which he/she was appointed by the Executive Committee. Each Editor-in-Chief's total term of office, including reappointments, cannot exceed 8 years. No person shall serve as an elected or appointed member of the Executive Committee for more than 12 years total, except that a person who has served already for 8 years would be allowed to run for President and, if elected, serve for 4 years as President and a further 4 years as Past-President.

5.6. Election and appointment process

(a) The President, Secretary, Treasurer, and the Members-at-Large are elected by the member societies in accordance with the following process:
   (i) Not less than 1 year before the end of the Fiscal Period, the Executive Committee shall elect three delegates to serve as a nomination committee under the chairmanship of the Past-President (the "Nomination Committee").
   (ii) The Nomination Committee shall invite nominations from the member societies for the offices of President, Secretary, Treasurer, and the Members-at-Large to hold office for the following Fiscal Period. Having ascertained the willingness of the candidates to serve, the Past-President, as chairman of the Nomination Committee shall submit their names to a ballot vote of the member societies, and inform the Secretary of the result of the ballot. Each member society has the same number of votes to which it is entitled in the General Assembly. The ballot is to be sent to the Delegate (as defined below) of the member society who is responsible for returning the ballot by the specified date.
   (iii) In establishing the slate of candidates for election, the Nomination Committee shall adhere to the following guidelines to ensure geographical and disciplinary balance in the composition of the Executive Committee:

      Geographical areas are (1) North and South America, Australasia and Japan and (2) Europe, Asia (except Japan) and Africa. At the time of their nomination, nominees should be given a disciplinary designation of electroencephalographer or electromyographer by the nominating society. The designation should be justified on the basis of practice or research. The Nominating Committee should approve the designation. If the designation is disapproved, the decision may be appealed to the Executive Committee whose decision is final. The disciplinary designation cannot be changed during a voting cycle. Even if a society is not eligible to vote, it may still nominate persons for any position, and its members remain eligible for nomination. The President and Past-President should preferably be from different geographical regions, and cannot be from the same geographical region in more than two consecutive elections. The Secretary and Treasurer should be from different geographical regions. The two Members-at-Large should be from different geographical regions and from countries different from that of the President, Past-President, Treasurer and Secretary. Concerning disciplinary balance, the Executive Committee shall at all times be comprised of no more than five representations from one discipline.
   (iv) Voting for members of the Executive Committee should occur in the following sequence: first round, President and Treasurer; second round, Secretary; third round, Members at Large. For each round of voting, voting should be by written ballot only (post or fax is permitted) and adherence to the deadline is mandatory. To declare an election valid, ballots must be received from at least 50% of the member societies eligible to vote. The deadline can be extended to achieve a quorum. Extension is limited to the

time when the quorum is achieved. To win an election, an absolute majority of the votes cast is required; and a run-off election between the top two candidates should be held if necessary. If a society ineligible to vote becomes eligible during an election, it may initiate participating in the voting when the next round of the election begins.

(v) The members of the Nomination Committee or the Executive Committee should not promote a particular candidate for any office. The Nomination Committee should report to the Executive Committee after each step of the election process. The report must include the number of votes for each candidate.

(b) The Editor(s)-in-Chief of the Journal are appointed by the Executive Committee. The Editor(s)-in-Chief cannot vote on their own reappointment, tenure or termination of appointment and may not be present at meetings of the Executive Committee when any such matter is discussed or put to a vote.

5.7. Vacancy

The office of any director and member on the Executive Committee shall be automatically vacated:

(a) if that director shall resign his office on the Executive Committee by delivery of a written resignation to the Secretary of the Federation, and in the case of a resigning Secretary to the President;
(b) if he/she is found by a court of competent jurisdiction to be of unsound mind;
(c) if he/she is convicted by a court of competent jurisdiction of a serious crime;
(d) if he/she becomes bankrupt; or
(e) upon death.

If a vacancy on the Executive Committee shall occur for any of the above reasons, the office may be filled by a qualified candidate appointed by the Executive Committee except that the office of President shall be immediately assumed by the immediate Past-President.

5.8. Conduct of meetings

The Executive Committee may hold meetings at any time and in any place which may be convenient to its members and may conduct its business by postal ballot or any other means of communication.

5.9. Remuneration

The members of the Executive Committee shall serve as such without remuneration and no member shall directly or indirectly receive any profit from his position as such, provided that a member of the Executive Committee may be paid reasonable expenses incurred by him in the performance of his duties.

5.10. Exoneration of liability vis-à-vis the Federation and third parties

Except as otherwise provided in the Act or in the Statutes of the Federation, no director or officer, commissioner or other person appointed to serve on behalf of the Federation, acting or having acted for or in the name of the Federation shall be held liable, in this capacity or in his capacity as agent of the Federation, whether it be vis-à-vis the Federation or third parties, for the acts, conduct, things done or allowed to be done, omissions, decisions made or not made, liabilities, undertakings, payment made, receipts given or discharges granted, negligence or the faults of any other director, officer, employee, clerk or representative of the Federation. Among other things, no director or officer shall be held liable vis-à-vis the Federation for any direct or indirect loss suffered by the latter for any reason whatsoever; in particular, he shall not be held liable either for the insufficiency or the deficiency of title to any property acquired by the Federation, or for or on its behalf, or for the insufficiency or the deficiency of any security or debt instrument in or by which any of the funds or of the assets of the Federation shall be or have been placed or invested or for any loss or damage resulting from the bankruptcy, the insolvency or the delictual act of any person, including any person with whom or with which funds, shares, assets or negotiable instruments shall be or have been placed or deposited. Furthermore, the directors or the officers shall not be held liable vis-à-vis the Federation for any loss or embezzlement, misappropriation or any other damage resulting from any dealings with respect to any funds, assets or shares or for any other loss, damage or misfortune whatsoever which may occur in the discharge of, or in relation to the discharge of, their duties unless the same shall occur owing to their failure to discharge the duties of their office prudently, diligently, honestly and faithfully in the best interests of the Federation or owing to the fact that the directors or the officers shall have placed themselves in a position of conflict of interest between their personal interest and that of the Federation. None of the above shall be interpreted in such a way as to relieve a director or an officer of his duty to act in accordance with the Act and its Regulations or of his joint and several liability for any breach thereof, in particular in the event of a breach of the specific provisions of the Act or its Regulations. Moreover, the directors or the officers shall not be held individually or personally liable vis-à-vis third parties during their term of office in respect of a contract, a decision made, an undertaking or a transaction, whether or not concluded, or with respect to bills of exchange, to promissory notes or to checks drawn, accepted or endorsed, to the extent that they are acting or they acted in the name, or on behalf, of the Federation, in the ordinary course of the performance of the powers which they have received, unless they acted prior to the incorporation of the Federation and unless their acts have not been ratified by the Federation after its incorporation within the time limit prescribed by the Act.

5.11. Right to compensation

The Federation shall compensate its directors, officers or its representatives in respect of all costs or expenses reasonably incurred by them in connection with the defense of an action, of a suit, or a petition, of a proceeding of a civil, of a criminal or of an administrative nature or of any other legal proceeding to which one or more of them were parties by reason of their duties or of their office, whether this action, this suit, this petition or this legal proceeding was instituted by or on behalf of the Federation or by a third party. Reasonable costs or expenses shall include, in particular, all damages or fines arising from the acts done by the directors, by the officers or by the representatives in the discharge of their duties as well as all amounts paid to settle an action or to satisfy a judgment. The right to compensation shall exist only to the extent that the directors, the officers or the representatives were substantially successful on the merits in their defense of the action, of the suit, of the petition or of the legal proceeding, that they acted prudently, diligently, honestly and faithfully in the best interests of the Federation, that they did not place themselves in a position of conflict of interest between their personal interest and that of the Federation, and, in the case of an action, of a suit, of a petition or of a proceeding of a criminal or of an administrative nature leading to the imposition of a fine, to the extent that they had reasonable grounds for believing that their conduct was lawful or to the extent that they were acquitted or freed. The Federation shall assume these liabilities in respect of any person who acts or acted at its request as a director, as an officer or as a representative of a body corporate of which the Federation is or was a member or a creditor. If such be the case, this compensation shall be paid to the heirs, legatees, liquidators, transferees, agents, legal representatives, successors, assigns or rightful claimants of the directors, of the officers or of the representatives, in accordance with the following.

5.12. Legal action by third party

Where an action, a suit, a petition, a proceeding of a civil, criminal or administrative nature or any other legal proceeding is instituted by a third party against one or more of the directors, officers or representatives of the Federation for one or more acts done in carrying out their duties, the Federation shall assume the defense of its agent.

5.13. Legal action by the Federation

Where an action, a suit, a petition, a proceeding of a civil, criminal or administrative nature or any other legal proceeding is instituted by the Federation against one or more of its directors, officers or representatives for one or more acts done in carrying out their duties, the Federation may pay compensation to the directors, officers or representatives if it loses its case and is a court of law or a tribunal so orders. If the Federation only wins its case in part, the court of law or the tribunal may determine the amount of the costs or of the expenses which the Federation shall assume.

5.14. Liability insurance

The Federation may purchase and maintain for the benefit of its directors, officers, representatives, of their predecessors as well as of their heirs, legatees, liquidators, transferees, agents, legal representatives, successors, assigns or rightful claimants insurance covering any liability incurred by them by reason of their acting or having acted as a director, officer or representative of the Federation or, at the request of the latter, of a body corporate of which the Federation is or was a member or a creditor. However, this insurance shall not cover the liability arising from the failure of the insured to act prudently, honestly and faithfully in the best interests of the Federation, nor the liability arising from a fault or from a personal offence severable from the discharge of their duties nor the liability arising from the fact that the insured shall have placed themselves in a position of conflict of interest between their personal interest and that of the Federation.

5.15. Compensation after end of term of office

The Compensation provided for in the preceding paragraphs may be obtained even after the person has ceased to hold the office of director, officer or representative of the Federation or, if such be the case, of a body corporate of which the Federation is or was a member or a creditor. In the event of death, the compensation may be paid to the heirs, legatees, liquidators, transferees, agents, legal representatives, successors, assigns or rightful claimants of such person. Such compensation may also be combined with any other recourse which the director, officer or representative, one of his predecessors as well as his heirs, legatees, liquidators, transferees, agents, legal representatives, successors, assigns or rightful claimants may have.

5.16. Determination of conditions prior to compensation

In the event that a court of law or a tribunal has not made a finding on the matter, the compliance or the non-compliance of the conduct of a director, officer or representatives with the standards of conduct set out in paragraph 5.11 above, or the question of whether a case was won in part of whether a person was substantially successful on the merits in his defense of the action, of the suit, of the petition or of the legal proceeding shall be determined in the following manner: (a) by a simple majority vote of the directors who are not parties to such action, suit, petition or legal proceeding, if a quorum exists; or (b) by way of opinion from an independent legal counsel if such a quorum of the directors cannot be attained, or, even if attained, if a quorum of the directors who are not parties to such action, suit, petition or legal proceedings so decides; or, failing the above, (c) by decision of the simple majority of the members of the Federation.

5.17. Place of action

The powers and the duties of the Federation with respect to the compensation of any director, officer or representatives shall apply regardless of the place where the action, the suit, the petition or the legal proceedings shall have been instituted.

6. The General Assembly

6.1. Composition

The General Assembly is composed of the Executive Committee and the delegates and additional representatives of each member society, or their specified alternates. Each member society has one delegate that is the principal person serving as a liaison between the Federation and the member society. The number of additional representatives of each member society who are eligible to sit in the General Assembly corresponds to the number of dues-paying members of that society as follows:

1–99 members = 1 additional representative
100–399 = 2 additional representatives
400 or more = 3 additional representatives

Each delegate is appointed by his member society to represent his society and to be the point of communication with the Federation. In the absence of a delegate from a meeting of the General Assembly an alternate shall be appointed by the member society for the duration of the meeting of the General Assembly. The names of its current delegates or, if required, its alternates shall be forwarded by each member society to the Secretary and the Secretary shall at all times maintain a list of all current delegates and alternates. In addition, the names of additional representatives shall be notified to the Secretary prior to a meeting of the General Assembly.

6.2. Frequency of meeting

The General Assembly is bound to meet at the place and date fixed for the session of the Congress.

6.3. Business of General Assembly

The General Assembly shall:
(a) propose the place and date of the next International Congress of Clinical Neurophysiology (the "Congress");
(b) vote on the proposals for memberships of the Federation submitted to it by the Executive Committee;
(c) vote on the budget for the following Fiscal Period proposed and presented by the Executive Committee; and
(d) vote upon all other resolutions relating to the fulfillment of the purposes of the Federation placed before it by the Executive Committee.

6.4. Those entitled to vote

All persons registered at the Congress may attend the General Assembly, but only members of the Executive Committee and delegates, alternates and additional representatives whose names appear on the list maintained by the Secretary (each a member of the General Assembly) may speak and vote at the General Assembly. Exceptionally, the chairman of the General Assembly (normally the President, or in his absence the Past-President of the Federation), with the approval of the General Assembly, may invite persons other than members of the General Assembly to speak.

6.5. Required vote

Each member of the General Assembly has one vote. In all cases a simple majority (50% plus one vote) is required except:
(a) a two-thirds (2/3) majority is required for the election of an Honorary Fellow (as defined above), for the amalgamation or dissolution of the Federation and for the amendment of these Statutes; and
(b) a three-quarters (3/4) majority is required for the expulsion of a member society from membership in the Federation.

In all cases the requisite majority is of those voting either in person or by ballot.

6.6. Tie-vote

A tie-vote on a simple (for/against) motion is lost. In the case of a tie-vote concerning a choice between courses of action or between candidates, the Chairman of the General Assembly has the deciding vote, whether or not he has already voted.

6.7. Quorum

A quorum of the General Assembly is one delegate of each of one-third (1/3) of the member societies together with the President and two other members of the Executive Committee. The Chairman of the General Assembly shall be the President. The Secretary of the General Assembly shall, if present, be the Secretary, otherwise shall be such other member of the Executive Committee as appointed by the President.

7. Organization of congress

7.1. Establishment of organizing committee

The organization and conduct of the Congress approximately every 4 years is vital to the operation and advancement of the objectives of the Federation. Not less than 3 years before the end of the current Fiscal Period an organizing committee (the "OCIC") shall be established for the purpose of organizing all aspects of the next congress.

7.2. Composition of the OCIC

The Organizing Committee of the International Congress (OCIC) shall be comprised of the President, Past-President, Secretary, Treasurer, one Editor-in-Chief, and four appointees of the member society in charge of the Congress as chosen at the last General Assembly. The President shall be the Chairman of the OCIC and the appointees of the member society shall act as Convener, Secretary, Treasurer of the OCIC, and the Scientific Program Committee Chairperson.

7.3. Delegation

The OCIC may establish sub-committees to conduct the different affairs of the Congress and the other persons may be co-opted as members of the OCIC.

7.4. Honorary President

Not less than 2 years before the end of the current Fiscal Period the member society in charge of the Congress shall recommend an Honorary President(s) of the Congress to the OCIC.

8. Financial year end and annual proceedings

8.1. Financial year and annual proceedings

The financial year end of the Federation shall be December 31. Within 6 months of the most recently completed financial year end the Treasurer shall, through the Secretariat, mail the following to all member societies:

(a) audited financial statements for the most recently completed financial year, with the auditor's report thereon; and
(b) a disapproval form which may be completed by any member society, disapproving of the audited financial statements; the appointment of the auditor of the Federation for the ensuing financial year, or both. A completed disapproval form is to be sent to the Secretariat Federation no later than 8 months following the most recently completed financial year.

8.2.1. Disapprovals
In the event that the Secretariat receives disapproval forms from member societies representing more than 50% of the eligible vote, the Executive Committee shall immediately call a meeting to be conducted by ballot vote for the purpose of: (i) approving the financial statements for the most recently completed financial period, and

(ii) appointing the auditors of the Federation for the ensuing financial year.

8.2.2. Finance matters
The Executive Committee determines all matters of finance such as the site of the Treasury and the making of grants and loans, except that the amounts of dues levied on the Member Society are determined by the General Assembly.

9. Fiscal period

For the purposes of these Statutes, the Fiscal Period shall mean the period commencing at the end of one congress and ending at the completion of the next congress, normally 4 years. In no case shall a Fiscal Period of the Federation exceed 6 years.

10. The minutes of Executive Committees

The minutes of the Executive Committee shall not be available to the general membership of the Federation but shall be available to the members of the Executive Committee, each of whom shall receive a copy of such minutes.

11. Amendment of Statutes

The Statutes of the Federation not embodied in the Letters Patent may be replaced or amended by a Bye-Law enacted by a majority of the Executive Committee and sanctioned by the affirmative vote of at least two-thirds (2/3) of the members of the General Assembly, provided that the repeal or amendment of such Statutes shall not be enforced or acted upon until the approval of the Minister of Industry has been obtained.

12. Books and records

The Secretary shall see to it that all necessary books and records of the Federation required by the Statutes of the Federation or by any applicable statute or law are regularly and properly kept.

13. Operational Bye-Laws

13.1. Rules and regulations

The Executive Committee may, on its own or upon the recommendation of the Rules Committee, propose such rules and regulations, to be termed "Operational Bye-Laws", not inconsistent with these Statutes relating to the management and operation of the Federation as they deem expedient, provided that such Operational Bye-Laws shall not have force and effect until approved by the General Assembly.

14. Committees

14.1. Rules Committee

At the beginning of the "Fiscal Period" a Rules Committee of five members shall be set up by the Executive Committee. The Rules Committee shall constantly review the Statutes and any other Bye-Laws of the Federation and make recommendations, if necessary, for their amendment to the Executive Committee. Questions regarding the interpretation of existing Statutes and Bye-Laws may be referred to the Rules Committee by the President, and its decisions shall be final.

14.2. Special committees

Special committees may be appointed by the President of the Federation and ratified by the Executive Committee. A Special Committee may act through representatives duly appointed.

15. Special commissions

On recommendations of the Executive Committee, with the approval of the General Assembly, special commissions may be set up, each to represent a special branch of Neurophysiology. Each special commission shall be composed of three members, one of whom shall be designated

Chairman; they will be proposed by the Nomination Committee and elected by the member societies similarly to the members of the Executive Committee. The Chairman will be a member of the Executive Committee and will advise it of the interest of his specialty. The members will be members of the General Assembly. The President may delegate tasks, such as the organization of specialized meetings, to the appropriate special commissions.

16. Chapters

On recommendation of the Executive Committee and the approval of the General Assembly, Chapters may be set up, each to represent the member societies located in a particular region. Each Chapter is governed by its own Bye-Laws. Those Bye-Laws are considered to be Bye-Laws of the Federation. These Bye-Laws must be compatible with these Statutes, reviewed by the Executive Committee and approved by the General Assembly. The Federation Rules Committee serves as the Rules Committee of each Chapter.

17. Interpretation

In these Statutes and in all other Bye-Laws of the Federation hereafter passed, unless the context otherwise requires, words importing the singular number or the masculine gender shall include the plural number or the feminine gender, as the case may be, and vice versa, and references to persons shall include firms and corporations.

18. Dissolution or amalgamation

As specifically provided for in the Federation's Application for Incorporation:

(a) The Federation may be dissolved or may amalgamate with another body having similar objectives, on the proposal of the Executive Committee, ratified by a two-thirds (2/3) majority vote of the General Assembly.

(b) In the event of its dissolution the assets of the Federation may not be divided among its members and shall be transferred to another international body, or bodies, of like interests, agreed to by the General Assembly.

International Federation of Clinical Neurophysiology Bye-Laws

1. General policies

The Secretary should keep a book containing the current Bye-Laws and in which all such modifications are entered as they are made. The Bye-Laws may conveniently be grouped under the titles of the topics to which they refer, and in relation to the Statutes to which they are addenda.

1.1. Member societies

1.1.1. (Statutes 2.1)
Any national society for the study of a branch of clinical neurophysiology and its related sciences may apply for membership, but the Federation will give preference to those societies which encompass all branches of clinical neurophysiology. A society can be formed by three members (President, Secretary and Treasurer), but a minimum of 10 members is required to apply for IFCN affiliation and to maintain membership once approved. In the event of application being made by a society from a country in which there is already a member society of the Federation, the Executive Committee shall discuss with the societies concerned the possibility of their amalgamation. If this should prove impossible the Federation may accept the application from the second society, provided that its main sphere of interest differs from that of the first. Not more than two national societies from any country can simultaneously be members of the Federation.

Societies which exclude suitably qualified non-medical scientists from full voting membership shall be urged to make their inclusion possible in consideration of their contributions to clinical neurophysiology.

If a professional is excluded from membership in a national society, that society may officially support such excluded persons for ICNS membership.

1.2. Executive Committee

1.2.1. Conduct of meetings (Statutes 5.8)
The meetings must be convened by the President who, however, is not compelled to be present. Those who cannot attend may express their views by letter or other available methods. At the meeting the opportunity may be taken, at the discretion of the President or, in his absence, of the Chairman of the meeting, of hearing the views of persons who are not members of the Executive Committee, although such persons are not entitled to vote.

1.2.2. No person may hold, at one time, more than one office by virtue of which he is a member of the Executive Committee.

1.3. Delegates

1.3.1. Each Delegate is appointed by his member society to serve continuously during the Fiscal Period of the Federation.

1.3.2. The appointment of the Delegate for the new Fiscal Period must be made by each member society prior to the International Congress of Clinical Neurophysiology and his name given to the Secretary of the Federation before the Congress. The responsibilities of the new Delegate commence with the beginning of the new Fiscal Period.

Should any member society not give the name of a new or re-appointed Delegate, the Delegate for the previous Fiscal Period shall be the responsible Delegate for that society. The member society will be so informed by the Secretary of the Federation.

1.3.3. In case of appointment by a member society of a new Delegate during the Fiscal Period, the name of this Delegate must be immediately forwarded to the Secretary of the Federation.

1.3.4. In the event of a Delegate being unable to attend a meeting of the General Assembly, an alternate to attend may be appointed by the member society for the duration of the meeting only. The name of this alternate shall be submitted in writing to the Secretary of the Federation prior to the meeting.

1.3.5. One Delegate or alternate may represent only one member society at any one time, and may not be a member of the Executive Committee.

1.3.6. No person may hold, at any one time, more than one office by virtue of which he is a member of the General Assembly.

1.4. Special commissions

1.4.1. (Statutes 15.1)
The Executive Committee for any reasons which it deems sufficient, may propose to the General Assembly that a Special Commission be discontinued. The General Assembly shall be informed of the reasons for and against the action. If the proposal receives the assent of a two-thirds majority of the General Assembly, the Commission shall be discontinued at the end of the Fiscal Period in which General Assembly action is taken unless an earlier date is specified.

1.4.2. Commissions shall have powers of co-option by majority vote but co-opted members shall have no voting rights.

1.5. Committees

1.5.1. Rules Committee (Statutes 14.1)
The Rules Committee can be terminated only by the Fiscal Period but the Executive Committee shall fill vacancies in its composition as they arise and, at the beginning of a new Fiscal Period, must reconstitute the Committee with the same or altered membership.

1.5.2. Special Committees (Statutes 14.2)

The composition of a Special Committee set up by the President is determined by him, and he nominates a Chairman and, if necessary, a Secretary; these appointments must be notified to the Executive Committee, whose assent is assumed in the absence of any counter-proposal within reasonable time, allowing for postal delays. Such a Committee may be disbanded whenever the President is satisfied that it has completed its task, normally when it has made a definitive report. When it is terminated by the end of a Fiscal Period the new President may reconstitute it immediately or later, with the same or altered membership and terms of reference.

Special Committees, with the exception of the Rules Committee, shall have powers of co-option by majority vote but co-opted members shall have no voting rights.

2. General Assembly

2.1. Officers

These shall be the Chairman, the Secretary and the Procedural Counselor.

2.1.1. THE CHAIRMAN of the Assembly shall be the President of the Federation. In the absence of the President the immediate Past-President shall act as the Chairman. In the absence of both, the Chairman must be appointed by agreement between those members of the Executive Committee present.

2.1.2. THE SECRETARY shall be the Secretary of the Federation. In the absence of the Secretary an alternate must be appointed by agreement between those members of the Executive Committee present.

2.1.3. THE PROCEDURAL COUNSELOR shall be appointed by the Executive Committee prior to the meeting of the General Assembly. He shall normally be a member of the Rules Committee but not of the Executive Committee.

2.1.4. Other members of the Executive Committee will not be officers of the General Assembly. They may vote as members of the General Assembly.

2.2. The duties of the officers

2.2.1. The chairman

The Chairman shall officially open and close the General Assembly. He shall direct discussion, decide right and order of speaking, advice regarding the form of motions, rule on points of order and limit the length of discussion or the number of times a discussant speaks.

He shall pronounce or cause to be pronounced to the General Assembly the final form of any motion or amendment.

He shall be responsible for maintaining audibility of proceedings and of keeping order in the General Assembly.

The Chairman, as President of the Federation, shall present his report to the General Assembly.

The Chairman may propose deferments and amendments on his own initiative. He shall reintroduce deferred motions at the appropriate time in the General Assembly. The Chairman may vote if he so wishes.

2.2.2. The secretary

The Secretary shall be responsible for notifying all Delegates of the proposed date, time and place of the General Assembly, at least 1 month before the Congress. He shall also be responsible at the beginning of the Congress for displaying visually and notifying verbally to the members the exact date, time and assembly hall of the General Assembly.

The Secretary shall draw up the Agenda and be responsible for its presentation to the members of the General Assembly. He shall record the motions, their proposers and seconders, the results of the voting and the number of votes cast for and against, if counted. He shall briefly record the trend of the discussion.

The Secretary shall report to the General Assembly on his work since the last Congress. A report of the previous General Assembly published in the Journal "Clinical Neurophysiology" shall be taken as read.

The Secretary shall be responsible for the publication of a report on the meeting of the General Assembly, approved by the Executive Committee, in the Journal "Clinical Neurophysiology." The minutes of the General Assembly, approved by the Executive Committee, shall be approved by the Delegates of national societies by e-mail, fax or airmail.

The Secretary shall maintain a list of all members of the General Assembly. The Secretary may discuss, move and vote. He may have assistants who may, or may not, be members of the General Assembly.

2.2.3. The procedural counselor

The Procedural Counselor shall be responsible for assisting the Chairman in interpretation of points of order and Rules of Order. He shall assist the Chairman before and during the General Assembly. When the ruling of the Chairman is challenged by a motion from the floor, the ruling of the Procedural Counselor shall be final for that General Assembly.

The Procedural Counselor can only discuss, he cannot move or vote unless he should also be a member of the General Assembly as a Delegate or Officer of a member society.

2.3. The agenda

2.3.1. The agenda of the General Assembly, when convenient, shall follow this sequence:

i. The report of the President of the Federation.
ii. The report of the Secretary.
iii. The report of the Treasurer on past expenditures.
iv. The report of the Editor(s)-in-Chief of the Journal.
v. The reports of the Chairmen of Special Commissions.
vi. The report of the Chairman of the Nominating Committee.
vii. The reports of Chairmen of other Committees.
viii. Proposal of budget for the forthcoming Fiscal Period.
ix. Election of Honorary Fellows.
x. Selection of time and place of next Congress.
xi. Amendments of Statutes.
xii. Further business relating to the Federation.
xiii. Roll call of member societies and introduction of Delegates for the new Fiscal Period.
xiv. Closure of meeting.

2.3.2. All reports may be pre-circulated. Each individual must present his report, have it caused to be presented or request that it be taken as read. No vote of acceptance or rejection is necessary. Discussion of points in any report shall be made immediately after the giving of the report.

Motions made on a report may be made immediately after the report or under the item of "Further business relating to the Federation" (item 2.3.1 xii of these Bye-Laws). Deferment for later discussion may be moved by the Chairman, on his own initiative, or by a seconded motion from the floor; it shall then be voted on.

2.3.3. The proposed budget shall be presented by the Treasurer or alternate appointed by the Executive Committee and voted on. In the case of rejection an amendment shall be proposed and voted on. Failure of this requires resubmission of the budget in modified forms until it is accepted.

2.4. Motions

2.4.1. Mechanisms of proposal

i. Proposed by the Chairman acting on the request of the Executive Committee.

ii. If the Executive Committee recommends acceptance of a proposal from a Delegate the Chairman may call on that Delegate or an alternate to propose the motion. No seconder shall be required.

iii. A motion proposed from the floor without prior notification shall be seconded. The Chairman shall have the motion repeated in the official languages.

2.4.2. Withdrawal

A motion may be withdrawn by the proposed with agreement of the seconder.

2.4.3. Amendments

Amendments may be proposed by the Chairman on his own initiative, on the request of the Executive Committee, or from the floor. A seconder shall be required in the latter case.

A motion that is withdrawn cannot be amended.

The amendment shall be voted on before the motion is voted on.

Amendments to amendments shall not be permitted. In cases where further amendments are desired the Chairman may request the proposer of the first motion to withdraw it and resubmit it in the amended form.

The relevance of amendments may be challenged on a point of order.

2.4.4. Deferment

A motion before the General Assembly may be moved to be deferred for later discussion by the Chairman on his own initiative, or from the floor. In the latter case a seconder is required. The deferment can only be to some appropriate time in the same General Assembly. The motion of deferment, with or without amendment, shall be voted on in the normal manner before any further business is conducted.

2.4.5. Relevance

When following a report the motion must be relevant to the contents of the report, otherwise it must be deferred to an appropriate point in the Agenda. Amendments must be relevant to the motion on the floor. Relevancy may be challenged by the Chairman or as a point of order from the floor without seconding.

2.4.6. Discussion

This shall always be directed through the Chairman. When a question is asked from the floor, providing it is relevant, the Chairman may direct any appropriate person to answer it. Discussion itself must be relevant to the motion being presented. The relevancy may be challenged by the Chairman or as a point of order from the floor unseconded.

2.4.7. Voting

Votes shall normally be indicated by a show of hands. Votes for the motion first, against last. In cases of doubt of majority the Chairman may move or it may be moved and seconded from the floor that there be an exact count of votes. This motion does not require to be voted on and cannot be denied by the Chairman.

At the discretion of the Chairman or by seconded motion from the floor a secret ballot may be moved. This motion does not require to be voted on and cannot be denied by the Chairman.

A member abstaining may request his abstention to be recorded.

2.4.8. Majority (Statutes 6.5)

In all cases a simple majority (more than 50%) is required except that a two-thirds (2/3) majority is required for the election of an Honorary Fellow, for amalgamation or dissolution of the Federation, or for amendment of the Statutes.

2.4.9. Subject of motions

i. *Specific subjects*: The General Assembly is normally expected to pass, amend, or reject motions pertaining to subjects raised in the reports of the President, the Secretary, the Treasurer, the Editor(s)-in-Chief of the Journal and the Chairmen of Commissions and Committees. The General Assembly approves proposals for the date and place of the next Congress, the election of Honorary Fellows, and changes in the Statutes.

ii. *General subjects*: The General Assembly is expected to vote on other items on the Agenda submitted by the Chairman and on written or verbal proposals intended to fulfill the purposes of the Federation as outlined in the Statutes (Statutes 1.1–1.3).

2.4.10. Precedence of motions

i. The motions of the Chairman take first precedence, those of the Officers of the Federation or the various Chairmen second precedence, and verbal motions last. Nevertheless, verbal motions take precedence for an amendment, deferment, calling for a secret ballot, interpretation of a point of order, vote count or introducing a Rule.
ii. Only one motion can be considered at any one time except when there is a motion of amendment, deferment, call for secret ballot, point of order, vote count or introducing a new Rule. When any of these latter are presented they must be voted in the order of the last presented first, last but one second, and so on.

2.5. Requests

These may be made by any member of the General Assembly including the Chairman. They require no seconding. They take immediate precedence and must be acted on immediately:

a. for improving audibility;
b. for maintaining order;
c. for interpretation of a point of order;
d. for translation into an official language.

All other procedures must be in the form of motions.

2.6. Points of order

These shall include challenge of relevancy and of interpretation of the Rules of Order. The Chairman must decide immediately on the relevancy of the point or the interpretation of the Rules of Order. If the Chairman's ruling is challenged it must be as a seconded motion from the floor and thereupon voted on. The Chairman shall then consult the Procedural Counselor whose ruling shall be final for the meeting.

When a situation arises for which no Rule exists, the Chairman or any other member may propose a Rule in the manner of a motion, which must thereupon be voted on. This Rule shall hold for the duration of the Assembly only.

2.7. Validity

Should these Rules of Order be incorrectly implemented and the fact not challenged, nevertheless all decisions passed by the requisite majority shall be valid.

2.8. Selection of the time and place of a subsequent international congress

Selection of the time and place of the International Congresses should be made at least 4 years in advance. Nominations may be made by any member society. Preference should be given for successive congresses to be in different geographical areas. Nominations must be less than 10 min each and should include both oral and written information about the proposed Organizing Committee, the congress venue, the hotel arrangements and a preliminary budget. General information about the city or country of the nomination cannot exceed 5 min of the presentation time.

The final selection should be by majority vote, each member of the General Assembly casting one vote. After the first round of voting, should no nomination receive a majority, a second round should consider only those nominations receiving the four highest number of votes. After the second round of voting, should no nomination receive a majority, a third round should consider only those nominations receiving the two highest number of votes.

3. Organization of a congress

3.1. The OCIC, constituted as indicated in Statute 7.1, shall have responsibility to organize all aspects of the International Congress. A budget shall be created consistent with standard accounting practices and appropriate fiscal assumptions. Responsibility for any net financial deficit of the congress shall be decided explicitly at least 2 years prior to the Congress. Fiscally responsible organizations shall be presented with accounting reports and budget estimates at least twice each year through the time of the Congress.

3.2. The OCIC will set aside congress program time for three honorary lectures, named the Berger, Adrian and Kugelberg lectures. The OCIC will invite distinguished speakers to present these lectures.

3.3. The OCIC will budget to set aside as uncommitted funds 15% of the congress registration fee from all active members of constituent societies, excluding junior members. If the congress runs a budget deficit, these uncommitted funds will be used to cover the deficit. If uncommitted funds still remain or if the congress has a net profit, these uncommitted funds will be transferred to the IFCN to defray costs of a fellowship program to help young clinical neurophysiologists attend congresses.

3.4. Other international meetings

3.4.1. In addition to the International Congress of Clinical Neurophysiology the Federation may organize or sponsor interim meetings on any other subject related to clinical neurophysiology. The President of the Federation shall be the Chairman of the Organizing Committees of such meetings, but may delegate authority to organize a meeting to two members of the Executive Committee with the cooperation of the host society.

3.4.2. The financial arrangements for such meetings shall be subject to 3.1 of these Bye-Laws.

3.5. Finance

3.5.1. The Treasurer of an Organizing Committee shall keep proper accounts of the expenses and receipts of the Congress or meeting. Any excess shall be deposited in the Treasury of the Federation.

3.5.2. In the case of any symposium or meeting sponsored jointly by the Federation and another body any profit or loss shall be born in such proportions as shall have been previously agreed.

4. Journal

4.1. (Statutes 5.6 (b))

The Executive Committee appoints the Editor(s), assigns to them their functions and defines their relationships. If there are two Editors-in-Chief, they should be from different geographical areas. It appoints the Consulting Editors from nominees submitted by the Editor(s)-in-Chief based upon scientific merit and willingness to serve. Except for the Editor(s)-in-Chief, all these appointments may be for an indefinite period. All these appointments may be subject to review at any time and shall not be terminated by the end of the Fiscal Period.

4.2. The Executive Committee advises the Editor(s)-in-Chief on matters of general policy and arbitrates on matters referred to it by the Editor(s)-in-Chief, but leaves the day to day conduct of, and responsibility for, the Journal entirely to the Editor(s)-in-Chief, in conjunction with the Publishers.

4.3. The Editorial Staff may consist of one or two Editor(s)-in-Chief, several Associate Editors as necessary, a Review Editor, a Consultant for Supplements and such others as the Executive Committee may decide. At any time any of these posts may be in abeyance, and any two or more may be combined at the discretion of the Executive Committee.

4.4. The function of the Consulting Editors is to give critical evaluation of, and to correct when necessary, manuscripts submitted to them by the Editor(s). Nevertheless, the Editors are free to make use of the services of other experts. The number of Consulting Editors may be increased or decreased at any time by the Executive Committee.

4.5. The contract for the publication of the Journal "Clinical Neurophysiology" is made between the Executive Committee, acting for the Federation, and the Publishers (Elsevier Science Publishers).

Statutes of the European Chapter of the International Federation of Clinical Neurophysiology

1. Purpose

The European Chapter of the International Federation of Clinical Neurophysiology (EC-IFCN) is created and shall be governed by the present statutes.

2. Aims of the EC-IFCN

The EC-IFCN has the following goals:

- To organize the European Congress of (the Societies of) Clinical Neurophysiology.
- To promote and support pre- and postgraduate educational programs in Clinical Neurophysiology in Europe, as well as regional educational courses suggested by National Societies and approved by the EC-IFCN ExCo.
- To foster and encourage European scientific research in Clinical Neurophysiology. This includes promoting and organizing Research projects.
- To establish, maintain and encourage efficient collaboration within Europe in order to promote education and good practice in Clinical Neurophysiology. This includes the promotion of an important role of Clinical Neurophysiology in European Public Health Plans.
- EC-IFCN shall not engage in any activity contrary to the statutes of the IFCN.

3. EC-IFCN society members

Membership of EC-IFCN will be those national societies for Clinical Neurophysiology which are members of the IFCN and are situated in the European geographic region, as well as Societies affiliated to this region.

Exceptions from the geographical rule can be decided by the General Assembly.

European Societies for Clinical Neurophysiology intending to join the IFCN may be granted the status of Candidate Society of the EC-IFCN pending the outcome of their application to the IFCN. They may attend the meetings of the EC General Assembly but will not have the right to vote. If, for any reason, one of the societies is excluded from IFCN its membership to the EC-IFCN will cease.

4. EC-IFCN finances

1. EC-IFCN will receive any surplus funds from the European Congresses. It has the right to accept and administer gifts, legacies, movable and immovable properties, donations and assets of any kind.
2. EC-IFCN will receive support from the International Federation dependent on IFCN-ExCo finances and policy.
3. The assets of the EC-IFCN shall be used for its own operation and in a general way to provide for the attainment of its purposes. In particular, they shall be used for the material organization of the European Congress and other scientific and educational Chapter activities. Any excess shall be deposited in the treasury of the EC-IFCN. No portion of the assets of the EC-IFCN shall be paid directly or indirectly to any member society or any officer of the EC-IFCN except for reimbursement for direct expenses (reasonable payment for services actually rendered), or of expenses incurred in the EC-IFCN. Officers, delegates, committee members and other professionals

serving the chapter do so on a voluntary basis and are not reimbursed for their own professional time spent. The assets of the EC-IFCN are kept in a separate account by the IFCN Treasurer. Any of the reimbursements mentioned above will be sent out through the treasurer of the IFCN. The expenses will be audited and controlled according to the rules of the IFCN. The IFCN Treasurer will deliver an annual report of the account of the EC-IFCN to the Executive Committee of the EC-IFCN (EC-ExCo). The Treasurer of the IFCN has final responsibility, but EC-IFCN has its own account and the right to spend an appropriate amount of money to be proposed by the EC-IFCN Secretary/Treasurer and to be decided by the EC-IFCN General Assembly.

4. The EC-IFCN may be dissolved by a two-thirds majority vote of the EC-General Assembly. In the event of its dissolution the treasury of the EC-IFCN shall be transferred to the IFCN.

5. Executive Committee of the EC-IFCN

1. The EC-ExCo consists of the Chairman, the Secretary/Treasurer, the Liaison Officer of the IFCN and two Members-at-Large. These members are to be proposed and elected by the member societies except for the Liaison-Officer which is an IFCN-ExCo member and appointed by the ExCo of the IFCN. Except for the Liaison Officer, members of the EC-ExCo cannot serve at the same time on the IFCN-ExCo.
2. Election of EC-ExCo officers will be performed, preferably, during the European Congress of Clinical Neurophysiology (ECCN), by the vote of the Delegates during the EC General Assembly. However, should the 4-year term of office of one or several of the ExCo members expire more than 6 months before the next EC General Assembly, an electronic ballot will be held to ensure the replacement, before expiry of (an) officer's(s') terms and in a time scale which allows his/her/their replacement in time. To this aim, national societies will be contacted by the EC-ExCo and prompted to nominate candidates for each of the positions to be renewed (Chairman, Secretary/Treasurer or Member-at-Large). A period of at least 1 month will be allotted for individuals to bid as candidates, and for national societies to proceed with nominations to EC-ExCo.

   Only national societies can nominate, and they can nominate only one person for each office, from their own or a different country. When making nominations national societies should be aware that the successful candidates for each of the EC-ExCo positions must come from different countries. Therefore, if any of the top three candidates declared eligible for two or more EC-ExCo positions after the first ballot are from the same country (in terms of the affiliated national society to which they are entitled to belong), then the final ballot will be carried out sequentially in two or three steps to ensure that no country's national society will be represented by more than one Officer or Member-at-Large in the EC-ExCo. The voting should then occur in the following sequence: first round President, second round Treasurer/Secretary, third round Members-at-Large.

   After the EC-IFCN Secretary has received nominations, ExCo will ensure that nominees are willing to run for the position, and then accepted nominations shall be communicated to all national societies via their Delegates, so that an electronic (e-mail) vote can take place. A first ballot of all candidates will take place on a one society one vote method. After this the top three candidates in votes will participate in the second and final vote under the same method. Each national Society will send their votes to the

Secretary/Treasurer of the EC-ExCo. The results will then be communicated by e-mail to all National Societies and to the IFCN ExCo, and will be posted in the Web site of the EC-IFCN. The candidate with the most votes will be elected. The quorum of the electronic ballot is one-half of the European CN Societies. It is hoped to have voting for each office within a month. In the event of more than one officer retiring voting will be sequential to ensure officers are from different countries.

3. Elected EC-ExCo officers will serve a term of 4 years and will be eligible for re-election once. The maximum term of office for EC-ExCo officers and Members-at-Large is thus 8 years no matter if served consecutively or in non-consecutive years. Within this maximal term of office EC-ExCo officers are re-eligible for any of the positions in the EC-ExCo. The Officers and the Members-at-Large should be from different countries and reflect the whole geographical area. The IFCN Liaison Officer can also be appointed only for a maximum term of 8 years and must be a European (and is voted for within IFCN elections).
4. Most of the work and decisions of the EC-ExCo shall be made by fax and e-mail. The regular EC-ExCo meetings will be held by teleconferences or computerized connections as well as at every ECCN and, if necessary, during world congresses of the IFCN (ICCN).
5. The Chairman of the EC-IFCN shall organize and chair the EC General Assembly and is the official representative of the EC-IFCN. He coordinates the activities of the EC-ExCo. He shall submit a Chairman's report to each EC General Assembly. The Chairman and the Secretary/Treasurer should summarize the activities of the chapter every other year in a written report which should be delivered to the delegates and the IFCN officers. The Chairman shall keep close contact with the IFCN preferably during the IFCN-ExCo meetings in Europe. If the Chairman's and Secretary/Treasurer's terms are expiring 6 months before the next General Assembly, a complete report will be circulated in parallel with the election procedures and approved by e-mail by the Delegates.
6. The Secretary/Treasurer shall be responsible for correspondence, keeping archives for the EC-ExCo, notifying delegates of the EC General Assembly and for circulating the agenda at least 1 month before the ECCN and Advanced Courses. The Secretary/Treasurer of the EC-IFCN is responsible for the assets of the society. He/she shall keep proper accounts of the expenses and receipts and shall give a report and submit a budget for the next fiscal period at the EC General Assembly.
7. The Liaison Officer shall represent the IFCN.
8. The Members-at-Large can perform all other duties of the EC-IFCN in order to fulfill the aims of the EC-IFCN.

6. The European Congress of Clinical Neurophysiology

1. The ECCN should be held by the EC-IFCN, if possible, every 2 years. National Societies can apply to host the next congress at least 2 months before the preceding congress with an informal application (including the place of the congress and the convener) to the EC-IFCN Chairman. The EC General Assembly will decide on the place and date of the next congress. The EC General Assembly appoints the convener of the next ECCN. The convener should not be an elected member of the current EC-ExCo.
2. The Organizing Committee of the ECCN consists of the Convener, the Secretary/Treasurer of the Congress, three additional members to be determined by the National Society organizing the ECCN, the officers of the EC-IFCN and two IFCN officers including the Liaison Officer of the IFCN. Budget

and spending decisions have to be made by a two-thirds majority.

3. The International Scientific Committee consists of the delegates of the EC-IFCN Member Societies and additional members approved by the convener of the next ECCN together with the EC-ExCo.
4. The program of the ECCN will be proposed by the Organizing Committee and will be circulated among the members of the International Scientific Committee for further suggestions and comments. The Journal *"Clinical Neurophysiology"* is the official journal for the congress.
5. The National Society being appointed is responsible for the financial success of the congress. The EC-IFCN will help the hosting National Society with its assets.
6. The IFCN will provide a fixed amount of money for Fellowships for the ECCN and other Chapter's activities. The EC-ExCo is responsible for the election of the Fellows receiving grants. It will be paid out through the IFCN Treasurer. The EC-IFCN can provide additional Fellowships if resources are available. The amount of each fellowship will be decided by the EC-IFCN. The rules for receiving Fellowships will be the same as for the IFC Fellowships to the IFCN congresses. The ECCN will reimburse the IFCN for the cost of the Fellowships out of congress profits (if any).

7. The EC General Assembly

1. The EC General Assembly is composed of the EC-ExCo officers and of the delegates of each member society (according to a representative ratio as detailed in Article 7.4 of the present Bye-Law). The delegates or their substitutes should be the same for the IFCN and for the EC-IFCN.
2. The EC General Assembly decides the place and date of the next congress on the basis of bids presented by individual National Societies. It appoints the convener of the next European Congress. It discusses and approves, if deemed fit, the financial statement and accounts for the current fiscal period, submitted, duly audited, by the Treasurer of the EC-IFCN. It votes on the budget of the following fiscal period proposed by the EC-ExCo. It discusses and votes upon all resolutions and decisions taken to fulfil the purposes of the Federation and on all questions appearing on the agenda.
3. The EC General Assembly is bound to meet at each ECCN Congress. It is chaired by the Chairman of the EC-IFCN or his specified deputy. If one or more EC-ExCo officers arrive at term of mandate at the Congress, or less than 6 months earlier, the EC General Assembly elects the members to be replaced. If officers arrive at term more than 6 months before the next General Assembly, an electronic ballot is set in place according to the rules in Article 5.2 of the present Bye-Laws.
4. The number of delegates of each Member Society who are eligible to sit in the EC General Assembly is based on the number of the Society members paying dues to the IFCN as follows: 1–99: 1 delegate, 100–399: 2 delegates, >400: 3 delegates. Written identification of all the delegates or their substitutes must be submitted in advance to the secretary or the EC-IFCN by each Member Society. All those registered at the EC-IFCN Congress may attend the EC General Assembly, but only members of the Assembly may speak and vote.
5. The quorum of the EC General Assembly is one-half of the delegates or their substitutes, together with the Chairman and Secretary/Treasurer, or their specified deputies and one other EC-ExCo officer.
6. Each delegate and EC-ExCo officer has one vote. Vote by proxy is not allowed.
7. On the second request of one delegate a secret ballot shall be organised on any point of the agenda.

8. If not otherwise stated here, the EC General Assembly will be conducted according to the “Bye-Laws for the conduct of the General Assembly of the IFCN”.
9. Amending of Bye-Laws. The Bye-Laws can be modified by a majority vote of the EC member societies, either during the EC General Assembly or through an electronic ballot, and subsequent ratification of the Bye-Laws by the IFCN ExCo. An electronic ballot will be held only if modification of the Bye-Laws are urgent as judged by the EC-ExCo. To this aim, national societies will be contacted by the EC-ExCo and prompted to discuss, via e-mail, the Bye-Law modifications proposed by the EC-ExCo. A period of at least 3 weeks will be allotted for this discussion. Subsequently, the EC-ExCo will make such adjustments to the Bye-Law modifications that have gained substantial support during the discussion and present the final version for an electronic ballot.

Statutes of the Latin-American Chapter of the International Federation of Clinical Neurophysiology

1. Definition

The Latin-American Chapter of the International Federation of Clinical Neurophysiology (CLA-IFCN) is a federation of all Latin-American societies affiliated to IFCN.

CLN-IFCN was founded by the representatives of the Latin-American societies at Guatemala City in October 1995 and officially accepted as a chapter of the Federation in Kyoto, Japan in October 1995.

2. CLA-IFCN societies members

(a) All Latin-American societies ordinarily affiliated to IFCN are eligible to CLA membership.
(b) Admission of new societies to CLA can only occur after they have become members of IFCN. However, while waiting IFCN application approval, the new societies may apply for CLA membership. During this interim period these societies may participate in CLA General Assembly, but are not entitled to vote and cannot be officially accepted into the chapter.
(c) Societies that lose their IFCN affiliation also will lose CLA membership.
(d) CLA shall submit these Bye-Laws and any future amendments or changes in these Bye-Laws to IFCN for review and to IFCN’s council for ratification.

3. Aims of CLA-IFCN

(a) To promote, in accordance with IFCN, the creation, organization and development of Clinical Neurophysiology and encourage the formation of Clinical Neurophysiology Societies in Latin-America.
(b) To promote and encourage education and scientific research in Clinical Neurophysiology in Latin-America.
(c) To help establish and define equipment specifications and organize guidelines and minimal practice requirements for Clinical Neurophysiology.
(d) To promote, organize and announce, in accordance with IFCN, Clinical Neurophysiology meetings, congresses and advanced courses in Latin-America. These may occur in country members of CLA-IFCN and follow or precede other local national or international events. It is advisable that the society in charge of organizing such meeting receives help from other member societies. Information on local meetings and congresses should be shared among every CLA members to facilitate international collaboration in Latin America.
(e) CLA-IFCN shall not engage in activities contrary to IFCN Statutes.

4. CLA-IFCN organization and directory

(a) The administrative address of CLA is that of the current President.

(b) CLA-IFCN Executive Committee (CLA-ExCo) consists of: the President, the Past-President, the Secretary/Treasurer, the Liaison member of IFCN and two Members-at-Large.

(c) These members are to be proposed and elected by the society members, except for the Liaison member, who is an IFCN member, appointed by the IFCN's ExCo. Except for the Liaison member, other members of CLA-IFCN cannot serve at the same time on the IFCN-ExCo.

(d) Elected CLA-ExCo members will serve a 4-year term and will be eligible for re-election only once. The maximum term of office for CLA-ExCo members is 8 years, either served consecutively or non-consecutively. To maintain continuity in the chapter's leadership half of the CLA-ExCo will be replaced every 2 years as detailed in Section 5h. CLA-ExCo members should belong to different societies, reflecting geographical diversity. The Liaison member may also serve an 8-year term.

(e) The chapter is administered by the ExCo composed of the President, the immediate Past-President, the Secretary/Treasurer, two Members-at-Large and the Liaison member of IFCN. CLA-ExCo may hold meetings at any time and in any place that may be convenient to its members. It may also conduct its business by postal ballot or teleconference. It shall have full authority to formulate Bye-Laws, subject to ratification by the General Assembly.

(f) CLA-IFCN will have a permanent statute committee, composed by three elected members that will serve a 4-year term. The members of the committee are eligible for re-election only once.

(g) CLA-IFCN General Assembly is composed by the delegates of each member society, or their specified alternates. The General Assembly will meet every 2 years, during the Latin-American Clinical Neurophysiology Congress, meeting or advanced course.

(h) Communication among CLA-ExCo members and with IFCN will be done through various means including: mail, e-mail, fax, telephone, etc.

(i) The CLA President's duties are: (1) coordination of CLA activities; (2) preparation, together with the Secretary/Treasurer, of the General Assembly agenda; (3) chairing the ExCo; (4) convene and chair the General Assembly; (5) report the activity of the ExCo and the chapter.

(j) In the event of prolonged incapacity or death of the President, the immediate Past-President assumes his/her office and duties for the remainder of the Fiscal Period.

(k) The CLA Secretary/Treasurer's duties are: (1) preparation of a summary of CLA activities, informing both the delegates of society members and the IFCN through the Liaison member; (2) organization of CLA mailing and archives; (3) preparation, together with the President, of the General Assembly agenda; (4) dissemination of information of CLA societies of the General Assembly agenda and date, at least 2 months before its occurrence; (5) dissemination of information to CLA General Assembly delegates of the finances report.

(l) The Liaison member represents IFCN and constitutes the officer in charge of communication between CLA and IFCN.

(m) The Members-at-Large perform the designated tasks of CLA-IFCN in order to accomplish the aims of CLA-IFCN.

(n) Official CLA languages are Spanish and Portuguese.

(o) CLA may be dissolved by a two-thirds majority of valid votes in an Extraordinary General Assembly especially created for this purpose. In this case, all financial resources and properties will be transferred to IFCN.

(p) These statutes may be modified by vote majority in the General Assembly, pending IFCN-ExCo approval.

5. CLA General Assembly

(a) Every 2 years, during CLA congresses or courses, a General Assembly will take place. The General Assembly and its agenda shall be informed by CLA-ExCo at least 2 months prior to the meeting.

(b) Every CLA member may participate in the General Assembly, but only the delegates of society members of CLA will be allowed to vote.

(c) CLA societies shall send to the Secretary/Treasurer of the chapter, before the General Assembly the name of the designated delegate(s) that is their representatives. The name of the delegate(s) or an alternate in his/her absence shall be appointed by each society at least 2 months in advance of the General Assembly.

(d) CLA General Assembly quorum is equal to half the number of designated delegates added to the members of CLA-ExCo.

(e) The number of votes per society shall be proportional to the number of members of the society, according to the following rules: (1) less than 49 members = 1 vote; (2) from 50 to 149 members = 2 votes; (3) more than 150 members = 3 votes. A member society may entrust by proxy all its votes (1–3) to only one delegate. However at least one delegate per member society must be present to the meeting to cast the vote.

(f) By proposal of any delegate, seconded by another, a secret ballot shall be organized on any point of the agenda.

(g) The General Assembly will discuss: (1) the President's report; (2) the Secretary/Treasurer's report, including the financial report; (3) reports of other members of CLA-ExCo; (4) the agenda previously prepared. The reports must be approved by the General Assembly. The General Assembly has the right to introduce new items at the assembly.

(h) At each General Assembly part of CLA-ExCo will be elected; the President and one Member-at-Large are elected in one General Assembly. After 2 years, a next election will choose the Secretary/Treasurer and the other Member-at-Large. The Liaison member is selected by IFCN-ExCo.

(i) The General Assembly proposes the place and date of next congress and/or course, and also appoints the local convener. The local society must accept the selection of the General Assembly.

(j) When the congress or advanced course takes place in a country that is not a member of CLA-IFCN, the General Assembly will appoint a committee of representatives of CLA members to help in the organization of the meeting.

(k) In all cases a proposal is approved by a simple majority (more than 50%) with the exception for the dissolution of the chapter or for amendment of the Bye-Laws. In these two cases a two-thirds majority is required.

(l) Not less than 1 year before the end of the biennial CLA congress or course, the CLA ExCo shall select three delegates to serve as a Nomination Committee under the chairmanship of the immediate Past-President. Should the immediate Past-President be incapacitated for a prolonged period of time or dead the President will appoint a member of the ExCo to serve as a chair of the nominating committee. Members of the nominating committee shall not be eligible for nomination for the fiscal period they select the nominees.

(m) The Nomination Committee shall invite nominations from the delegates of each member society and from all the members of the CLA ExCo. As half of the officers will be elected every 2 years, the nominees are for the position of President and one Member-at-Large at one meeting and for the Secretary/Treasurer, and one Member-at-Large at the next meeting. It is desirable that the officers belong to different societies reflecting geographical diversity. The President and the Past-President cannot be from the same country. Having ascertained the willingness to serve, the Chairman of the Nomination Committee shall submit their names to the postal vote of the member societies, and inform the Secretary/Treasurer of the results of the ballot. Each society has the number of votes to which it is entitled in the General Assembly.

6. CLA finances

(a) The CLA Fiscal Period is defined as a 4-year period starting at the end of one CLA meeting to the end of the second CLA meeting 4 years hence. The Fiscal Period defines the term of the Executive Committee and its members, the term of the General Assembly and all special committees or commissions.
(b) CLA will receive any surplus funds generated by the CLA congresses and advanced courses.
(c) The CLA shall have the right to accept and administer gifts, legacies, donations of any kind, without restriction as to the amount of value.
(d) CLA is a non-profit charitable organization.
(e) CLA assets shall be used for its own administrative operation and to provide for its educational and research accomplishment as described in its Bye-Laws. In particular, they shall be used for the organization of CLA congresses and advanced courses. Any excess shall be deposited in CLA treasury. No portion of CLA assets shall be paid directly or indirectly to any member, society or officer of CLA-IFCN, except for reimbursement of direct authorized expenses, incurred in the interest of CLA-IFCN. Officers of CLA-ExCo and delegates serve the chapter on a voluntary basis and are not reimbursed for their own professional time spent on behalf of the chapter.
(f) The Secretary/Treasurer shall keep proper books of account.
(g) CLA expenses will be audited and controlled according the rules of IFCN at the end of each Fiscal Period.

7. CLA clinical neurophysiology congresses and advanced courses

(a) Latin-American clinical neurophysiology congresses or advanced courses should be held every other year (biennial). National societies can apply to host the next congress or advanced course at least 2 months before the preceding congress, with a written application to CLA-ExCo.
(b) The organizing committee of the CLA congress or advanced course consists of the Convener, the Secretary/Treasurer of the congress, three Members appointed by the National society and two officers of CLA-ExCo, including the Liaison member of IFCN. The convener and local society hold the responsibility for the scientific and local arrangements. The local society is responsible for financial aspects of the congress and/or courses. Whenever possible, CLA will help in this organization.
(c) The convener, together with CLA-ExCo, will appoint the international scientific committee. The scientific program shall be proposed by the international committee

and receive evaluation of CLA-ExCo and delegates of societies. All these processes will be supervised by IFCN through the Liaison member.

(d) IFCN will provide funds for fellowship during CLA congresses and advanced courses. Requests for fellowship will be submitted in writing to the IFCN ExCo at least 1 year prior to the meeting. These monies will be paid out through the IFCN Treasurer. CLA-IFCN can provide additional fellowships, if resources are available. CLA-ExCo will be responsible for selection of the fellows receiving grants. The rules for the award of these fellowships shall be the same as the rules of IFCN in awarding grants for IFCN congresses.

(e) At the biennial CLA meeting and/or course, the ExCo will set up the organization for the next chapter meeting.

Statutes of the Asian and Oceanian Chapter of the International Federation of Clinical Neurophysiology

1. Purpose

The Asian and Oceanian Chapter of the International Federation of Clinical Neurophysiology (AOC-IFCN) is created and shall be governed by the Statutes.

2. Aims of the AOC-IFCN

The AOC-IFCN has the following goals:

- To organize the Asian and Oceanian congress of clinical neurophysiology (AOCCN) and the educational courses in clinical neurophysiology.
- To promote and support pre- and postgraduate educational programs in clinical neurophysiology in Asia and Oceania.
- To foster and encourage scientific research in clinical neurophysiology in Asia and Oceania.
- To establish, maintain and encourage efficient collaboration among countries in Asia and Oceania in order to promote education and good practice in clinical neurophysiology.
- AOC-IFCN shall not engage in any activity contrary to the Statutes of the IFCN.

3. AOC-IFCN society members

Membership of the AOC-IFCN will be those national or regional societies for clinical neurophysiology which are members of the IFCN and are situated in the Asian and Oceanian geographic region.

None of the national or regional societies for clinical neurophysiology which belongs to another regional chapter can be a member of AOC-IFCN.

Asian and Oceanian Societies for Clinical Neurophysiology intending to join the IFCN may be granted the status of Candidate Society of the AOC-IFCN pending on the outcome of their application to the IFCN. They may attend the meetings of the General Assembly but will not have the right to vote. If, for any reasons, one of the societies is excluded from IFCN, its membership to the AOC-IFCN will cease.

4. AOC-IFCN finances

4.1. AOC-IFCN will receive any surplus funds of the Asian and Oceanian congress and the educational course. It has the right to accept and administer gifts, legacies, movable and immovable properties, donations and assets of any kind.

4.2. The assets of the AOC-IFCN shall be used for its own operation and in a general way to provide for the attainment of its purposes. In particular, they shall be used for the material organization of the congress and the educational courses. Any excess shall be deposited in the treasury of the AOC-IFCN. No portion of the assets of the AOC-IFCN shall be paid directly or indirectly to any Member Society or officer of the AOC-IFCN except for reasonable payment for services actually rendered, or repayment of expenses incurred in the interest of the AOC-IFCN.

4.3. The AOC-IFCN may be dissolved by a two-thirds majority vote of the General Assembly. In the event of its dissolution the treasury of the AOC-IFCN shall be transferred to the IFCN.

5. Executive Committee of the AOC-IFCN (AOC-ExCo)

5.1. The AOC-ExCo consists of the Chairperson, the Secretary/Treasurer, and the Liaison officer of the IFCN. These members are to be proposed and elected by the Member Societies except for the Liaison officer who is appointed by the ExCo of the IFCN.

5.2. At each Asian and Oceanian congress, the AOC-ExCo except for the Liaison officer is elected by the General Assembly. Elections shall be held by the General Assembly at the Asian and Oceanian Congress at intervals of not more than 4 years.

5.3. Elected AOC-ExCo officers will normally serve a term of 4 years and will be eligible for reelection once. The maximum term of office for AOC-ExCo officers is thus 8 years. Within this maximal term of office the ExCo officers are re-eligible at any of the positions in the AOC-ExCo. The officers should be from different countries. The Liaison officer can also be appointed only for a maximum term of 8 years. The Liaison officer of the IFCN must be from the Asian and Oceanian Societies of IFCN.

5.4. Most of the work and decisions of the AOC-ExCo shall be made by mail, fax and e-mail. The regular AOC-IFCN meetings will be held at every AOCCN Congress and if necessary during the World Congresses of the IFCN.

5.5. The Chairperson of the AOC-IFCN shall organize and chair the General Assembly and is the official representative of the AOC-IFCN. He/she coordinates the activities of the AOC-ExCo. He/she shall submit a Chairperson's report to each General Assembly.

5.6. The Secretary/Treasurer shall be responsible for correspondence, keeping archives for the AOC-ExCo, notifying delegates of the General Assembly and for circulating the agenda at least 1 month before the AOC-IFCN Congress. The Secretary/Treasurer of the AOC-IFCN is responsible for the assets of the society. He/she shall keep proper accounts of the expenses and receipts and shall give a report and submit a budget for the next fiscal period at the General Assembly.

5.7. The Liaison officer shall represent the IFCN.

6. The Asian and Oceanian Congress of Clinical Neurophysiology and educational courses

6.1. The AOCCN is to be held by the AOC-IFCN every 4 years. National societies can apply to host the next congress at least 2 months before the preceding congress with an informal application (including the place of the congress and the convener) to the AOC-IFCN Chairperson. The General Assembly will decide on the place and date of the next congress. The General Assembly appoints the Convener of the next AOCCN.

6.2. The Organizing Committee of the AOCCN consists of the Convener, the Secretary/Treasurer of the Congress, additional members to be determined by the National Society organizing the AOCCN and the officers of the AOC-IFCN.

6.3. The International Scientific Committee consists of the delegates of the AOC-IFCN member societies and additional members approved by the Convener of the next AOCCN together with the AOC-ExCo.

6.4. The National Society being appointed is responsible for the financial success of the congress. The AOC-IFCN will help the hosting National Society with its assets.

7. The General Assembly

7.1. The General Assembly is composed of the ExCo officers and of the delegates of each member society.

7.2. The General Assembly proposes the place and date of the next congress. It appoints the Convener of the next Asian and Oceanian congress. It discusses and approves, if deemed fit, the financial statement and accounts for the current fiscal period, submitted, duly audited, by the Treasurer of the AOC-IFCN. It votes on the budget of the following fiscal period proposed by the AOC-ExCo. It discusses and votes upon all resolutions and decisions taken to fulfill the purposes of the Federation and on all questions appearing on the agenda.

7.3. The General Assembly is bound to meet once every 4 years at the place and date fixed for the AOCCN. It is chaired by the Chairperson of the AOC-IFCN or his/her specified deputy. The General Assembly elects the AOC-ExCo in the following sequence: (1) Chairperson (2) Secretary/Treasurer.

7.4. Each member society has one vote. Written identification of all the delegates or their substitutes must be submitted in advance to the secretary of the AOC-IFCN by each member society. All those registered at the congress may attend the General Assembly, but only Members of the Assembly may speak and vote.

7.5. The quorum of the General Assembly is one-half of the delegates or their substitutes, together with the Chairperson and Secretary/Treasurer, or their specified deputies.

7.6. Each delegate and AOC-ExCo officer has one vote. Vote by proxy is not allowed.

7.7. On the seconded request of one delegate a secret ballot shall be organized on any point of the agenda.

7.8. If not otherwise stated here, the General Assembly will be conducted according to the Bye-Laws for the conduct of the General Assembly of the IFCN.

North American Chapter Bye-Laws of the International Federation of Clinical Neurophysiology

1. Membership

There will be three society members of the North American (NA) Chapter of the IFCN: the American Association of Neuromuscular and Electrodiagnostic Medicine (AANEM), the American Clinical Neurophysiology Society (ACNS), and the Canadian Society of Clinical Neurophysiologists (CSCN).

2. Chapter board of directors

2.1. Board of directors

The Board of Directors of the chapter will consist of three Directors and one Treasurer. The Directors and Treasurer are appointed as follows:

Director – the designated AANEM Delegate to the IFCN (currently Dr. Donald Sanders);

Director – the designated ACNS Delegate to the IFCN (currently Dr. John Ebersole);

Director – the designated CSCN Delegate to the IFCN (currently Dr. M. George Elleker);

Treasurer – chosen by the other directors.

2.2. Terms

The term for each Director will begin effective the date this document is signed below and the term shall end when a new IFCN delegate is appointed by the member society. The Treasurer shall be voted on by the other Directors each year and serve through December of the year elected to serve. Each society must notify the AANEM when a new IFCN Delegate is appointed for their organization.

2.3. Treasurer's duties

The Treasurer shall oversee the financial aspects of the NA Chapter. He/she will with the assistance of the AANEM Executive Director maintain an itemized account of receipts and disbursements. He/she shall oversee and direct the AANEM Executive Director in the receipt and disbursement of funds as approved by the NA Chapter Board of Directors and shall report the results after each year to the Chapter Board of Directors.

3. Members' meetings

The Board of Directors of the North American Chapter shall hold a regular meeting annually to discuss the administration of the funds received by the IFCN. The specific time and place will be designated by the Board members. Meeting may be held via conference call or other electronic means.

4. Mission and objectives

The mission of the NA Chapter of the IFCN is to strive to promote education and the attainment of the highest level of knowledge and understanding in the field of clinical neurophysiology by:

(a) providing fellowships to physicians in disadvantaged countries to attend the meetings of NA member societies,
(b) providing educational opportunities within disadvantaged countries,
(c) distributing educational material to disadvantaged countries, and
(d) providing networking opportunities for physicians from disadvantaged countries.

The primary intent of the NA Chapter of the IFCN is to provide educational opportunities for physicians from disadvantaged countries. Physicians from these countries should receive special consideration. In addition, the funds can be used to support travel to meetings of the AANEM, ACNS, or CSCN for individuals in training or early in their careers who are not from disadvantaged countries.

The NA Chapter member societies acknowledge that the meeting held by each society currently provides excellent educational opportunities for physicians from disadvantaged countries and that there is no need for the NA Chapter to hold an additional educational meeting. This does not limit the opportunity for member societies to hold a joint meeting in the future. Each society is encouraged to discuss this possibility for the future.

5. IFCN funds

5.1. Allocation of initial IFCN distribution

The IFCN has agreed initially to distribute US $100,000 to the NA Chapter over a 4-year fiscal period beginning in 2007 and ending 2010. The IFCN will send these funds to the AANEM. The AANEM will maintain a separate interest bearing account for the funds. If the entire US $100,000 is distributed to the AANEM by the IFCN in a lump sum, interest earned (less a US $1000 annual administrative fee to the AANEM) will be reported to the NA Chapter Board of Directors each year and will be allocated based on the allocation proportion listed below, that has been agreed to by all three chapter member societies. Earned interest will be allocated in the same allocation proportion as listed below and will be available for distribution the following year. If the IFCN distributes US $50,000 or less during the 4-year period, the AANEM will retain any interest earned (if any) to cover the administrative expenses of handling the funds. Each of the member chapters will receive a portion of the funds. The proportions are as follows:

Allocation proportion:

AANEM	60% (US $15,000/year);
ACNS	25% (US $6250/year);
CSCN	15% (US $3750/year).

5.2. Allocation of future IFCN distributions

Should the IFCN determine to issue further funds to the NA Chapter, the funds will be allocated as described in Section 5.1 above (including payment to AANEM of administration fees), and the same approval and disbursement procedures as listed in Sections 5.3 and 5.4 below will be followed.

5.3. Approval

Each of the three member societies should prepare a Project Plan for the use of the allocated funds (including a budget). The Project Plan should identify which of the missions listed in Section 4.0 above is being addressed. Project Plans and fund requirements should be submitted no later than January 31 of the year the money is to be spent to the NA Chapter Board of Directors via e-mail with a copy to the AANEM Executive Director. In 2007, if a chapter member plans to expend funds, the Project Plan including budget requirements should be submitted by July 1, 2007.

The Board of Directors will review and approve or reject each Project Plan via e-mail. A majority of the Board of Directors must approve each Project Plan. If a Director of the Board has concerns about a Project Plan, he/she must articulate the areas of concern. If a majority of the Board of Directors does not approve a member society's Project Plan, the Director who represents that member society must notify his/her society of these concerns and seek clarification or changes to the Project Plan that address the concerns of the other members of the board. This new information should then be provided to the NA Chapter Board of Directors. The Board will reconsider their decision and vote again on the Project Plan. If a majority of the Board of Directors does not approve the revised plan, further opportunity will be allowed for changes to the Plan until a majority vote can be reached. At any time, a member of the Board of Directors can call for a meeting of the group via teleconference or other mutually agreed upon methods. Each Director is responsible for coordinating approval requests with his/her society.

5.4. Disbursement

After a fund-sponsored event, but no later than December 1 of the year in which the Project Plan was approved, the member society shall submit to the AANEM the actual expenditures for the Project Plan for that year. The NA Chapter Treasurer, with the assistance of the AANEM Executive Director, will assure that the submitted expenditures align with the approved Project Plan. Checks will be disbursed within 30 days of receipt of the request. In the event that less money is spent than budgeted, only the expended funds will be disbursed, and the remaining funds will be added to the monies available to that chapter society for the following year. In the event that the actual expenses exceed the budgeted amount, the full amount will be paid only if funds owed to the society are available in the account. The excess payment will reduce the monies available the next year unless there was carryover from prior years. If no additional funds exist in that society's account, only the budgeted amount will be paid. Chapter member societies may resubmit any unpaid bills for payment after another IFCN distribution is received, if any.

6. Parliamentary authority

The rules contained in the current edition of *Robert's Rules of Order Newly Revised* shall govern the Chapter in all cases to which they are applicable and in which they are not inconsistent with these Bye-Laws.

7. Amending Bye-Laws

These Bye-Laws may be amended by majority vote of the Board of Directors at any scheduled meeting. All proposals, however, must be submitted in final written, adoptable form to the Treasurer at least 10 days before the meeting. The Bye-Laws may be amended via mail, e-mail, facsimile, or any other appropriate communication method. Each Director must receive approval from their respective society for the amendment prior to amending these Bye-Laws. After the changes are approved by the North American Board of Directors, the amended Bye-Laws must be approved by the IFCN Rules Committee and ratified by the IFCN General Assembly before the change is final.

8. Notices

Any notices should be sent to the following:

American Association of Neuromuscular & Electrodiagnostic Medicine (AANEM)
Attention Shirlyn Adkins, JD Executive Director
2621 Superior Drive NW
Rochester, MN 55901
USA
sadkins@aanem.org

American Clinical Neurophysiology Society (ACNS)
Attention: Jackie Coleman, Executive Director
One Regency Drive
PO Box 30
Bloomfield, CT 06002
USA
jcoleman@ssmgt.com

Canadian Society of Clinical Neurophysiologists (CSCN)
Attention: Dan Morin, Chief Executive Officer
Canadian Neurological Sciences Federation
7015 MacLeod Trail SW, Suite 709,
Calgary, AB T2H 2K6
Canada

These Bye-Laws were duly adopted by a unanimous vote of the NA Directors. Each signatory below verifies that their respective society Board of Directors has approved and authorized their agreement to these Bye-Laws.

Statutes of the International Clinical Neurophysiology Society (ICNS)

1. Mission statement

The ICNS (for members of non-affiliated countries) is a professional association dedicated to fostering excellence in clinical neurophysiology and furthering the understanding of nervous system function in health and disease through education, research and the provision of a forum for discussion and interaction. This society is designated for members from countries that do not have an affiliated society membership in the IFCN.

2. Name

The name of the society shall be "International Clinical Neurophysiology Society (for members of non-affiliated countries)." The name shall be abbreviated to ICNS.

3. Purposes

The purposes of the society shall be:

- To promote personal contact between investigators and clinical neurophysiology and closely related fields, between the society and other similar societies throughout the world through the IFCN, thus facilitating of exchange of scientific and professional information and opinions.
- To further the greater understanding and knowledge of clinical neurophysiology and disorders for which it is applied.
- To arrange for the exchange of journals or other written materials in these fields.
- To assist in the formation of committees for evaluation of standards, techniques, procedures, education, training or qualification of physicians or technologists.

- To achieve high standards for clinical practice of clinical neurophysiology.

4. Members

The society shall consist of honorary fellows, fellows, members and junior members from non-affiliated countries. Additional members may be from countries with an affiliated society if the individual cannot be a member of that affiliated society, and that society provides written support for the individual's request for ICNS membership.

Only honorary fellows, fellows and members shall vote on any question concerning the society. Each person is entitled to one vote.

Should the number of members in any one country exceed 10, it is expected that they will apply to the IFCN for affiliation. Should affiliation take place, the individual members of the ICNS from that country will be transferred to the new affiliated National Society. In that case, individual memberships in ICNS shall be discontinued. Also, if the ICNS President or Council Members-at-Large are from a society so converted to full IFCN membership, his or her service on the ICNS Council shall be discontinued effective 1 year after his or her membership in ICNS is discontinued.

5. Officers

5.1. Only fellows and members shall be eligible to hold elected office.

5.2. The officers of the society shall be a President, Secretary and Treasurer. The President shall be nominated by the IFCN Executive Committee. The Secretary and Treasurer shall be the IFCN Secretary and IFCN Treasurer.

5.3. The ICNS Council will consist of eight members. These include the three ICNS officers, three Members-at-Large, and the two most recent ICNS Past-Presidents. The Members-at-Large will be chosen from among the ICNS membership at the time of the election of officers.

6. Meeting of the society

6.1. The society shall meet at the time and location of the International Congress. For installation of officers, the transaction of such business may come forward and presentation of any scientific or educational program.

6.2. Council may call special meetings of the society whenever it is expedient.

7. Rules of consistency

The IFCN Rules Committee will review any issues arising out of conflicting rules or opinions about ICNS rules, or between the ICNS rules and other IFCN organizations' rules. Decisions of the IFCN Rules Committee shall be final. These ICNS Bye-Laws shall be considered to be Bye-Laws of the IFCN.

8. IFCN membership

The ICNS shall be considered to be a member society of the IFCN. It shall be allowed to apply for membership in IFCN Chapters. It shall elect a Delegate to the IFCN General Assembly and is entitled to votes and representatives in the IFCN General Assembly consistent with its membership numbers.

9. Effective date

9.1. These statutes will become effective upon acceptance by at least 15 prospective ICNS members, and after acceptance by the IFCN in accordance with its rules for acceptance of IFCN Bye-Laws.

9.2. These ICNS Statutes may be amended in accordance with proposals initiated by ICNS Council or by petitions signed by at least 15 members of the society. Such proposals shall be placed on the agenda for general discussion at the next meeting. If approved at the meeting, a final adoption will be made by mail ballot sent to all members of the society. Changing the Statutes requires responses from a majority of eligible voters, with at least two-thirds of the voting members voting in favor of the proposed amendment. All amendments to the Statutes shall take effect immediately after both the necessary two-thirds vote and ratification by the IFCN in accordance with its rules for acceptance of IFCN Bye-Laws.

10. Bye-Laws

10.1. Members

Honorary fellows are distinguished workers in the field of clinical neurophysiology. Honorary fellows do not pay fees for dues.

Fellows are experienced individuals in the field of clinical neurophysiology, including physicians, neuroscientists, and others who have distinguished themselves in the field. Fellows pay dues, vote, and can hold appointive office in the society.

Members are other individuals who support the aims of the society and who are professionally active in the field of clinical neurophysiology, allied fields, neurophysiology technologists, allied health professionals or others, whose work advances the goal of the society. Members pay dues, vote and may hold appointive office.

Junior members work in clinical neurophysiology or closely related fields. These are generally pre-doctoral or post-doctoral trainees. Junior membership shall be limited to a period of 5 years. Junior members pay dues, but do not vote or hold office. Applications for membership for any category of membership shall be made in writing to the societies' secretary along with any documentation required by policies and procedures of the society. Acceptance for membership or change in membership status shall be made by majority vote of the council.

Any member who fails to pay dues for three successive years shall be considered to have withdrawn from the society, and his or her membership will be discontinued. The individual may, however, reapply for membership in the normal manner.

Any individual considered to have acted in a manner unworthy of membership in the society may be dismissed from membership by a three-fourths vote of council members, confirmed by a majority vote of society members present at the next meeting. The individual shall have the right to appear before the council, hear the charges and argue in defense, with witnesses if desired. Expenses for this will be borne by the accused.

10.2. Officers

The President shall preside at all business meetings of the society and at the council meetings. The President shall be allowed to vote in all matters before the society and the council. The President shall appoint members to the standing committees of the society, except for a nominating committee. The President appoints members of the nominating committee only after a majority vote of the council. The President may act as the delegates to the IFCN General Assembly.

The IFCN Secretary shall serve as Secretary to the ICNS Council and to the Society and shall ensure that a true and careful record of the meetings of the society and council is kept. The Secretary shall ensure that members are kept informed of society activity, proposed annual meetings, educational opportunities, process for applications for membership and other appropriate duties.

The Secretary shall also keep a listing of the members with their addresses and other contact information. This information shall be distributed to officers and other council members upon request.

The IFCN Treasurer shall be empowered to receive and hold in trust or otherwise such funds, personal or real property received by gift, bequest or otherwise, and to invest or reinvest, expend, convey or otherwise dispose of such funds or property in a manner as appropriate to accomplish the purposes of the society. Such actions will be under the control and within the appropriate policies and procedures as established by the council. The Treasurer shall pay all fees, bills or other obligations of the society and for that purpose shall sign checks or drafts in payment. The Treasurer shall be responsible for collecting fees or dues.

The ICNS Council shall be responsible for conducting the affairs of the society and have direction over all officers and all appointed committee members. It shall act on all questions of general policy and administration, and have final authority regarding policies and procedures of the society and expenditures of money and budgeting. The council shall approve of all appointees to a nominating committee. It shall approve the date and place of the next meeting, and announce its decision to members of the society. Council will choose a delegate to the IFCN, who may be the same as one of the society officers. Council shall determine the annual dues, or waive dues as needed, or make other special assessments. A quorum of the council to conduct business shall consist of a majority of the members of the council.

10.3. Elections

The ICNS Council shall set forth the policies and procedures for the timing and conduct of the elections. However, the elections must be held at least as often as the IFCN elections for officers. The Secretary shall ensure that mail ballots are sent out to the voting members of the society. The candidates for Members-at-Large receiving the largest number of ballots cast shall be elected. In the case of a tie vote by mail, those receiving the number of tying votes shall be voted in a second round election. In the case of a tie vote on the second round, the President of the society shall cast a deciding vote.

The Council has authority to establish a Nominating Committee to prepare a slate of proposed new Members-at-Large for the society in advance of the time of the elections.

10.4. Amendments to the Bye-Laws

Amendments to the Bye-Laws may be initiated by the Council or by a petition signed by at least 15 voting members of the society. Bye-Law amendments will be proposed to the voting members either by mail ballot or at the time of the annual meeting. A majority vote is needed to adopt the proposal.

Amendments must be ratified by the IFCN General Assembly before they can become effective.

10.5. Proposed dues

Dues for individual members from non-affiliated countries initially should be US $4.00.

Wave Length and Action Potentials: History of the IFCN
(Supplements to Clinical Neurophysiology, Vol. 61)
By: M.R. Nuwer and C.H. Lücking

Appendix 11

Historical photographs of IFCN meetings, 1985–2010

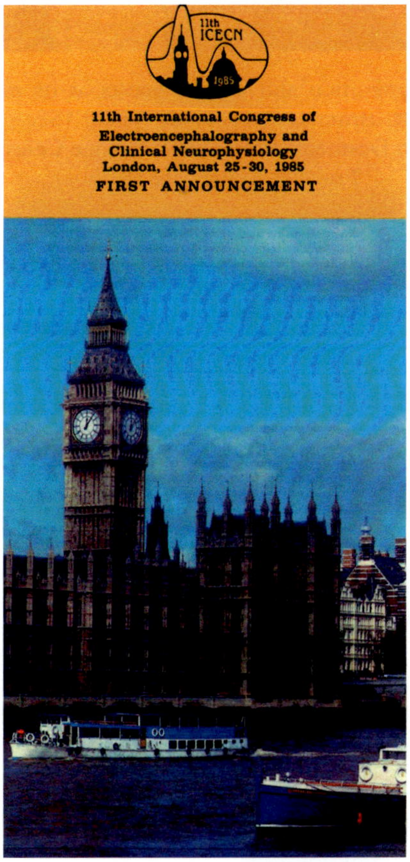

Fig. 1. First announcement for the 1985 London International Congress, cover page for the flier.

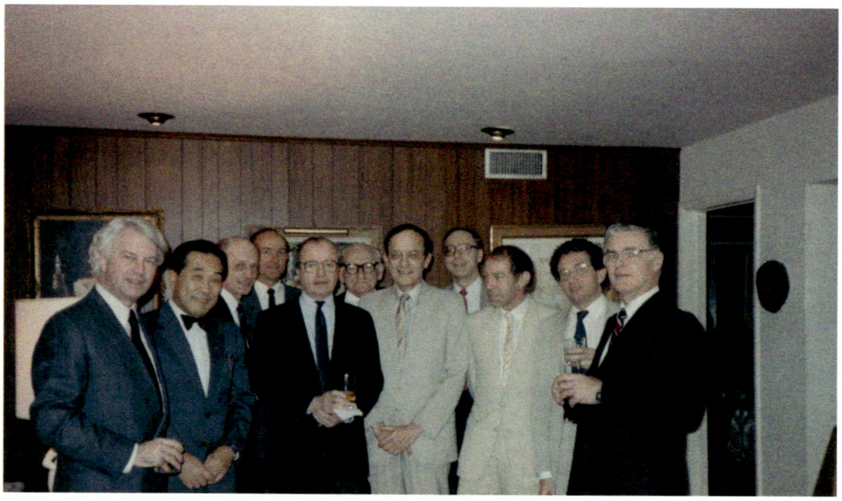

Fig. 2. The Federation Executive Committee and invited guests at its meeting in Miami 1988. The Executive Committee members are, from the left: Bram Ongerboer de Visser (Secretary), Juhn Wada (Member-at-Large), Robert Ellingson (Past-President), John Desmedt (President), Gastone Celesia (Editor), Manuel Meyer (Treasurer), François Mauguière (Editor).

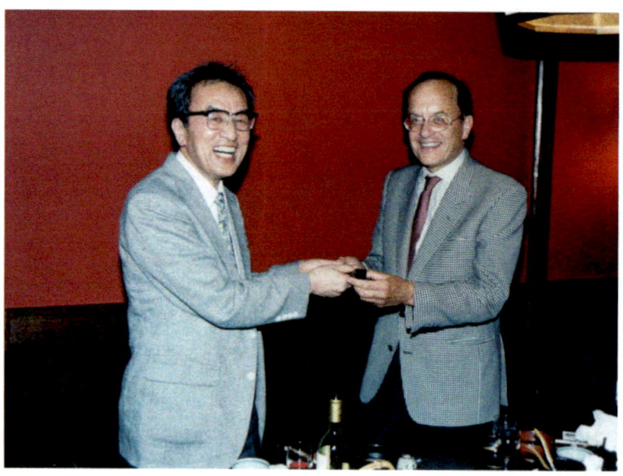

Fig. 3. Past-President John Desmedt presenting the Federation's honorary gavel, Nyoi-Bo, to President Jun Kimura.

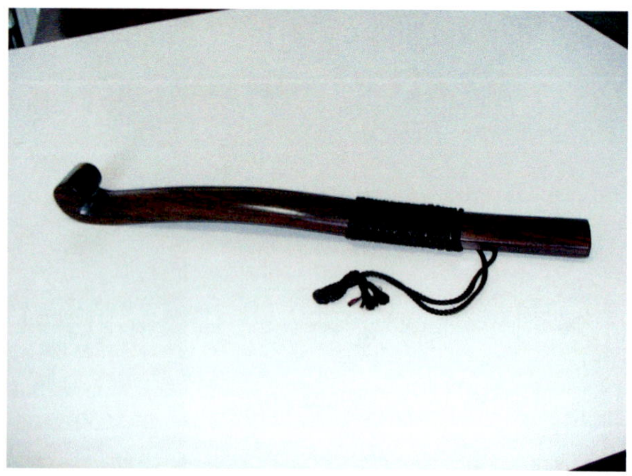

Fig. 4. The Nyoi-bo was described in an ancient Chinese tale, Saiyuhki. It was used by an ape warrior, Songoku, to help a Chinese priest travel from China to India to obtain the Buddhist Bible. During the journey the Nyoi-bo empowered the monkey to accomplish miracles to protect the priest. Nyoi-bo is neither a sceptre nor a gavel but rather a magical tool to help one accomplish what one needs to do. In the Federation, it symbolizes both the power and the hope of accomplishment placed in the authority of the President. Each President keeps it for the duration of his term.

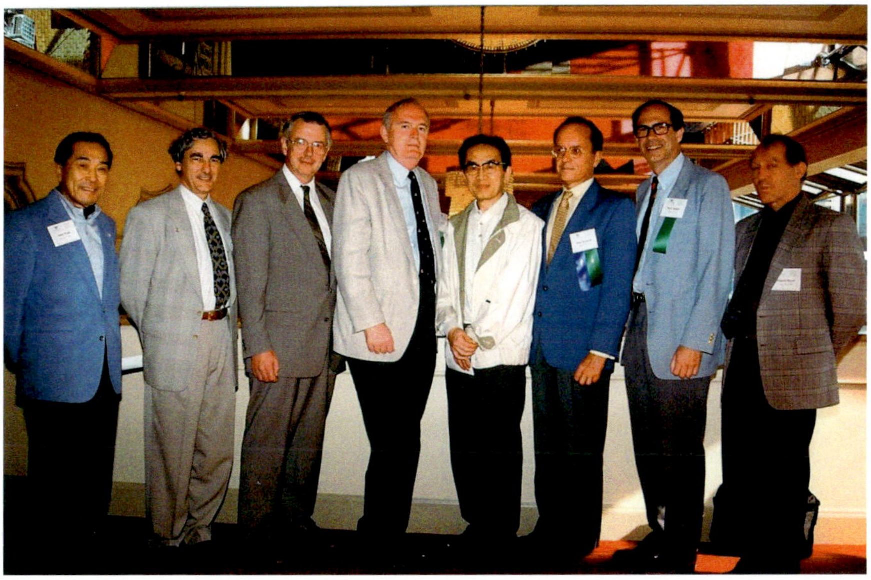

Fig. 5. Organizing Committee of the Vancouver 1993 International Congress just prior to the opening ceremony. From left to right: Juhn Wada (Convener), Andrew Eisen (Secretary), William Weber (Dean of Medicine, Univ. British Colombia), Barry Tharp (Secretary), Jun Kimura (President), John Desmedt (Past-President), Mark Hallett (Treasurer), and Manuel Meyer (Treasurer). Dr. Weber spoke at the Opening Ceremony.

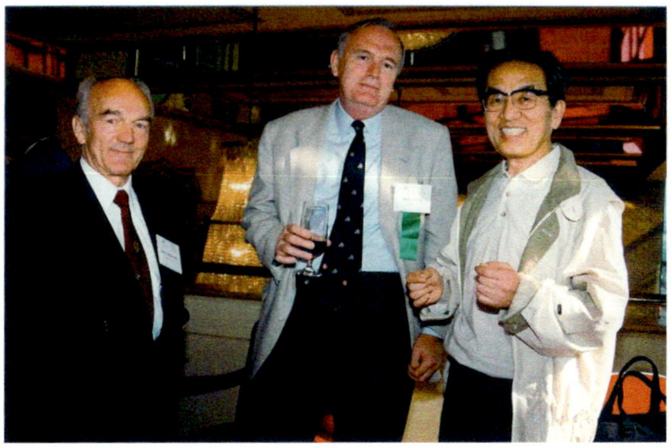

Fig. 6. At the Vancouver 1993 International Congress Opening Ceremony reception. From the left: Executive Committee Member-at-Large Jerzy Majkowsky, Secretary Barry Tharp, and President Jun Kimura.

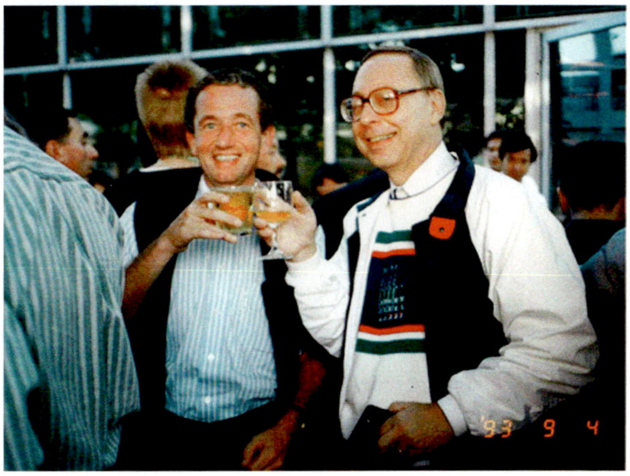

Fig. 7. A social event at the Vancouver 1993 International Congress had the theme of lumberjack and other outdoor activities typical of the Canadian west coast. Editors-in-Chief Gastone Celesia and François Mauguière toast the Congress's success.

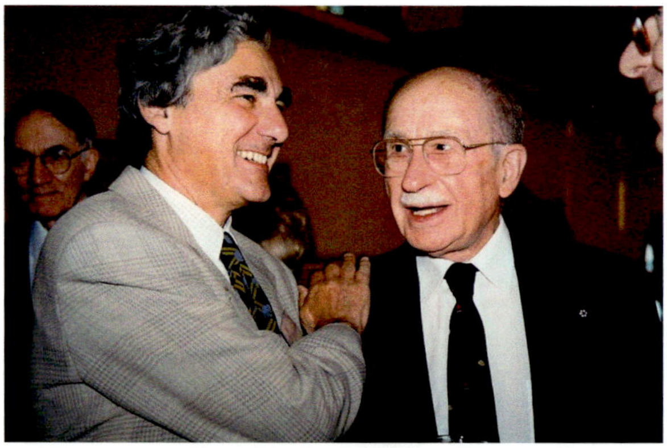

Fig. 8. Vancouver Congress organizer Andrew Eisen welcomes founding Federation President and fellow Canadian Herbert Jasper to the 1993 International Congress.

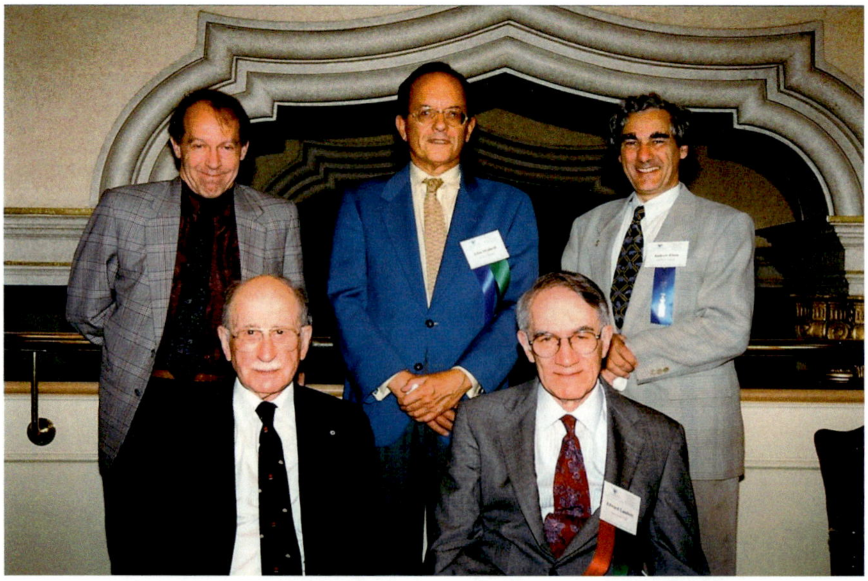

Fig. 9. Vancouver Congress Organizers and Congress Honorary Presidents. Back row left to right: Manuel Meyer (Federation Treasurer), John Desmedt (Federation Past-President), Andrew Eisen (Congress Organization Secretary). Front row: Honorary Presidents Herbert Jasper and Edward Lambert.

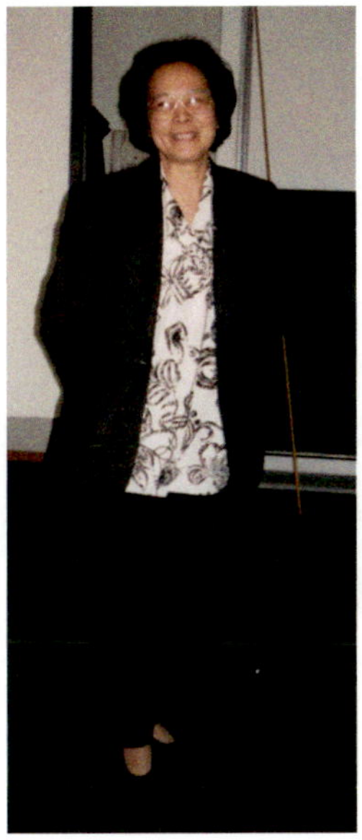

Fig. 10. Xiao-Fu Tang at an Executive Committee meeting in Freiburg, Germany, 1994. She served as an Executive Committee Member-at-Large from 1993 to 1997, Organizer of the Beijing 1996 Asian Symposium of Clinical Neurophysiology, and Founding President of the Asian–Oceanian Chapter.

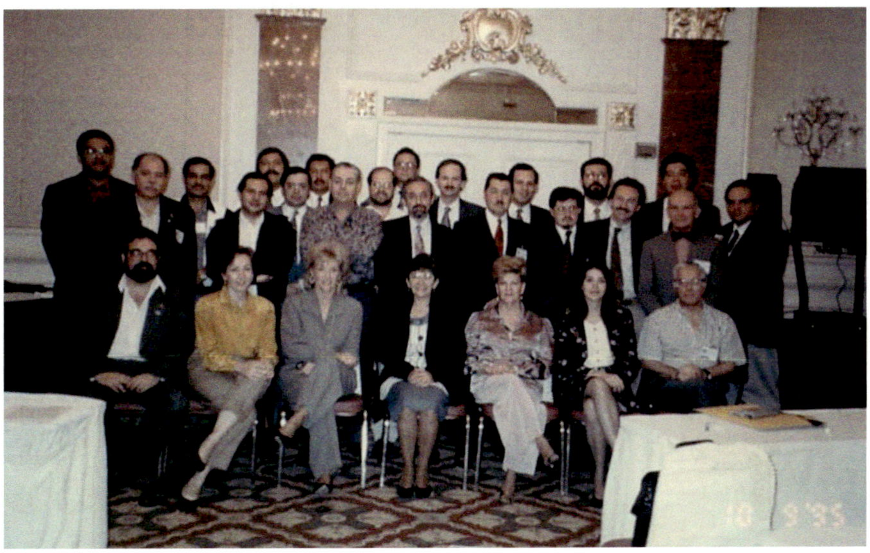

Fig. 11. The 1st Latin American Congress of Clinical Neurophysiology and founding meeting of the Latin American Chapter in Guatamala City in 1995. Principal organizer Nelly Chiofalo is seated in the front row, third from the left.

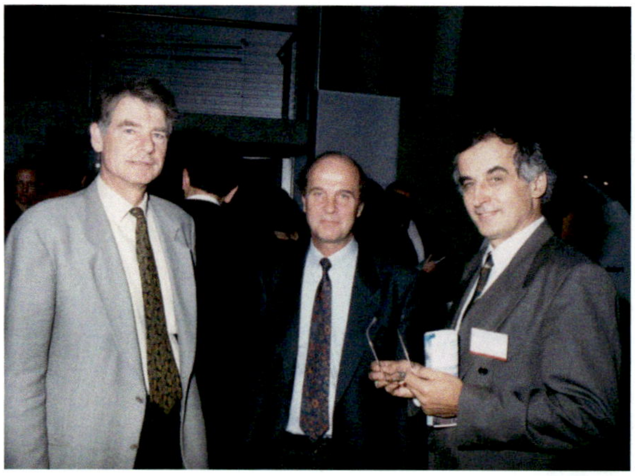

Fig. 12. At the VIII European Congress of Clinical Neurophysiology, Munich 1996. From the left: Honorary Lecturer W. Singer, IFCN President C. Lücking, and ECCN Convener B. Conrad.

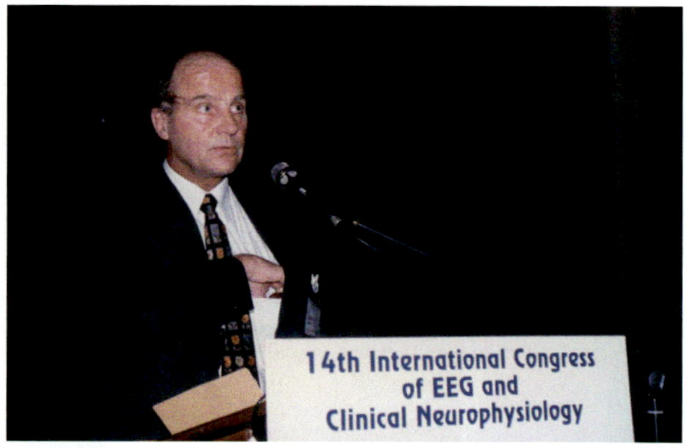

Fig. 13. Federation President Carl Lücking welcomes the audience to the 1997 Florence XIV International Congress Opening Ceremony.

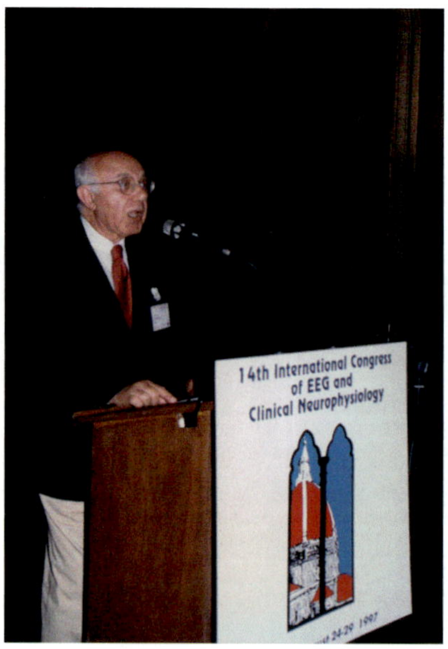

Fig. 14. Federation Secretary Giuseppe Caruso briefs the audience on congress activities, taken during the 1997 Florence XIV International Congress opening ceremony.

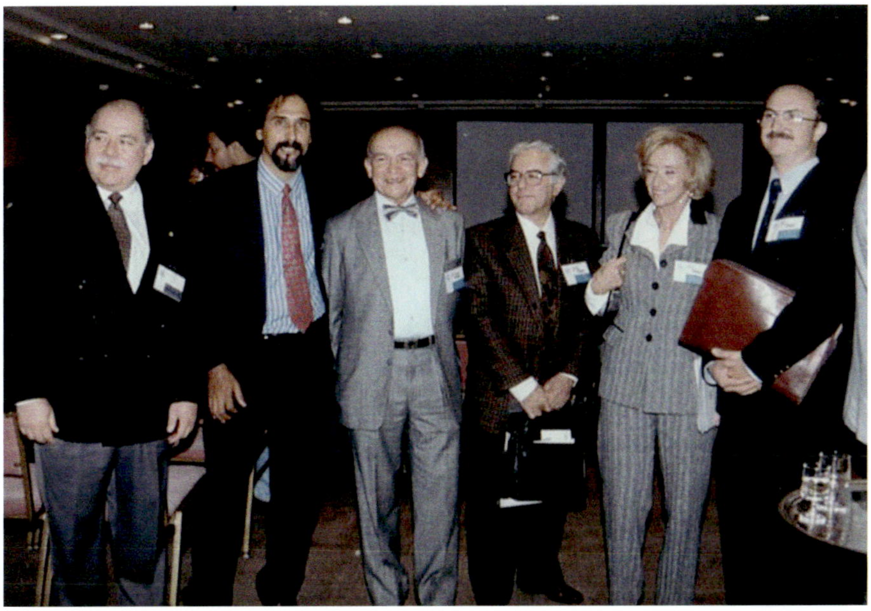

Fig. 15. Clinical neurophysiologists from across the Americas meet at a Latin American Symposium on Clinical Neurophysiology, Buenos Aires, Argentina 2001. Federation President Marc Nuwer is on the right standing next to Chapter Past-President Nelly Chiofalo.

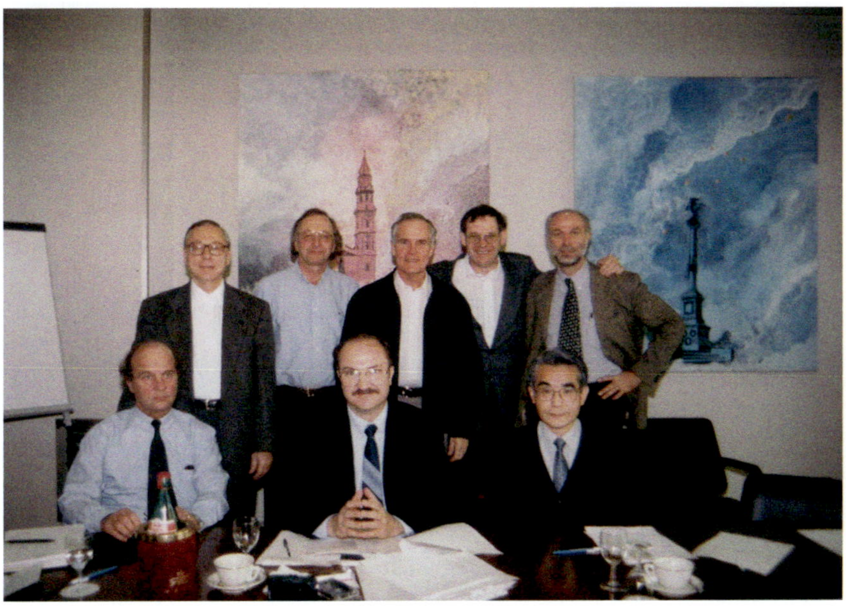

Fig. 16. The 1997–2001 Federation Executive Committee at their meeting in Naples 1998. Back row, left to right: Editor-in-Chief Gastone Celesia, Treasurer Paul Despland, Member-at-Large David Burke, Member-at-Large Guenther Deuschl, Editor-in-Chief Paolo Rossini. Front row, left to right: Past-President Carl Lücking, President Marc Nuwer, Secretary Hiroshi Shibasaki.

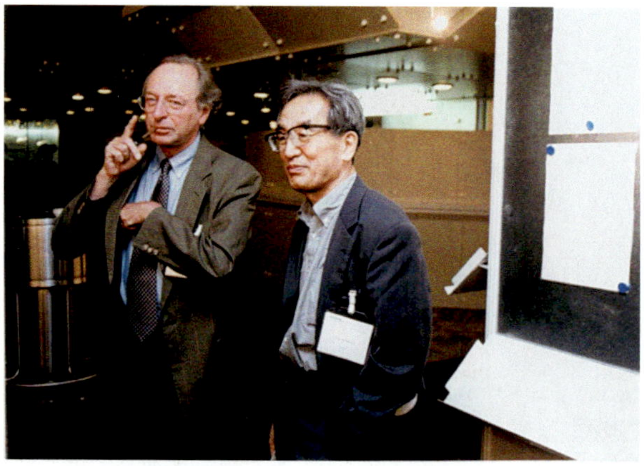

Fig. 17. Federation Treasurer Paul Despland and Past-President Jun Kimura take a break during the IX European Congress of Clinical Neurophysiology in 1998 in Ljubljana.

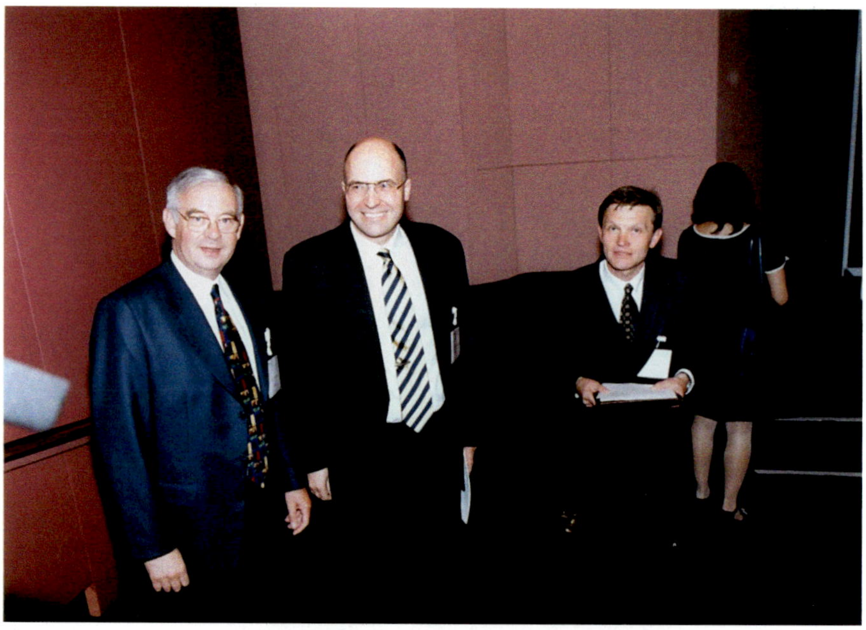

Fig. 18. European Chapter President Erik Stålberg, Prof. David Vodušek, and Congress Convener Janez Zidar prepare for the opening ceremony at the 1998 IX European Congress of Clinical Neurophysiology in Ljubljana, Slovenia.

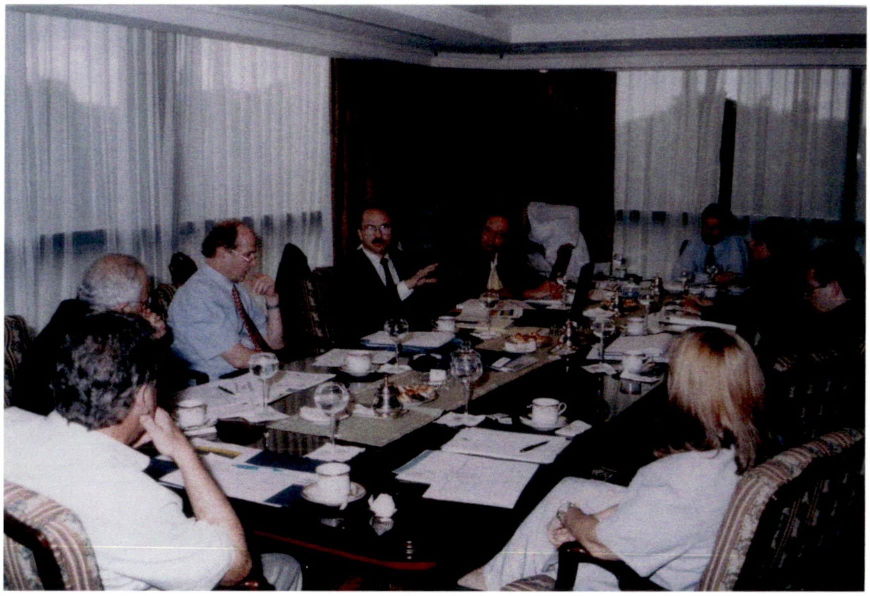

Fig. 19. The Organizing Committee for the International Congress meets in Buenos Aires in 1999, working on preparations for the 2001 International Congress. Faces visible to the camera from the left: Federation Past-President Carl Lücking, President Marc Nuwer, Treasurer Paul Despland, and Congress Secretary Ricardo Reisin.

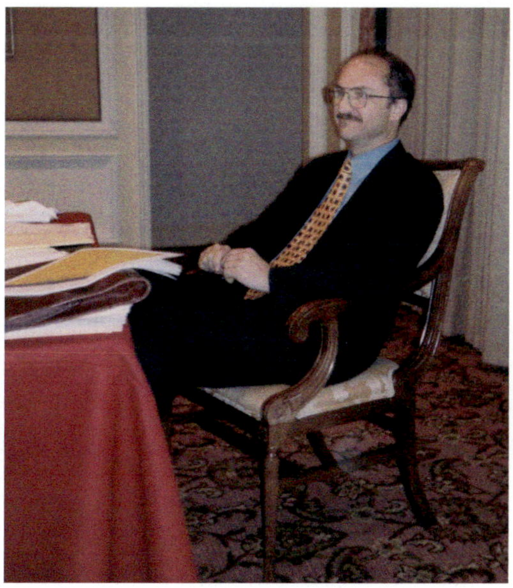

Fig. 20. Federation President Marc Nuwer chairs an Executive Committee meeting in Prague during the XI International Congress of EMG and Clinical Neurophysiology.

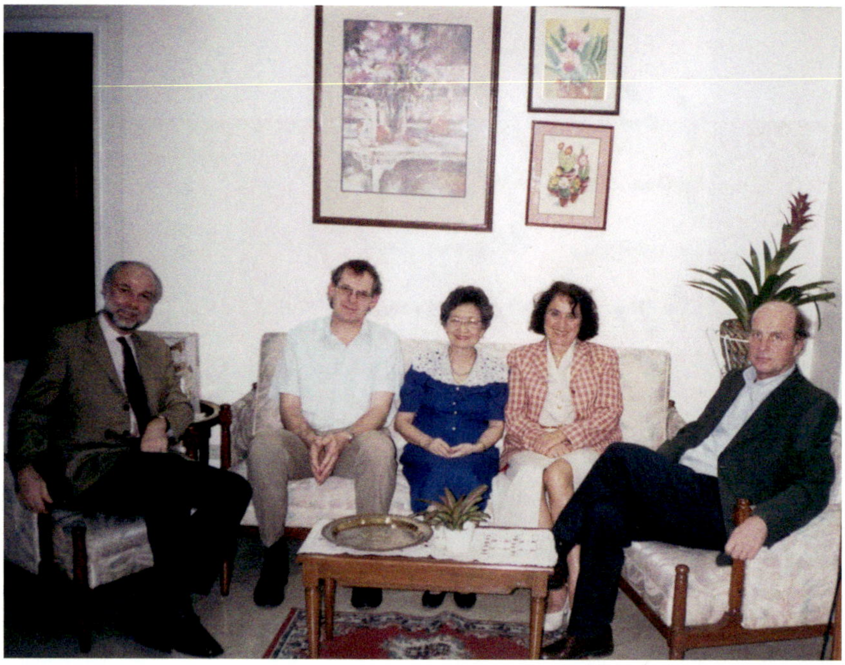

Fig. 21. During the Manila 2000 2nd Asian–Oceanian Congress of Clinical Neurophysiology Federation Executive Committee members meet at the Philippine society president's home. From left to right: Editor-in-Chief Paolo Rossini, Member-at-Large Guenther Deuschl, Philippine Society of Clinical Neurophysiology President Zenaida Bagabaldo, Merula Lücking, and Federation Past-President Carl Lücking.

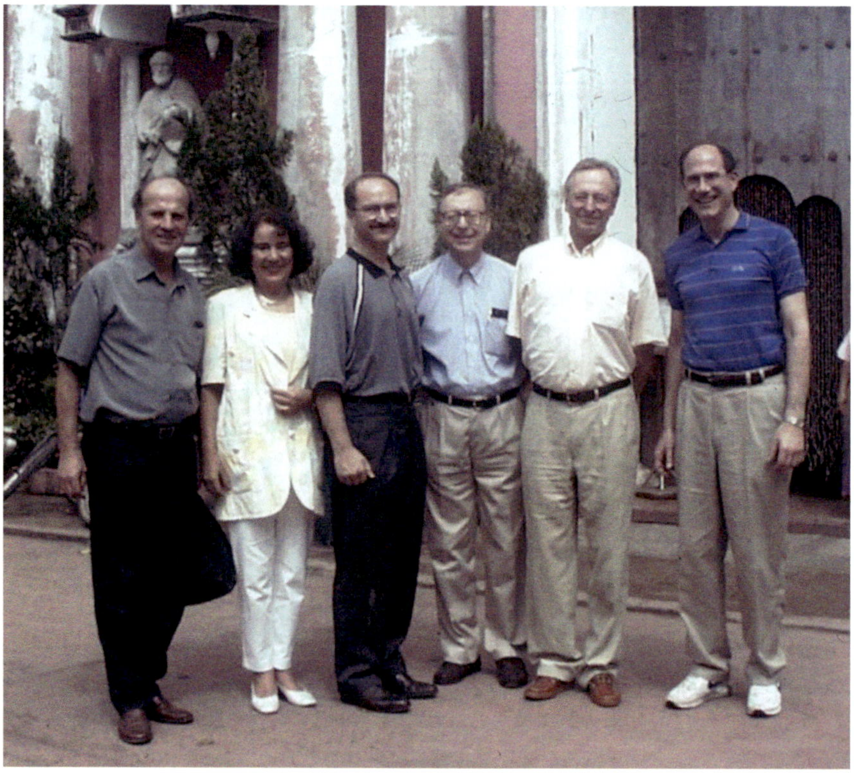

Fig. 22. On a city tour during the Manila 2000 2nd Asian–Oceanian Congress of Clinical Neurophysiology, Executive Committee members and guest from the left: Carl Lücking, Merula Lücking, Marc Nuwer, Gastone Celesia, Paul Despland, and Mark Hallett.

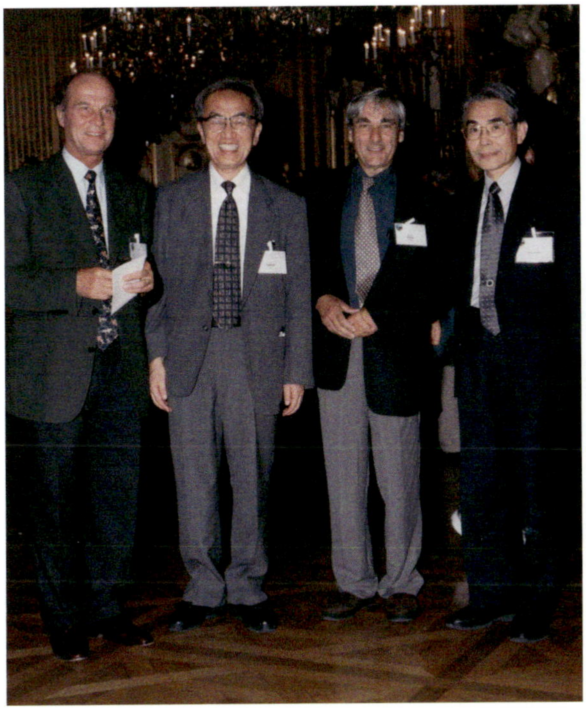

Fig. 23. At the X European Congress of Clinical Neurophysiology in Lyon 2000, from the left: IFCN Past-President Carl Lücking, former IFCN President Jun Kimura, Andrew Eisen, and IFCN Secretary Hiroshi Shibasaki.

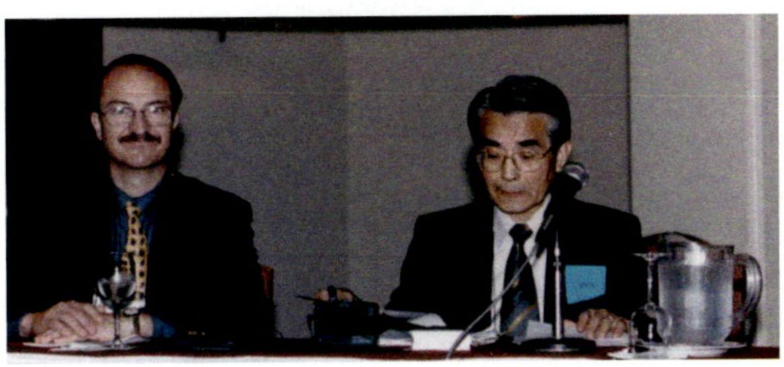

Fig. 24. The General Assembly meeting at the XV International Congress of Clinical Neurophysiology, Buenos Aires, 2001. At the front table are Federation President Marc Nuwer and Secretary Hiroshi Shibasaki.

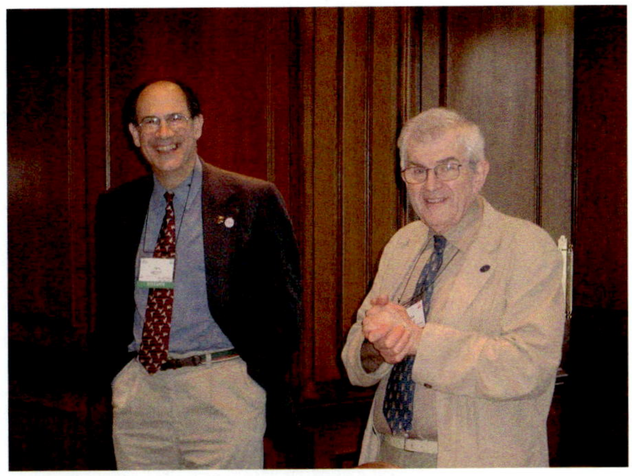

Fig. 25. At the first meeting of the new Executive Committee in Buenos Aires, 2001, Editor-in-Chief Mark Hallett and new Secretary Graham Harding prepare to get to work on Federation activities.

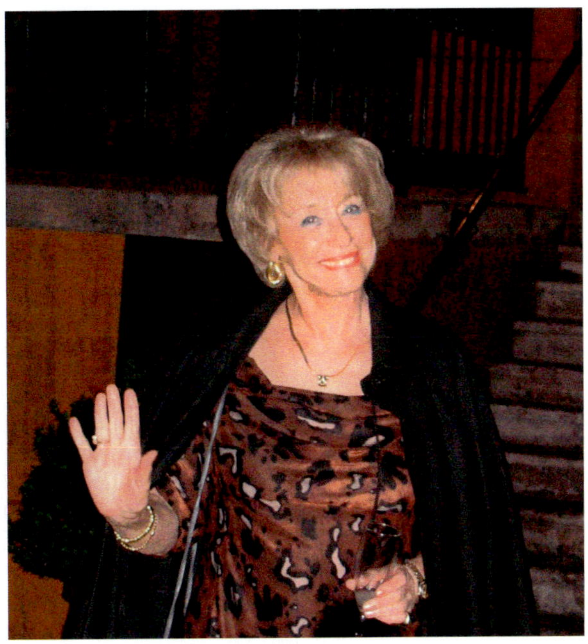

Fig. 26. Long-time Federation Delegate and founding Latin American Chapter President Nelly Chiofalo greets guests as the local host at the social event for the 2004 IV Latin American Symposium of Clinical Neurophysiology in Santiago, Chile.

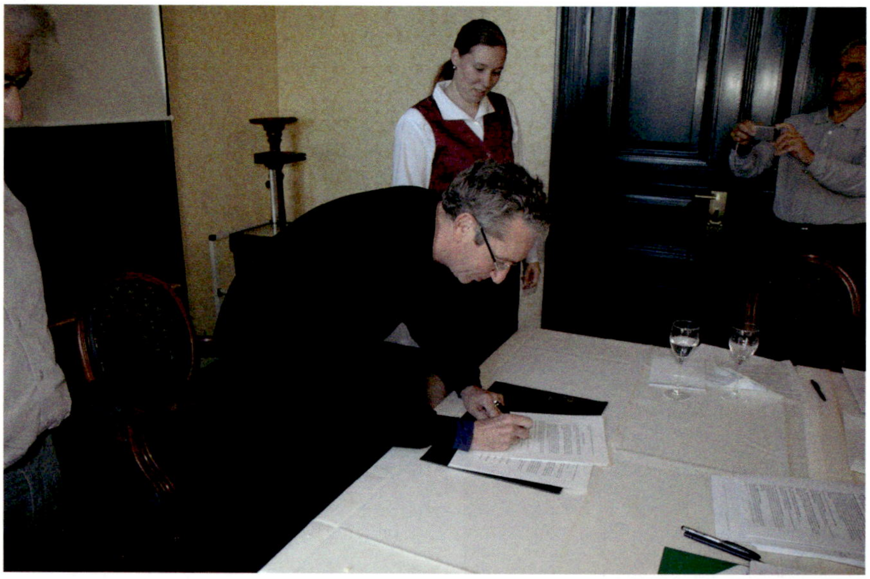

Fig. 27. During a key Executive Committee meeting in Aachen, Germany and Vaals, The Netherlands, President François Mauguière signs the incorporation papers for the new Canadian organization.

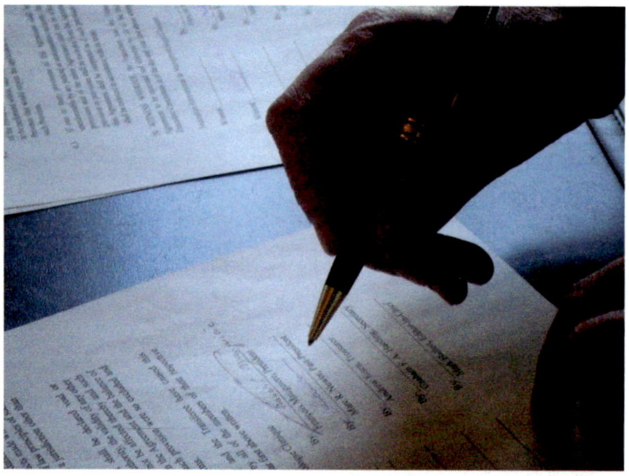

Fig. 28. Signing the formal incorporation papers for the Canadian organization of the Federation – two signatures down, five to go.

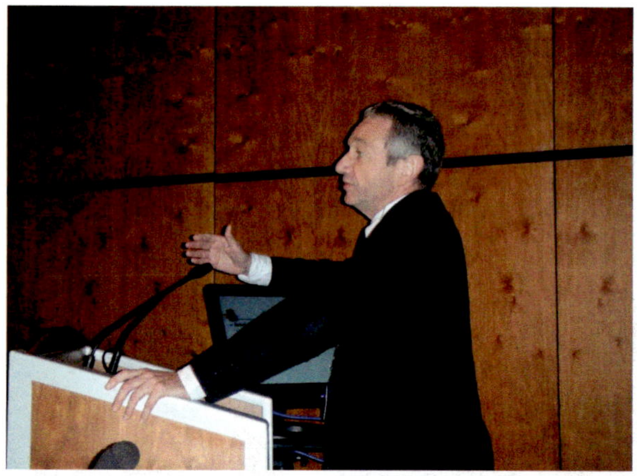

Fig. 29. Federation President addresses the General Assembly at the 2006 Edinburgh International Congress.

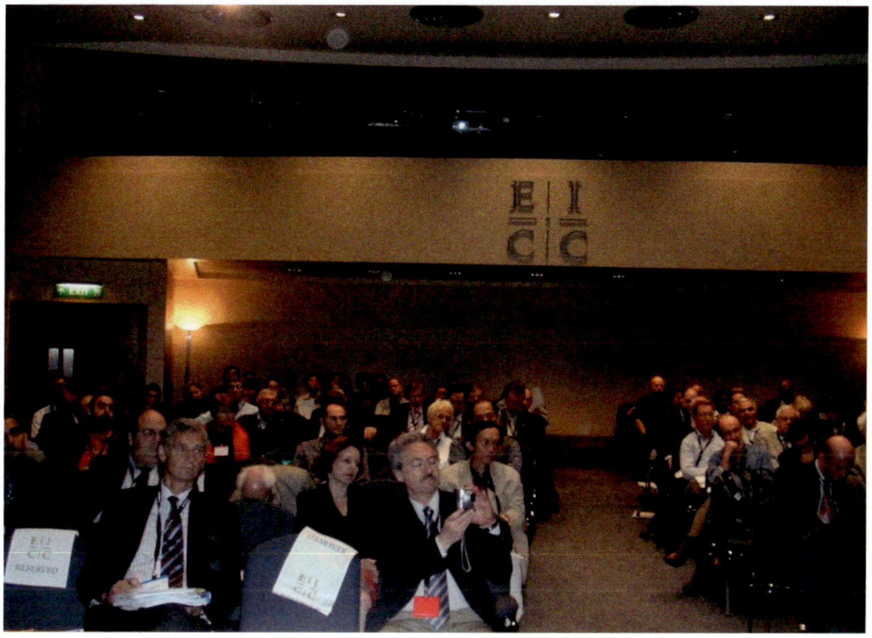

Fig. 30. 2006 Edinburgh General Assembly as it prepares formally to vote to close the Federation's French Registration organization. The subsequent vote was unanimous.

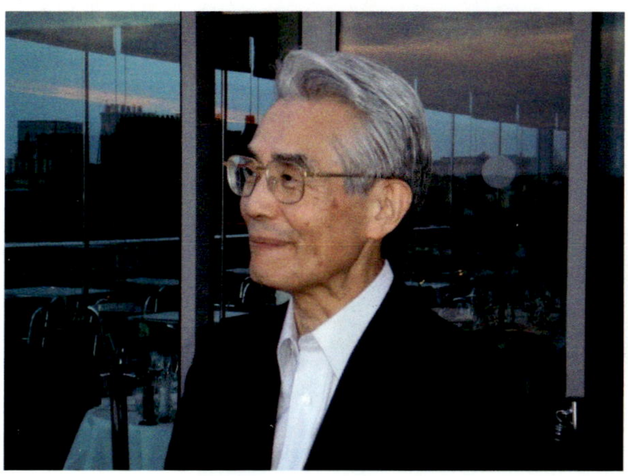

Fig. 31. New Federation President Hiroshi Shibasaki at a joint dinner of the old and new Executive Committees at a restaurant overlooking the Edinburgh city center and castle.

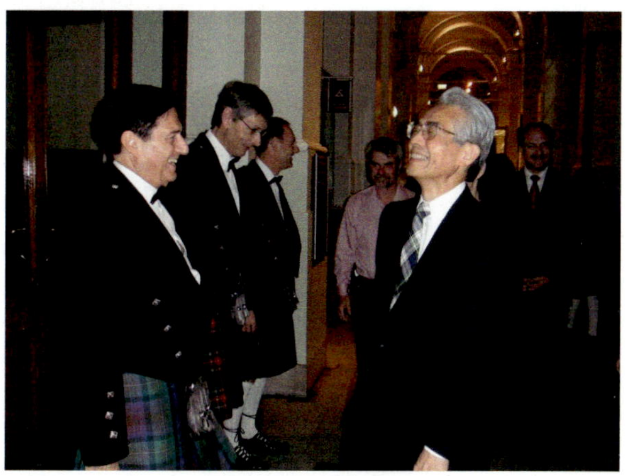

Fig. 32. New Federation President Hiroshi Shibasaki being welcomed at the official greeting line for the traditional Scottish gala dinner and Ceilidh, the gala social event for the Edinburgh 2006 ICCN. Note that the local organizing committee adhered to the formal Scottish dress customs.

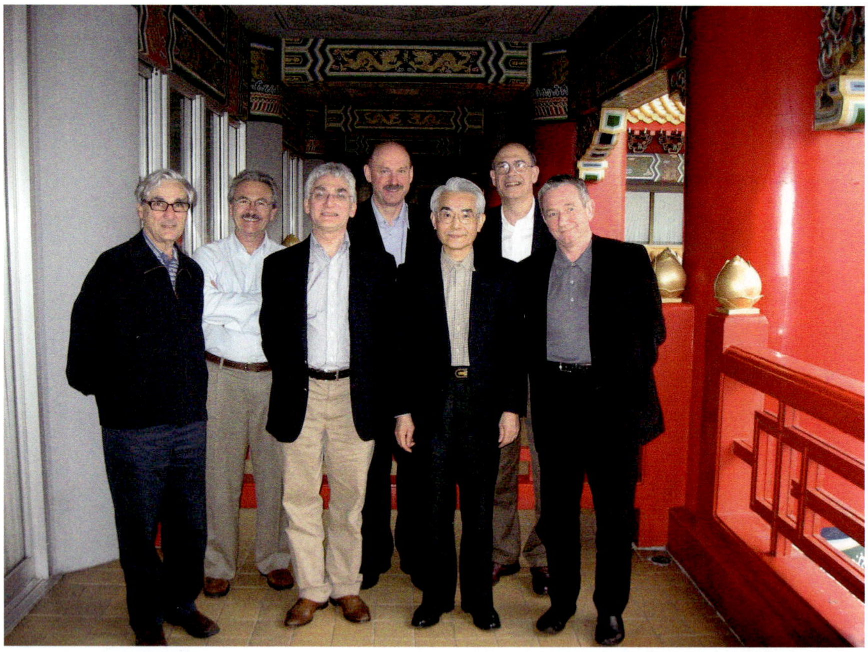

Fig. 33. The 2006–2010 Federation Executive Committee at their meeting with the Taiwan Clinical Neurophysiology Society in Taipei. From left to right: Treasurer Andrew Eisen, Members-at-Large Daniel Cibils and Kerry Mills, Secretary Reinhard Dengler, President Hiroshi Shibasaki, Editor-in-Chief Mark Hallett, and Past-President François Mauguière.

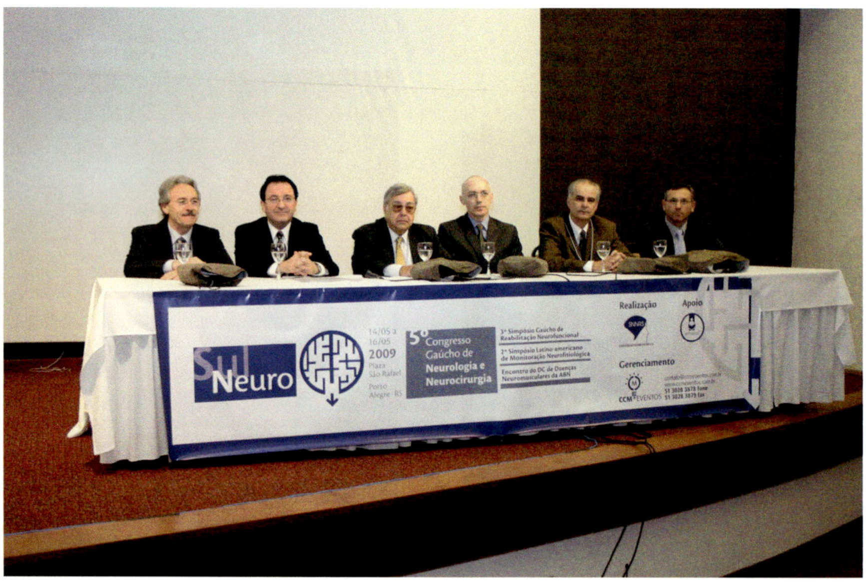

Fig. 34. Organizers at the Opening Ceremony for the Latin American Symposium of Neurophysiologic Monitoring, a part of the Neurology do Sul Congress in Porto Alegre, Brazil. From left to right: Daniel Cibils (Member-at-Large IFCN), Ricardo Ferreira (organizer of the Latin American Symposium of Neurophysiologic Monitoring), José Xavier de Castro (President of the Latin American Chapter of the IFCN), Francisco Tellechea Rotta (President of the Neurological and Neurosurgical Society of Rio Grande do Sul), Carlos Silvado (President of the Brazilian Society of Clinical Neurophysiology), Carlo Domenico Marrone (Coordinator of the Neuromuscular Scientific Department, Brazilian Academy of Neurology).